Current Review of

Interventional Cardiology

Current Review of

Interventional Cardiology

Third Edition

David R. Holmes, Jr., MD
Professor of Medicine
Cardiovascular Diseases
Mayo Medical Center;
Consultant
Division of Cardiovascular Diseases
Mayo Clinic
Rochester, Minnesota, USA

Patrick W. Serruys, MD, PhD, FACC, FESC
Professor of Interventional Cardiology
Department of Interventional Cardiology
Erasmus University;
Research Director
Catheterization Laboratory
Thoraxcenter
Dijkzigt Hospital
Rotterdam, the Netherlands

With 40 contributors

CHURCHILL LIVINGSTONE

Developed by Current Medicine, Inc.
Philadelphia

Current Medicine, Inc.
400 Market Street, Suite 700
Philadelphia, PA 19106

Managing Editor: **Lori J. Bainbridge**
Developmental Editors: **Gloria Klaiman, Elise Paxson, and Danielle Shaw**
Editorial Assistant: **Scott Thomas Hurd**
Art Director: **Paul Fennessy**
Design and Layout: **Christine Keller and Lisa Weischedel**
Illustration Director: **Ann Saydlowski**
Illustrators: **Liz Carrozza and Debra Wertz**
Production: **Lori Holland**
Indexing: **Dorothy A. DiRienzi**

ISBN: 0-443-07951-X

ISSN: 1068-4115

Although every effort has been made to ensure that drug doses and other information are presented accurately in this publication, the ultimate responsibility rests with the prescribing physician. Neither the publishers nor the authors can be held responsible for errors or for any consequences arising from the use of information contained herein. Products mentioned in this publication should be used in accordance with the prescribing information prepared by the manufacturers. No claims or endorsements are made for any drug or compound at present under clinical investigation.

Printed in the United States by Edwards Brothers
5 4 3 2 1

DISTRIBUTED WORLDWIDE BY CHURCHILL LIVINGSTONE, INC.

CONTRIBUTORS

SERGEI AIRIIAN, MD
Cardiologist
Department of Interventional Cardiology
Thoraxcenter
University Hospital Rotterdam
Rotterdam, the Netherlands

R. DAVID ANDERSON, MD
Cardiology Fellow
Division of Cardiology
Department of Medicine
Johns Hopkins University School of Medicine
Baltimore, Maryland, USA;
Fellow, Duke University Medical Center
Durham, North Carolina, USA

Y.E.A. APPELMAN, MD
Fellow, Department of Cardiology
University of Amsterdam;
Resident, Academical Medical Centre
Amsterdam, the Netherlands

DAVID C. AUTH, PHD
Affiliate Professor
Department of Bioengineering
University of Washington School of Medicine
Seattle, Washington, USA;
Consultant, Boston Scientific Corporation
Northwest Technology Center
Redmond, Washington, USA

ANDREAS BAUMBACH, MD
Department of Cardiology
University of Tübingen Medical School;
Division of Cardiology
University of Tübingen Medical Clinic
Tübingen, Germany

JOEL S. BENNETT, MD
Professor, Department of Medicine
University of Pennsylvania School of Medicine
Philadelphia, Pennsylvania, USA

JOHN A. BITTL, MD
Associate Professor
Department of Medicine
Harvard Medical School;
Director of Interventional Cardiology
Brigham and Women's Hospital
Boston, Massachusetts, USA

SORIN J. BRENER, MD
Clinical Instructor of Medicine
Department of Medicine
Case Western Reserve University School of Medicine;
Staff, Interventional Cardiology
Cleveland Clinic Foundation
Cleveland, Ohio, USA

PIM J. DE FEYTER, MD, PHD
Department of Interventional Cardiology
Thoraxcenter
University Hospital Rotterdam
Rotterdam, the Netherlands

NEAL EIGLER, MD
Associate Professor of Medicine
Department of Cardiology
University of California, Los Angeles, School of Medicine;
Co-director, Cardiovascular Intervention Center
Cedars-Sinai Medical Center
Los Angeles, California, USA

PETER J. FITZGERALD, MD, PHD
Assistant Professor of Medicine
Department of Cardiovascular Medicine
Stanford University Medical Center
Stanford, California, USA

GEERT H.M. GIJSBERS, PHD
Director, Laser Laboratory
Thoraxcenter
Dijkzigt Hospital
Rotterdam, the Netherlands

KENTON GREGORY, MD
Assistant Professor
Division of Cardiology
Oregon Health Sciences University;
Director, Providence St. Vincent Hospital and Medical Center
Oregon Medical Laser Center
Portland, Oregon, USA

VICTOR GUETTA, MD
Interventional Fellow
Cleveland Clinic Foundation
Cleveland, Ohio, USA

Karl K. Haase, MD
Associate Professor
Department of Cardiology
University of Tübingen Medical School;
Division of Cardiology
University of Tübingen Medical Clinic
Tübingen, Germany

Jaap N. Hamburger, MD
Cardiologist
Department of Interventional Cardiology
Thoraxcenter
University Hospital Rotterdam
Rotterdam, the Netherlands

Jean-Paul R. Herrman, MD
Catheterization Laboratory
Erasmus University
Thoraxcenter
Dijkzigt Hospital
Rotterdam, the Netherlands

David R. Holmes, Jr., MD
Professor of Medicine
Cardiovascular Diseases
Mayo Medical School;
Consultant, Division of Cardiovascular Diseases
Mayo Clinic
Rochester, Minnesota, USA

Yasuhiro Honda, MD
Department of Cardiovascular Medicine
Stanford University Medical Center
Stanford, California, USA

Mun K. Hong, MD
Director, Experimental Physiology and Pharmacology
Washington Cardiology Center/Cardiology Research Foundation
Washington, DC, USA

Karl R. Karsch, MD, FESC, FACC
Professor of Medicine
Department of Internal Medicine
University of Tübingen Medical School;
Division of Cardiology
University of Tübingen Medical Clinic
Tübingen, Germany

Kenneth M. Kent, MD, PhD
Clinical Associate Professor
Department of Medicine
Georgetown University Medical Center;
Director, Washington Cardiology Center/Cardiology Research Foundation
Washington, DC, USA

Stephen L. Kopecky, MD
Assistant Professor of Medicine
Department of Cardiovascular Diseases
University of Texas Medical School at Houston
Houston, Texas, USA;
Consultant, Division of Cardiovascular Diseases
St. Mary's Hospital
Rochester, Minnesota, USA

Iftikhar J. Kullo, MD
Fellow, Division of Cardiovascular Diseases
Mayo Medical Center
Rochester, Minnesota, USA

Martin B. Leon, MD
Clinical Associate Professor
Department of Medicine
Georgetown University Medical Center;
Director, Cardiovascular Research and Education
Washington Cardiology Center/Cardiology Research Foundation
Washington, DC, USA

A. Michael Lincoff, MD
Assistant Professor
Health Science Center
Ohio State University College of Medicine
Columbus, Ohio, USA;
Staff, Cleveland Clinic Foundation
Cleveland, Ohio, USA

Frank Litvack, MD
Associate Professor of Medicine
Department of Cardiology
University of California, Los Angeles, School of Medicine;
Co-director, Cardiovascular Intervention Center
Cedars-Sinai Medical Center
Los Angeles, California, USA

Raj Makkar, MD
Senior Interventional Fellow
Department of Cardiology
University of California, Los Angeles, School of Medicine;
Cardiologist, Cedars-Sinai Medical Center
Los Angeles, California, USA

Michael E. McClurken, PhD
Medical Device Development Consultant
Ramsey, Minnesota, USA

Gary S. Mintz, MD
Director, Intravascular Ultrasound Program
Washington Cardiology Center/Cardiology Research Foundation
Washington, DC, USA

Shaker A. Mousa, PhD, MBA, FACC
Research Fellow
Dupont Merck Pharmaceutical
Wilmington, Delaware, USA

Merle Myerson, MD, EdD
Resident, Department of Medicine
Duke University Medical Center
Durham, North Carolina, USA

E. Magnus Ohman, MD
Assistant Professor of Medicine
Division of Cardiology
Department of Medicine
Royal College of Surgeons of Ireland
St. Laurence's
Dublin, Ireland;
Assistant Professor of Medicine
Duke University Medical Center
Durham, North Carolina, USA

J.J. Piek, MD
Associate Professor
Department of Cardiology
University of Amsterdam;
Cardiologist, Academical Medical Centre
Amsterdam, the Netherlands

Nicolaus Reifart, MD
Professor, Department of Medicine
University of Frankfurt;
Head, Department of Cardiology
Red Cross Hospital and Heart Center
Frankfurt, Germany

Mark Reisman, MD
Director, Cardiovascular Research and Cardiac Catheterization Laboratory
Swedish Medical Center
Seattle, Washington, USA

Robert S. Schwartz, MD
Professor of Medicine
Cardiovascular Diseases
Mayo Medical School;
Consultant, Division of Cardiovascular Diseases
Mayo Clinic
Rochester, Minnesota, USA

Patrick W. Serruys, MD, PhD, FACC, FESC
Professor of Interventional Cardiology
Department of Interventional Cardiology
Erasmus University;
Research Director
Catheterization Laboratory
Thoraxcenter
Dijkzigt Hospital
Rotterdam, the Netherlands

Eric J. Topol, MD
Chairman and Professor
Department of Cardiology
Director, Joseph J. Jacobs Center for Thrombosis and Vascular Biology
Cleveland Clinic Foundation
Cleveland, Ohio, USA

Robert A. VanTassel, MD
Clinical Associate Professor of Medicine
University of Minnesota Medical School–Minneapolis;
Consulting Cardiologist
Minneapolis Heart Institute
Minneapolis, Minnesota, USA

Patrick L. Whitlow, MD
Director, Interventional Cardiology
Department of Cardiology
Cleveland Clinic Foundation
Cleveland, Ohio, USA

Paul G. Yock, MD
Associate Professor
Department of Cardiovascular Medicine
Stanford University School of Medicine;
Acting Chief, Division of Cardiovascular Medicine
Stanford University Medical Center
Stanford, California, USA

PREFACE

The pace of change in interventional cardiology continues to accelerate. This is the result of several factors, including improved understanding of vascular biology and the response to arterial injury; advances in pharmacology with the introduction of new groups of drugs, for example, antithrombins and antiplatetlet agents; development of new devices that have expanded the pool of patients and lesions that can be treated with a percutaneous-based approach; and new diagnostic modalities such as intravascular ultrasound and intracoronary Doppler. These changes, coupled with creative and innovative interventional cardiologists, have greatly expanded the scope of the field.

It is difficult to remain abreast of all the new developments in the field. Diverse resources must be used, including international, national, and regional meetings; published papers; and dedicated editions that are up to date and presented in a directed fashion. The first two editions of *Current Review of Interventional Cardiology* provided detailed information on a variety of topics ranging from thrombolytic therapy for acute myocardial infarction to catheter-based therapies and coronary bypass surgery, and from some clinical aspects of molecular biology to current new drug treatment strategies. This third edition builds on the first two; it includes new information on alternative device strategies for common interventional procedures, including updates on rotational atherectomy and intravascular ultrasound–guided directional atherectomy. As well, it addresses new approaches to laser treatment, including saline flushing, multiplexing, and homogenous light distribution techniques. These techniques may result in a rebirth of interest in laser therapy. Finally, this edition includes new pharmacologic treatment information with recent advances in platelet receptor antagonists and antithrombins.

J. Edward Demming wrote: "You do not need to change; survival is not mandatory." The field of interventional cardiology is changing rapidly. Unless we change with it, we fall behind and fail to offer optimal treatment strategies to our patients. As we move from practical applications of older techniques to gain fundamental insights as to why the techniques work and when they should be applied, new information is greatly needed. It is the goal of this continuing series to fulfill this need.

David R. Holmes, Jr, MD

Patrick W. Serruys, MD, PhD, FACC, FESC

CONTENTS

Chapter 1

The Value of Intravascular Ultrasound Guidance in Directional Coronary Atherectomy

Yasuhiro Honda
Paul G. Yock
Peter J. Fitzgerald

Over the past several years the introduction of intravascular ultrasound (IVUS) into the interventional laboratory has provided significant and interesting new insights into the mechanisms and outcomes of directional coronary atherectomy (DCA). As experience with IVUS has grown, this method has begun to be used by many operators for guidance of the DCA procedure. Several trials are being conducted to revisit the issues of acute complications and restenosis rates with DCA in the context of "optimal atherectomy" as assessed by IVUS. Ongoing technical developments—including a combined imaging/atherectomy device now entering clinical trials—offer the prospect of obtaining more selective and complete atherectomy than has been possible using angiographic guidance alone.

Mechanisms of Directional Coronary Atherectomy

Potential mechanisms responsible for the acute lumen gain achieved by DCA include plaque removal, vessel expansion, dissection, plaque compression, and plaque redistribution. Several IVUS studies have suggested that plaque reduction is in fact the primary mechanism for lumen gain (accounting for 60% to 80% of the increase in area) [1,2•,3–7]. Braden and colleagues [2•] reported that plaque reduction was more extensive in eccentric compared with concentric lesions. Using volumetric measurements rather than simple cross-sectional area determinations, Suneja and colleagues [1] determined that as much as 57% of the reduction in plaque volume was caused by compression (as opposed to plaque removal). Unfortunately, the current level of technology for making volumetric measurements is limited. These important studies will need to be repeated with more accurate analysis techniques using high-quality images and gated image acquisition methods.

Intravascular Ultrasound Guidance for Optimal Directional Coronary Atherectomy

Before Intervention

Assessment of lesion characteristics

Lesion characteristics important for DCA include plaque thickness, eccentricity, vessel compliance, plaque type (soft or fibrous), and calcification. Calcification of the plaque is among the most significant factors determining the outcome of DCA because it is difficult to cut calcified plaque using the current DCA device. It has been reported that presence of a calcium arc of more than 90° as seen by IVUS is associated with greater residual plaque [8]. Matar and colleagues [9••] identified by multivariate regression analysis that the preintervention lesion arc of calcium detected by IVUS was the most consistent predictor of the effectiveness and results of DCA.

Several studies have shown that IVUS detects calcium approximately twice as often as conventional coronary angiography does [10,11•,12]. The GUIDE (Guidance by Ultrasound Imaging for Decision Endpoints) trial showed that the significant target lesion calcium was observed in 62% of all cases by IVUS but only 35% by angiography [10]. Mintz and colleagues [11•] showed that the sensitivity for angiographic detection of calcium depends on the calcium arc, length, and location as seen by ultrasound imaging. In addition to detecting the presence of calcium, IVUS can provide detailed information about extent and location of the calcium—a difficult issue for conventional angiography. Fitzgerald and colleagues [13] reported that the tissue weight retrieved by DCA was significantly less in lesions with superficial calcium than in lesions with deep calcium or noncalcified lesions (Fig. 1-1). Moreover, the superficial rim of calcium at the luminal border, or so-called "napkin-ring lesion," generally prevents any tissue removal and sometimes provides great resistance to passing the rigid housing of the device. On the other hand, if calcification is layered deep in the plaque at the medial border, it will be a protective barrier against deep-wall excision and the plaque can be removed aggressively with minimal concern for perforation. Preinterventional scanning of the target segment may permit an efficient means to triage lesions that are particularly well suited or not well suited for DCA.

Calcium of the proximal and distal reference sites

Because of the size and stiffness of the DCA device, whether or not the operator can safely place the device precisely at the target lesion site depends on the vessel dimensions, degree of tortuosity, and vessel compliance. The most significant factor affecting vessel compliance is the degree of calcification, and delivery of the device can be influenced by the presence of either proximal or distal vessel calcification, even in the presence of angiographically silent calcification. As known from recent clinical studies, the reference vessel calcification is observed more often by IVUS than expected by conventional coronary angiography. Mintz and colleagues [11•] examined 1155 native coronary target vessels by IVUS and found that 32% of the reference segments contained calcium. Failure to appreciate the significant reference vessel calcification may lead to an increase of complication rates or waste of the expensive DCA device. As well as proximal vessel injury due to aggressive device manipulation in diffusely diseased vessels, nose cone–induced trauma at the distal segment has been observed [14]. The risk of nose cone–induced trauma is higher if the distal segment has mild to moderate disease. In addition to nose

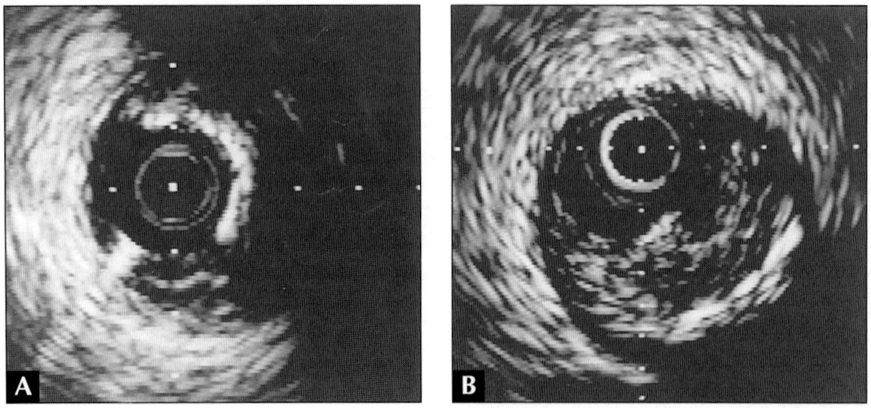

Figure 1-1. Superficial (**A**) versus deep (**B**) calcification within plaques. **A**, Superficial calcium is layered at the luminal surface, leading to acoustic shadowing behind it. **B**, An arc of calcium is positioned deeply adjacent to the media. The location of calcium significantly affects the procedural results of atherectomy.

cone–induced trauma such as dissection or thrombus formation, nose cone–induced spasm is also possible.

Primary device selection

Preinterventional IVUS imaging provides useful information in device selection by assessing 1) calcification of target lesion and proximal/distal reference site, 2) plaque eccentricity, and 3) lesion length. DCA is primarily used for debulking eccentric, noncalcified lesions in proximal, nontortuous vessels that are large enough to pass the DCA device. The only device that has been shown consistently to ablate calcium is rotational atherectomy. It causes partial-thickness calcium removal or fissuring of calcium deposits, and occasionally achieves full-thickness calcium removal. Excimer laser angioplasty does not ablate calcium but can cause shattering of the calcium. Preliminary observations suggest that DCA may be more efficient in debulking calcified lesions when combined with prior rotational atherectomy or laser angioplasty [15].

In eccentric lesions, pathologic studies have reported that balloon angioplasty works by stretching the normal wall opposite to the plaque and that this is followed by early recoil [16]. One of the advantages of the DCA device is its ability to address specific areas of the vessel wall by means of its side-directed cutting mechanism. Because of differential atheroablation, rotational atherectomy will also preferentially ablate the eccentric plaque as long as it is less compliant than the thinner portion of the lesion.

Lesion length can be accurately measured by IVUS using the automatic pullback device. This information is particularly helpful in choosing appropriate balloon size or stent length.

Orientation of the directional coronary atherectomy device

According to the previous pathologic study, greater than 70% of coronary lesions are eccentric [17]. Directing of the DCA device toward the thickest plaque accumulation is critically important to avoid the removal of normal vessel wall components. However, it is difficult to assess the distribution and amount of maximal plaque by conventional angiography alone. Several studies have reported that more than 50% of the DCA cuts retrieved the media and 30% reached the adventitia without IVUS guidance [18,19]. IVUS offers the significant potential for the safe and aggressive debulking of eccentric plaque providing detailed information about the rotational orientation. This requires that the operator be able to correlate the position of the plaque on the IVUS image with the position of the DCA device on fluoroscopy. The most effective current approach is to reference the position of the major plaque accumulation to the origin of a major branch near the stenosis (Fig. 1-2) [20].

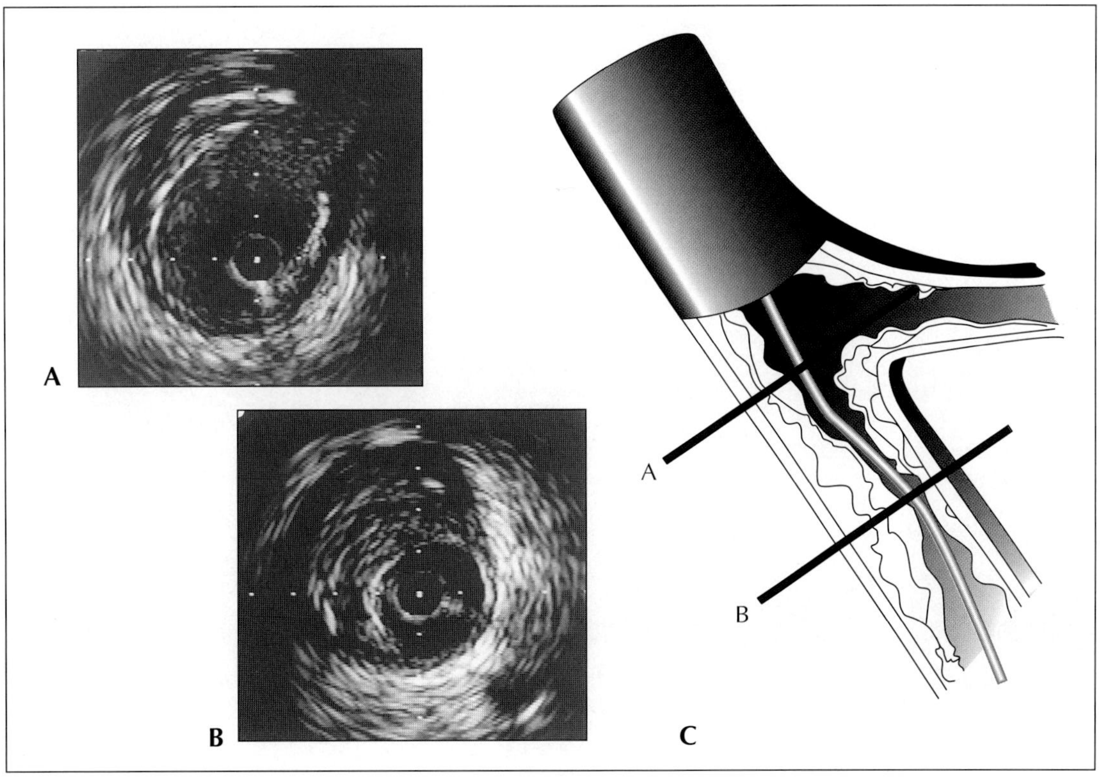

Figure 1-2. Intravascular ultrasound (IVUS) imaging for rotational device orientation. **A**, A major branch just proximal to the target lesion is identified at 1 o'clock on the IVUS image. **B**, Maximal plaque thickness is observed at 10 o'clock at the target lesion. The directional coronary atherectomy (DCA) cutter should be oriented 90° counterclockwise relative to the branch. **C**, Schematic representation of **A** and **B**.

Once this landmark is identified, the plaque is localized as being clockwise or counterclockwise from the origin of the branch by a certain amount of rotation. Then using an orthogonal projection of fluoroscopy, the housing of the DCA catheter can be correctly oriented toward the same predetermined number of degrees relative to the branch.

During and After Intervention

Assessment of endpoint achievement

Although contrast angiography can demonstrate the luminal improvement following intervention, it has several limitations in quantitative analysis of postinterventional results. Tomographic images by IVUS can more accurately define the luminal dimensions than planar silhouettes by angiography, especially in complex or asymmetrical lesions after the interventional procedures. Furthermore, vessel remodeling (compensatory enlargement) at the lesion site or significant plaque burden at the "normal" reference segment often lead the quantitative angiography to an underestimation of the lesion severity.

Recent preliminary studies suggested that percent plaque area immediately after the interventions may be a powerful predictor of long-term outcome [21]. In several IVUS studies, a significant amount of plaque remained within the target lesion following angiographically successful atherectomy [1,2•,22–24]. Residual plaque at the target lesion can be visualized directly by IVUS. Assessing the amount and location of residual plaque during DCA is especially important not only for the endpoint decision making but also for the reorientation of the DCA device toward residual plaque burden, upsizing the device, or changing the strategy (Fig. 1-3).

Adjunct device selection

The lesion morphology following atherectomy can be assessed by IVUS to determine whether adjunctive balloon dilatation or stenting would be helpful to achieve the optimal results and maximize lumen gain. In some cases, the reach of the DCA device itself becomes a limitation. Recent multicenter clinical trials have suggested that adjunctive balloon angioplasty following DCA with IVUS guidance can facilitate the achievement of larger lumens without increasing complications [25,26]. Whether this aggressive protocol has a significant impact on long-term outcome with DCA is now under investigation.

Extensive dissections that involve normal wall segments should be treated with stents. However, limited dissections within diseased plaque can be treated by adjunctive balloon angioplasty or further atherectomy (Fig. 1-4). The indications for adjunctive stents other than management of dissections have not been defined at this point. However, adjunctive stent deployment may prevent vessel shrinkage (negative remodeling) which may contribute significantly to the restenosis process following DCA [27–29].

Assessment of complications

The possible DCA complications other than perforation include 1) vasospasm, 2) dissection, and 3) thrombus formation. Angiographically "hazy" appearance often represents each or a combination of these conditions. The optimal treatment of these hazy lesions is based on the underlying causes [30,31], and IVUS imaging is quite helpful in assessing these conditions. Vasospasm can be diagnosed by a marked reduction in vessel dimensions. Usually spasms are transient and successfully treated by intracoronary nitroglycerin

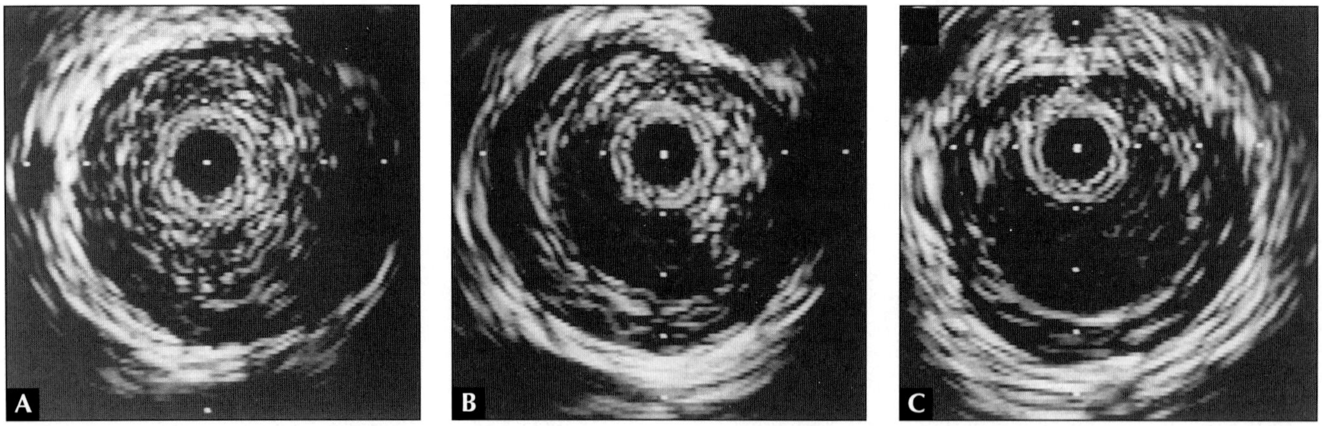

Figure 1-3. Intravascular ultrasound imaging for residual plaque burden assessment. **A**, Before intervention. **B**, After directional coronary atherectomy (DCA). A significant amount of residual plaque remains despite the luminal improvement by angiography. **C**, After adjunctive percutaneous transluminal coronary angioplasty (PTCA). Lumen area has significantly increased following PTCA.

or calcium antagonists. Significant dissection is also easily identified as a freely moving flap of tissue in the lumen, behind which blood flow can be seen. IVUS evaluation of the dissection size, depth, and localization is crucial to determine the need for treatment and the adjunct device selection (balloon angioplasty or stent deployment). Thrombus is usually difficult to differentiate from soft plaque by IVUS. The IVUS findings by which fresh thrombus is strongly suspected include irregular borders, scintillating or sparkling speckles, presence of microchannels, a lobulated or pedunculated appearance with projection into the lumen, and a mobile element with an undulating appearance in systole and diastole. Further advances of tissue characterization technique or higher frequency imaging may provide reliable information for identification of thrombus [32]. Persistent or recurrent thrombus formation should be treated by intracoronary thrombolytic agents as well as aggressive use of heparin. Combinations of a large amount of thrombus with dissections or recurrent vasospasms may demand an aggressive antiplatelet therapy following the intervention.

Clinical Trials

Two early randomized trials of DCA versus balloon angioplasty (CAVEAT [Coronary Angioplasty Versus Excisional Atherectomy Trial] and the CCAT [Canadian Coronary Atherectomy Trial]) failed to demonstrate a substantial and clinically significant reduction in late angiographic or clinical restenosis after DCA [33,34]. However, both series had minimal differences in acute results between the two treatments: residual diameter stenoses were 32% versus 38% in CAVEAT, and 31% versus 36% in CCAT, for DCA versus balloon angioplasty, respectively. Although few centers in CAVEAT used IVUS, it is assured that a large amount of residual plaque remained after the debulking—possibly more than 70%. Over the past several years, it has been reported that the late lumen diameter and the probability of restenosis after the interventions are influenced strongly by the lumen diameter immediately after the procedure rather than by the specific device used [33,35,36]. The GUIDE II trial also suggested that the residual percent plaque area was the significant predictor of restenosis [21]. These concepts led to great emphasis on aggressive plaque removal and on the use of adjunctive balloon angioplasty to achieve optimal atherectomy results. In the OARS (Optimal Atherectomy Restenosis Study) trial, which was designed to test the theory of optimal atherectomy, initial results yielded the low average residual stenosis of 7%, and this resulted in a lower binary restenosis rate at 6 months compared with CAVEAT (30% vs 50%) [37,38]. Despite the excellent initial results by angiography, IVUS imaging immediately following the procedure still revealed a significant amount of average residual plaque area of 58%. The ABACAS (Adjunctive Balloon Angioplasty following Coronary Atherectomy Study) is an ongoing prospective randomized multicenter trial in Japan to evaluate whether more aggressive debulking by IVUS-guided DCA followed by adjunctive balloon angioplasty can reduce the restenosis rate without any increase in complication rates. The preliminary report showed that the average residual plaque area was only 46% and 42% in

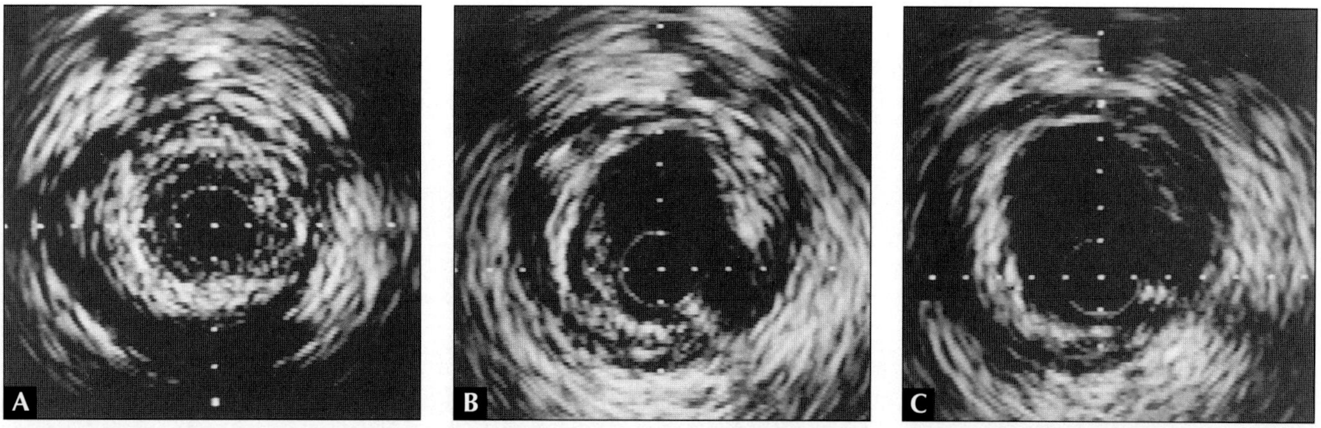

Figure 1-4. Intravascular ultrasound imaging in the context of adjunctive percutaneous transluminal coronary angioplasty (PTCA). **A**, Before intervention. **B**, After directional coronary atherectomy (DCA). IVUS reveals tissue protruding into the lumen at 7 o'clock. This flap can be successfully treated by adjunctive PTCA or further atherectomy because it is small and limited within the diseased plaque. **C**, After adjunctive PTCA. The flap is "tacked up" by adjunctive PTCA. A smoother luminal border is achieved as well as an improvement in lumen area.

the DCA group and adjunctive balloon group, respectively [26]. From these initial results, it may be expected that the restenosis rate should be much more favorable than that of the previous clinical trials.

Coronary artery remodeling is another current topic of IVUS study. It has been considered as a compensatory mechanism to maintain lumen area against plaque accumulation. The original concept of this compensatory vessel enlargement came from several pathologic studies [39–42]. Recent in vivo studies by high-frequency epicardial echocardiography or by IVUS have confirmed this phenomenon [43–48]. The significant change in vessel size has been also observed after coronary interventions [49,50•]. The SURE (Serial Ultrasound analysis of Restenosis) registry is a unique ongoing clinical trial with prospective serial IVUS and coronary angiography. It was designed to evaluate the relative contribution of intimal regrowth and geometric negative remodeling to late lumen loss after DCA and balloon angioplasty. In a preliminary report, geometric remodeling (vessel shrinkage) was demonstrated to be an important mechanism of restenosis after DCA [27]. On the other hand, our initial IVUS observations from the ABACAS registry revealed the vessel expansion at the lesion site after DCA in several follow-up cases. In the first consecutive 31 cases, deep cuts on the IVUS image (encroachment of sonolucent zone) were the only predictor of this observation (Figs. 1-5 and 1-6) [51]. Subsequent studies are needed to determine its clinical significance.

LIMITATIONS OF INTRAVASCULAR ULTRASOUND

IVUS enables interventionalists to obtain useful information that is not readily assessed by conventional angiography. However, there are several limitations to be considered:

1. The position of the imaging catheter relative to the vessel affects the geometric accuracy and backscatter of vessel wall components.
2. Some vessel characteristics, such as proximal vessel tortuosity or bendpoint at the lesion site, that influence the procedural success cannot be assessed by IVUS alone. At this point, IVUS is a powerful tool when used in conjunction with conventional contrast angiography that can provide an overview of the coronary tree. Further development of the three-dimensional reconstruction technique will define the spatial orientation.
3. Despite the technical improvement of the imaging catheter miniaturization, crossing curved segments or extremely tight lesions with calcification is still limited. Furthermore, the catheter itself may cause a certain amount of "dottering effect" of the vessel on preintervention imaging. Total occlusions are also impossible to assess by the current imaging catheters. Prototypes of imaging guidewires or forward-looking imaging catheters have been designed and tested to circumvent this problem [1,2•,22–24,52–55].
4. Failure of a uniform rotation of mechanical imaging catheter results in distortion of the image, termed "NURD" (nonuniform rotational distortion). If this occurs during an imaging orientation for DCA, there may be some inaccuracy in registering the precise position of the plaque.
5. Acoustic shadow or attenuation of ultrasound caused by calcification or dense fibrous tissue can make it impossible to evaluate vessel dimensions accurately. They may be also misinterpreted as dissections.
6. The delineation of luminal border is sometimes difficult in the segment with stagnant blood flow because blood echointensity with slower velocity becomes higher. Contrast injection may be helpful in such cases [56].

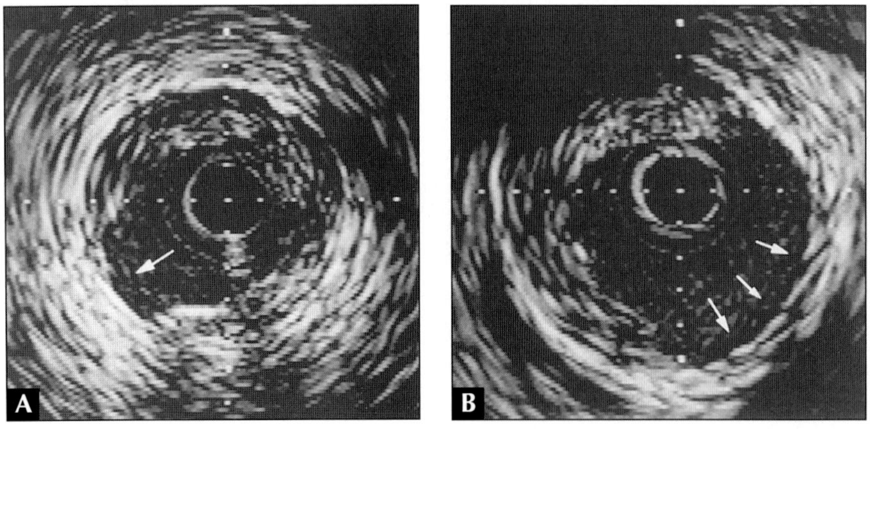

Figure 1-5. Two examples of sonographic "deep cuts" (*arrows*) after aggressive debulking by directional coronary atherectomy. The sonolucent zones are directly exposed to the blood speckles.

Future Directions

Combined Imaging/Directional Coronary Atherectomy Catheter

Intravascular ultrasound has significant potential to improve the outcome of DCA. Because information from the IVUS image is useful before, during, and after the atherectomy, IVUS-guided DCA requires an iterative process in which the DCA device and the IVUS catheter should be repeatedly exchanged. In order to make this process easier and to enhance the precision of IVUS-guided DCA, combined imaging/DCA catheters have been developed in recent years [24,57].

The prototype catheter is based on the Simpson Atherocath (Devices for Vascular Intervention, Inc., Redwood City, CA), and has a 30-MHz transducer mounted immediately behind the edge of the rotating atherectomy cutter (Fig. 1-7). Use of this combined device does not require a change in operation of the atherectomy catheter except for the imaging sequence. The transducer on the cutting element creates a 120°-sector image through the open window of the DCA housing providing real-time feedback about the rotational orientation of the device. By pulling back the cutter/imaging assembly in the housing, the operator is able to scan the entire segment of the target lesion that will be exposed to the cutter. In addition to the precise orientation of the DCA housing toward the maximal plaque accumulation, the depth of the potential cut can be also directly assessed; the tissue moving into the central gray zone on the IVUS image, which represents the cutting chamber, with the balloon inflation will be subjected to cutting (Fig. 1-8). If the pullback imaging sequence reveals any portion of too-deep cuts, the inflation pressure or the axial/rotational orientation of the device should be adjusted.

The initial results of in vitro study and animal experiments with this combination catheter suggest that the residual plaque burden was considerably reduced without medial injury (Fig. 1-9) [58••,59]. The image resolution was superior to stand-alone imaging catheters because of the relatively large aperture of the ultrasound transducer. The following preliminary clinical test on five patients in Brazil showed that a maximum residual plaque burden was only 40%, and that the subintimal resection was seen in only one of the five cases. Although a fixed-wire catheter configuration was selected in order to provide maximum rotational stability for imaging, the clinical feasibility of this catheter was acceptable. A commercially available combined imaging/DCA catheter is currently entering clinical testing for approval by the US Food and Drug Administration.

Three-Dimensional Reconstruction

Three-dimensional reconstruction of tomographic IVUS images has great potential for the quantitation of volumetric changes of lumen and plaque [60]. The measurements of plaque volume after three-dimensional reconstruction along the entire treated segment can provide a more reliable assessment of the mechanism of DCA [61]. This technique can also facilitate the spatial orientation of arterial structure, which currently requires an experienced mental conceptualization. Several reports have shown the usefulness of three-

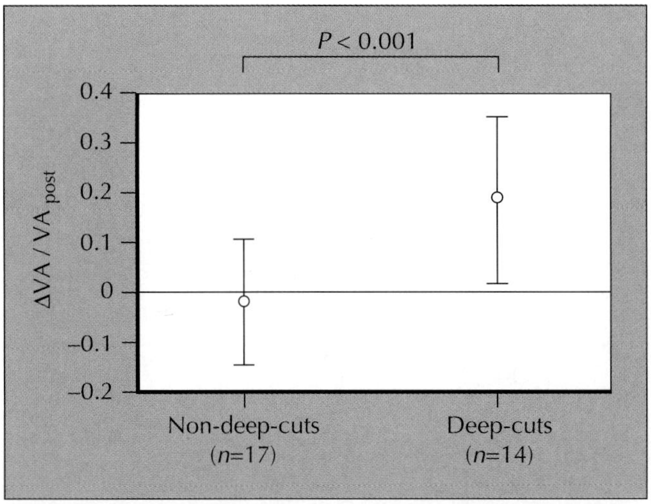

Figure 1-6. Comparison of vessel area changes at the lesion site 3 months after the atherectomy between the non–deep-cuts group and the deep-cuts group. FU—follow-up; POST—postintervention; VA—vessel area; $\Delta VA = VA_{FU} - VA_{post}$.

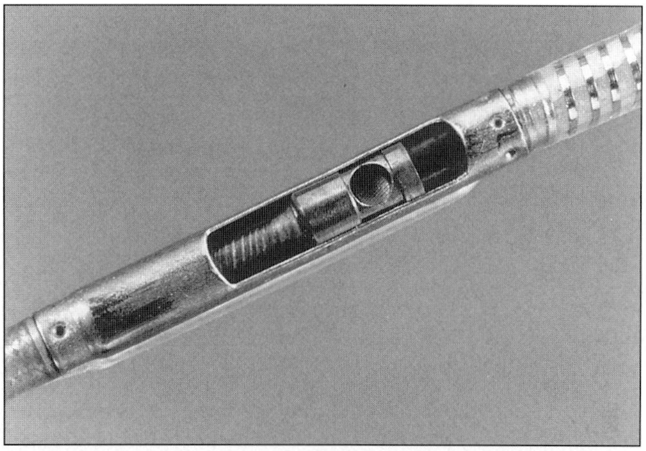

Figure 1-7. Prototype combined imaging/directional coronary atherectomy (DCA) catheter. A cylinder-shaped transducer is mounted just behind the edge of the cutting element within the body of the cutter. The atherectomy device consists of modified Atherocath (Devices for Vascular Intervention Inc., Redwood City, CA) with a fixed guidewire tip.

dimensional reconstruction or longitudinal view in the assessment of complications such as dissections [62–66]. One of the major limitations is a longitudinal image distortion due to a straight line reconstruction format. The combined use of biplane fluoroscopy for a spatial location system of the imaging catheter may be feasible in the near future [67]. A miniaturized receiving antenna located at the tip of the imaging catheter combined with external electromagnetic radiating antennas has also been proposed as a possible method to detect the orientation of the catheter [68,69]. Although several limitations must be solved, recent developments in computer technology have significantly increased the practicality of three-dimensional reconstruction as guidance for the intervention and for assessment of initial and long-term results.

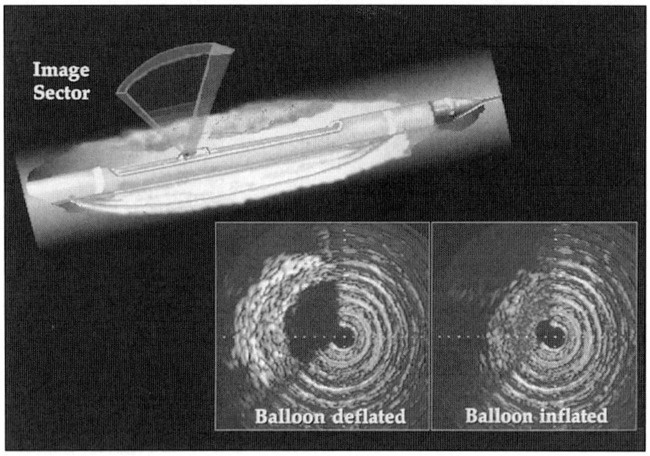

Figure 1-8. Example images by the prototype combined imaging/directional coronary atherectomy (DCA) catheter. The ultrasound image is limited to 120° through the open window of the DCA housing (from 8 to 12 o'clock in these images). The housing is represented by a series of rings that are reverberations from the strong reflection of the metal. As balloon is inflated, plaque is moving into the central gray disk corresponding to the cutting chamber, and operators are able to assess depth of excision.

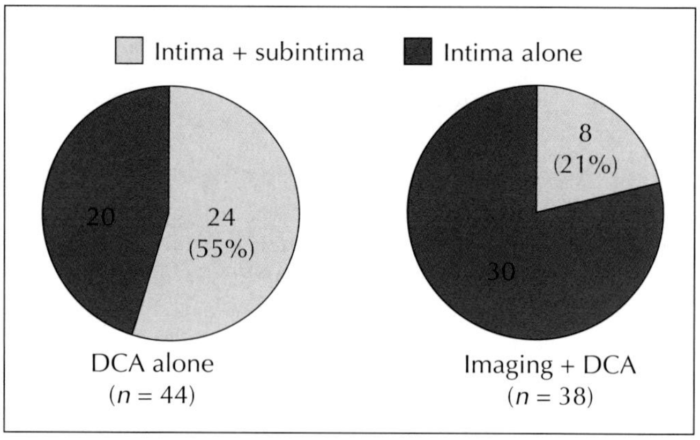

Figure 1-9. Difference in the incidence of subintimal resections between atherectomy with and without intravascular ultrasound guidance. In this initial in vitro study, debulking with the combined imaging/directional coronary atherectomy (DCA) catheter yielded only 21% of the tissue samples containing media, adventitia, or both. In contrast, 55% of the samples contained subintimal tissue in the atherectomy-alone group ($P < 0.001$). (*Data from* Fitzgerald and colleagues [58••].)

References and Recommended Reading

Recently published papers of particular interest have been highlighted as:

- • Of special interest
- •• Of outstanding interest

1. Suneja R, Nair RN, Reddy KG, *et al.*: Mechanisms of angiographically successful directional coronary atherectomy: evaluation by intracoronary ultrasound and comparison with transluminal coronary angioplasty. *Am Heart J* 1993, 126:507–514.

2.• Braden GA, Herrington DM, Downes TR, *et al.*: Qualitative and quantitative contrasts in the mechanisms of lumen enlargement by coronary balloon angioplasty and directional coronary atherectomy. *J Am Coll Cardiol* 1994, 23:40–48.

Intravascular ultrasound is systematically used to define the mechanisms of lumen enlargement by balloon angioplasty and directional atherectomy.

3. Di Mario C, Gil R, Camenzind E, *et al.*: Quantitative assessment with intracoronary ultrasound of the mechanisms of restenosis after percutaneous transluminal coronary angioplasty and directional coronary atherectomy. *Am J Cardiol* 1995, 75:772–777.

4. Tenaglia AN, Buller CE, Kisslo KB, *et al.*: Mechanisms of balloon angioplasty and directional coronary atherectomy as assessed by intracoronary ultrasound. *J Am Coll Cardiol* 1992, 20:685–691.

5. Nakamura S, Mahon D, Leung C, *et al.*: Intracoronary ultrasound imaging before and after directional coronary atherectomy: in vitro and clinical observations. *Am Heart J* 1995, 129:841–851.

6. Matar FA, Mintz GS, Farb A, *et al.*: The contribution of tissue removal to lumen improvement after directional coronary atherectomy. *Am J Cardiol* 1994, 74:647–650.

7. Umans VA, Baptista J, di Mario C, *et al.*: Angiographic, ultrasonic, and angioscopic assessment of the coronary artery wall and lumen area configuration after directional atherectomy: the mechanism revisited. *Am Heart J* 1995, 130:217–227.

8. Popma JJ, Mintz GS, Satler LF, *et al.*: Clinical and angiographic outcome after directional coronary atherectomy: a qualitative and quantitative analysis using coronary arteriography and intravascular ultrasound. *Am J Cardiol* 1993, 72:55E–64E.

9.•• Matar FA, Mintz GS, Pinnow E, *et al.*: Multivariate predictors of intravascular ultrasound end points after directional coronary atherectomy. *J Am Coll Cardiol* 1995, 25:318–324.

This article identifies the clinical, angiographic, procedural, and intravascular ultrasound predictors of directional atherectomy results assessed by intravascular ultrasound.

10. Fitzgerald PJ, Yock PG: Mechanisms and outcomes of angioplasty and atherectomy assessed by intravascular ultrasound imaging. *J Clin Ultrasound* 1993, 21:579–588.

11.• Mintz GS, Popma JJ, Pichard AD, *et al.*: Patterns of calcification in coronary artery disease: a statistical analysis of intravascular ultrasound and coronary angiography in 1155 lesions. *Circulation* 1995, 91:1959–1965.

Using intravascular ultrasound and coronary angiography, the authors describe the magnitude, location, and distribution of coronary artery calcification in a large number of patients.

12. Mintz GS, Douek P, Pichard AD, *et al.*: Target lesion calcification in coronary artery disease: an intravascular ultrasound study. *J Am Coll Cardiol* 1992, 20:1149–1155.

13. Fitzgerald PJ, Muhlberger VA, Moes NY, *et al.*: Calcium location within plaque as a predictor of atherectomy tissue retrieval: an intravascular ultrasound study [abstract]. *Circulation* 1992, 86:I-516.

14. Hinohara T, Robertson GC, Selmon MR, *et al.*: Directional coronary atherectomy complications and management. *Cathet Cardiovasc Diagn* 1993, 1:61–71.

15. Mintz GS, Pichard AD, Kent KM, *et al.*: Transcatheter device synergy: preliminary experience with adjunct directional coronary atherectomy following high-speed rotational atherectomy or excimer laser angioplasty in the treatment of coronary artery disease. *Cathet Cardiovasc Diagn* 1993, 1:37–44.

16. Hausmann D, Mugge A, Daniel WG: The form of atherosclerotic coronary plaques: pathoanatomic concepts and new insights using intravascular ultrasound [in German]. *Z Kardiol* 1994, 83:717–726.

17. Waller BF: Anatomy, histology, and pathology of the major epicardial coronary arteries relevant to echocardiographic imaging techniques. *J Am Soc Echocardiogr* 1989, 2:232–252.

18. Garratt KN, Edwards WD, Kaufmann UP, *et al.*: Differential histopathology of primary atherosclerotic and restenotic lesions in coronary arteries and saphenous vein bypass grafts: analysis of tissue obtained from 73 patients by directional atherectomy. *J Am Coll Cardiol* 1991, 17:442–448.

19. Safian RD, Gelbfish JS, Erny RE, *et al.*: Coronary atherectomy: clinical, angiographic, and histological findings and observations regarding potential mechanisms. *Circulation* 1990, 82:69–79.

20. Kimura BJ, Fitzgerald PJ, Sudhir K, *et al.*: Guidance of directed coronary atherectomy by intracoronary ultrasound imaging. *Am Heart J* 1992, 124:1365–1369.

21. The GUIDE Trial Investigators: IVUS-Determined predictors of restenosis in PTCA and DCA: an interim report from the GUIDE trial, phase II [abstract]. *Circulation* 1994, 90:I-23.

22. Nakamura S, Mahon DJ, Leung CY, *et al.*: Intracoronary ultrasound imaging before and after directional coronary atherectomy: in vitro and clinical observations. *Am Heart J* 1995, 129:841–851.

23. Suarez de Lezo J, Romero M, Medina A, *et al.*: Intracoronary ultrasound assessment of directional coronary atherectomy: immediate and follow-up findings. *J Am Coll Cardiol* 1993, 21:298–307.

24. Yock PG, Fitzgerald PJ, Sudhir K, *et al.*: Intravascular ultrasound imaging for guidance of atherectomy and other plaque removal techniques. *Int J Card Imaging* 1991, 6:179–189.

25. Leon MB, Kuntz RE, Popma JJ, *et al.*: Acute angiographic intravascular ultrasound and clinical results of directional atherectomy in the Optimal Atherectomy Restenosis Study [abstract]. *J Am Coll Cardiol* 1995 (February Special Issue):137A.

26. Aizawa T, Suzuki T, Kato O, *et al.*: Acute results from the ABACAS (Adjunctive Balloon Angioplasty following Coronary Atherectomy Study) trial. *J Invas Cardiol* 1996, 8:31.

27. Kimura T, Kaburagi S, Tashima Y, *et al.*: Geometric remodeling and intimal regrowth as mechanisms of restenosis: observations from Serial Ultrasound analysis of Restenosis (SURE) trial [abstract]. *Circulation* 1995, 92:I-76–I-77.

28. Mintz GS, Pichard AD, Dussaillant GR, *et al.*: Acute results of adjunctive stents following directional coronary atherectomy [abstract]. *Circulation* 1995, 92:I-328.

29. Mintz GS, Fitzgerald PJ, Kuntz RE, *et al.*: Lesion site and reference segment remodeling after directional coronary atherectomy: an analysis from the Optimal Atherectomy Restenosis Study [abstract]. *Circulation* 1995, 92:I-93.

30. Shurmur SW, Deligonul U, Rayner RW, *et al.*: Transverse coronary dissection resulting in abrupt vessel closure following directional coronary atherectomy: clinical, angiographic, and intracoronary ultrasound findings. *Cathet Cardiovasc Diagn* 1994, 32:174–177.

31. Popma JJ, Topol EJ, Hinohara T, *et al.*: Abrupt vessel closure after directional coronary atherectomy. *J Am Coll Cardiol* 1992, 19:1372–1379.

32. Komiyama N, Metz JA, Preuss P, *et al.*: Quantitative tissue characterization of atherosclerotic plaques and thrombus by intravascular ultrasound radio-frequency analysis [abstract]. *J Invas Cardiol* 1996, 8:77.

33. Topol EJ, Leya F, Pinkerton CA, *et al.*: A comparison of directional atherectomy with coronary angioplasty in patients with coronary artery disease: the CAVEAT Study Group [abstract]. *N Engl J Med* 1993, 329:221–227.

34. Adelman AG, Cohen EA, Kimball BP, *et al.*: A comparison of directional atherectomy with balloon angioplasty for lesions of the left anterior descending coronary artery. *N Engl J Med* 1993, 329:228–233.

35. Kuntz RE, Hinohara T, Safian RD, *et al.*: Restenosis after directional coronary atherectomy: effects of luminal diameter and deep wall excision. *Circulation* 1992, 86:1394–1399.

36. Kuntz RE, Safian RD, Carrozza JP, *et al.*: The importance of acute luminal diameter in determining restenosis after coronary atherectomy or stenting. *Circulation* 1992, 86:1827–1835.

37. Baim DS, Simonton CA, Popma JJ, *et al.*: Mechanism of luminal enlargement by optimal atherectomy: IVUS insights from the OARS study. *J Am Coll Cardiol* 1996, 27(2 suppl A):291.

38. Popma JJ, Baim DS, Kuntz RE, *et al.*: Early and late quantitative angiographic outcomes in the Optimal Atherectomy Restenosis Study (OARS). *J Am Coll Cardiol* 1996, 27(2 suppl A):291.

39. Beere PA, Glagov S, and Zarins CK: Experimental atherosclerosis at the carotid bifurcation of the cynomolgus monkey: localization, compensatory enlargement, and the sparing effect of lowered heart rate. *Arterioscler Thromb* 1992, 12:1245–1253.

40. Clarkson TB, Prichard RW, Morgan TM, *et al.*: Remodeling of coronary arteries in human and nonhuman primates. *JAMA* 1994, 271:289–294.

41. Glagov S, Weisenberg E, Zarins CK, *et al.*: Compensatory enlargement of human atherosclerotic coronary arteries. *N Engl J Med* 1987, 316:1371–1375.

42. Stiel GM, Stiel LS, Schofer J, *et al.*: Impact of compensatory enlargement of atherosclerotic coronary arteries on angiographic assessment of coronary artery disease. *Circulation* 1989, 80:603–1609.

43. Ge J, Erbel R, Zamorano J, *et al.*: Coronary artery remodeling in atherosclerotic disease: an intravascular ultrasonic study in vivo. *Coronary Artery Disease* 1993, 4:981–986.

44. Gerber TC, Erbel R, Gorge G, *et al.*: Extent of atherosclerosis and remodeling of the left main coronary artery determined by intravascular ultrasound. *Am J Cardiol* 1994, 73:666–671.

45. Hermiller JB, Tenaglia AN, Kisslo KB, *et al.*: In vivo validation of compensatory enlargement of atherosclerotic coronary arteries. *Am J Cardiol* 1993, 71:665–668.

46. Losordo DW, Rosenfield K, Kaufman J, *et al.*: Focal compensatory enlargement of human arteries in response to progressive atherosclerosis: in vivo documentation using intravascular ultrasound. *Circulation* 1994, 89:2570–2577.

47. McPherson DD, Sirna SJ, Hiratzka LF, *et al.*: Coronary arterial remodeling studied by high-frequency epicardial echocardiography: an early compensatory mechanism in patients with obstructive coronary atherosclerosis. *J Am Coll Cardiol* 1991, 17:79–86.

48. Wong CB, Porter TR, Xie F, *et al.*: Segmental analysis of coronary arteries with equivalent plaque burden by intravascular ultrasound in patients with and without angiographically significant coronary artery disease. *Am J Cardiol* 1995, 76:598–601.

49. Post MJ, Borst C, Kuntz, RE: The relative importance of arterial remodeling compared with intimal hyperplasia in lumen renarrowing after balloon angioplasty. *Circulation* 1994, 89:2816–2821.

50.• Isner JM: Vascular remodeling: honey I think I shrunk the artery. *Circulation* 1994, 89:2937–2941.

The author reviews the restenosis mechanisms after balloon angioplasty particularly in the context of vascular remodeling.

51. Honda Y, Schwarzacher SP, Suzuki T, *et al.*: Late vessel expansion after directional atherectomy: initial observation from the Adjunctive Balloon Angioplasty following Coronary Atherectomy Study (ABACAS) [abstract]. *J Invas Cardiol* 1996, 8:33.

52. Tenaglia AN, Kisslo K, Kelly S, *et al.*: Ultrasound guide wire-directed stent deployment. *Am Heart J* 1993, 125:1213–1216.

53. Tobis JM, Hall P, Maiello L, *et al.*: Clinical feasibility of an 0.018″ intravascular ultrasound imaging device. *Circulation* 1995, 92:I-400.

54. Evans JL, Ng KH, Vonesh MJ, *et al.*: Arterial imaging with a new forward-viewing intravascular ultrasound catheter: I. Initial studies. *Circulation* 1994, 89:712–717.

55. Ng KH, Evans JL, Vonesh MJ, *et al.*: Arterial imaging with a new forward-viewing intravascular ultrasound catheter: II. Three-dimensional reconstruction and display of data. *Circulation* 1994, 89:718–723.

56. Hausmann D, Sudhir K, Fitzgerald PJ, *et al.*: Contrast-enhanced intravascular ultrasound: validation of a new technique for delineation of the vessel wall boundary. *J Am Coll Cardiol* 1994, 23:981–987.

57. Crowley RJ, Hamm MA, Joshi SH, *et al.*: Ultrasound guided therapeutic catheters: recent developments and clinical results. *Int J Card Imaging* 1991, 6:145–156.

58.•• Fitzgerald PJ, Belef M, Connolly AJ, *et al.*: Design and initial testing of an ultrasound-guided directional atherectomy device. *Am Heart J* 1995, 129:593–598.

This paper describes initial in vitro testing of the prototype combined imaging and DCA catheter.

59. MacIsaac AI, Yock PG, Fitzgerald PJ, *et al.*: Initial in-vivo and in-vitro testing of an ultrasound-guided directional coronary atherectomy catheter [abstract]. *J Am Coll Cardiol* 1995 (February Special Issue):268–269.

60. Matar FA, Mintz GS, Douek P, *et al.*: Coronary artery lumen volume measurement using three-dimensional intravascular ultrasound: validation of a new technique. *Cathet Cardiovasc Diagn* 1994, 33:214–220.

61. Weissman NJ, Palacios IF, Nidorf SM, *et al.*: Three-dimensional intravascular ultrasound assessment of plaque volume after successful atherectomy. *Am Heart J* 1995, 130:413–419.

62. Rosenfield K, Losordo DW, Ramaswamy K, *et al.*: Three-dimensional reconstruction of human coronary and peripheral arteries from images recorded during two-dimensional intravascular ultrasound examination. *Circulation* 1991, 84:1938–1956.

63. Rosenfield K, Kaufman J, Pieczek A, *et al.*: Real-time three-dimensional reconstruction of intravascular ultrasound images of iliac arteries. *Am J Cardiol* 1992, 70:412–415.

64. Coy KM, Fishbein MC, Laas T, *et al.*: In vitro validation of three-dimensional intravascular ultrasound for the evaluation of arterial injury after balloon angioplasty. *J Am Coll Cardiol* 1992, 20:692–700.

65. Cavaye DM, White RA, Lerman RD, *et al.*: Usefulness of intravascular ultrasound imaging for detection of experimentally induced aortic dissection in dogs and for determining the effectiveness of endoluminal stenting. *Am J Cardiol* 1992, 69:705–707.

66. Schryver TE, Popma JJ, Kent KM, *et al.*: Use of intracoronary ultrasound to identify the "true" coronary lumen in chronic coronary dissection treated with intracoronary stenting. *Am J Cardiol* 1992, 69:1107–1108.

67. Klein HM, Guenther RW, Verlande M, *et al.*: 3D-surface reconstruction of intravascular ultrasound images using personal computer hardware and a motorized catheter control. *Cardiovasc Intervent Radiol* 1992, 15:97–101.

68. Aretz HT, Martinelli MA, LeDet EG: Intraluminal ultrasound guidance of transverse laser coronary atherectomy. *Int J Card Imaging* 1989, 4:153–157.

69. Aretz HT, Gregory KW, Martinelli MA, *et al.*: Ultrasound guidance of laser atherectomy. *Int J Card Imaging* 1991, 6:231–237.

THE STATUS OF THE ERBAC, STRATAS, AND DART TRIALS

Chapter 2

Sorin J. Brener
Nicolaus Reifart
Patrick L. Whitlow

Percutaneous rotational atherectomy is a second-generation coronary interventional device that has gained considerable popularity in the past 5 years. The Rotablator (Boston Scientific Northwest Technology Center [formerly Heart Technology], Redmond, WA) was designed by David Auth [1]. It consists of an abrasive diamond-coated elliptical burr welded to a flexible drive shaft that tracks along a central guidewire. The drive shaft is housed in a 4-F sheath connected to a high-pressure, air-powered turbine that rotates at speeds of up to 200,000 revolutions per minute (rpm). Continuous infusion of saline (with or without various vasodilatory drugs) is used to minimize arterial spasm and facilitate dissipation of the heat produced by the rotating drive shaft. Burr sizes range from 1.25 to 2.5 mm in diameter, necessitating 8- to 10-F sheaths.

Rotational atherectomy has been used for the entire spectrum of lesion morphology [2•], but has proven to be particularly effective in the treatment of calcified, ostial, and long lesions, for which balloon angioplasty is both ineffective and associated with high restenosis rates [3,4••]. Two aspects of this revascularization strategy appeal to the interventional cardiologist. First, lesions otherwise inaccessible to conventional balloon angioplasty can now be approached [5]. Second, rotational atherectomy selectively ablates atheromatous material without dissections or affecting the uninvolved portion of the vessel wall [6]. These two properties and the consistently obtainable enlarged lumen without haziness or dissection have led to an increased utilization of this device, in the hope of optimizing short-term results and reducing restenosis (Figs. 2-1 and 2-2).

As of January 1993, the Heart Technology Registry compiled 3424 rotablation procedures in 2499 patients, with an average age of 63 years. The procedural success was uniformly above 90%, regardless of the presence of adverse morphologic characteristics, such as calcification, bifurcation lesions, restenosis, or increased length.

Warth and colleagues [7] published a large observational report, summarizing the US experience in 709 patients, which confirmed the theoretical advantages described previously. The procedural success rate was extremely favorable (95% including the use of adjunctive balloon angioplasty). Despite a 10% incidence of angiographic dissection, the major complication rate was similar to that of other devices. Angiographic restenosis was 38% at 6 months.

MacIsaac and colleagues [4••] compared the outcome of rotational atherectomy in calcified and noncalcified lesions among 2161 patients with single-lesion procedures enrolled in the Heart Technology Rotablator Registry. The patients with calcified lesions were significantly older than those without calcifications, and had a higher incidence of unstable angina and multivessel involvement. Their lesions had significantly more adverse morphologic features, such as eccentricity, length greater than 10 mm, and excessive angulation. Despite these adverse clinical and angiographic characteristics, the procedural success rate was as good in patients with and without calcified lesions (94% vs 95%; $P = 0.32$). The rate of major complications (death, Q-wave myocardial infarction [MI], non–Q-wave MI, emergency coronary artery bypass graft [CABG]) in patients with calcified lesions was similar to that observed in patients without calcified lesions.

Important data on the evolution of the rotablation technique were reported recently by Stertzer and colleagues [8•]. Over a 4-year period, they observed a consistent decrease in the utilization of high-pressure (≥ 4 atm) adjunctive balloon angioplasty (36% to 14%) and an increase in the number of burrs used per lesion (2.0 to 2.7). Other technical refinements included the addition of verapamil and nitroglycerin to the flush solution, close monitoring of burr deceleration, and limitation of individual burr passage time to 10 to 20 seconds. With these refinements in technique, Stertzer and colleagues reported the almost complete abolition of slow flow and arterial spasm as complications. Collectively, these observations emphasize the urgent need for randomized trials designed to validate the role and efficacy of rotational atherectomy versus balloon angioplasty or other atherectomy devices. This article reviews three randomized trials of rotational atherectomy: the ERBAC (Excimer Rotational Balloon Angioplasty Comparison); STRATAS (the Study to Determine Rotablator and Transluminal Angioplasty Strategy); and the DART (Dilation versus Ablation Revascularization Trial).

The ERBAC Study

This study is the only completed randomized trial of rotational atherectomy versus alternative revascularization strategies to date. It was performed at a single institution in Frankfurt am Main, Germany, between October 1991 and December 1993.

Inclusion and Exclusion Criteria

A total of 615 symptomatic patients with 50% or greater *de novo* stenosis of a native coronary artery were randomly allocated to excimer laser (212 patients), rotational atherectomy (208 patients), and balloon angioplasty (195 patients) treatment. Data were analyzed and reported based on an intention-to-treat design. Angiographic inclusion criteria consisted of lesion types B or C (American Heart Association [AHA]/American College of Cardiology [ACC] classification) and potential treatment by all three devices. Lesions with excessive angulation or bifurcation morphology were excluded from enrollment. Patients who had MI or angioplasty within 4 months were also excluded.

General Procedural Aspects

Aspirin, nitrates, and heparin were used in all patients before and during the procedure, and aspirin was continued for at least 6 months after the procedure.

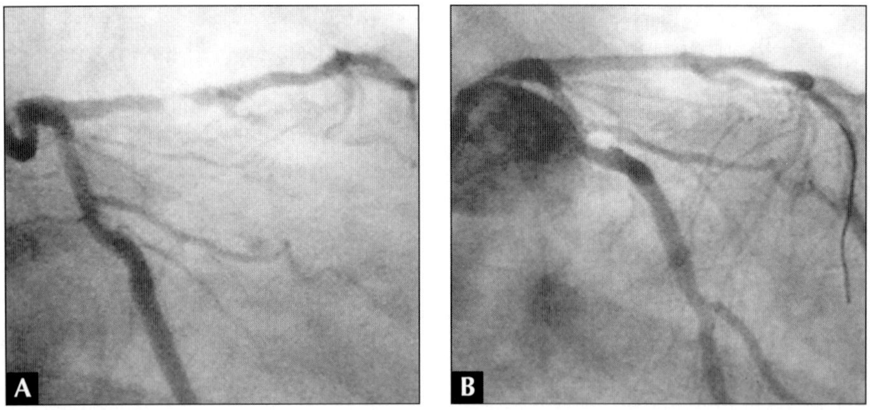

Figure 2-1. Angiographic appearance before (**A**) and after (**B**) rotational atherectomy and adjunctive balloon angioplasty of a proximal left anterior descending artery narrowing.

Creatine kinase (CK) measurement was performed 12 hours after the procedure and repeated if abnormal (> 2 × upper limit of normal). Independent core laboratory quantitative angiographic analysis was performed on images obtained before and after the procedure and at the 6-month follow-up catheterization.

Rotational Atherectomy

Rotational atherectomy was performed with burrs 1.25 to 2.25 mm in diameter. The starting burr size was chosen by the operator, and additional, larger burrs were used if angiographic results were unsatisfactory after a few passages. The planned maximal burr-to-artery ratio was 0.66 to 1. If residual stenosis was greater than 50%, adjunctive low-pressure (≤ 4 atm) balloon angioplasty was performed after ablation. The ablation sequences were limited to 20 s each to allow for particle dissipation. The flush solution contained saline, nitroglycerin (4 mg/1000 cc) and verapamil (10 mg/1000 cc).

Laser Angioplasty

Laser angioplasty was performed with two 308-nm xenon chloride excimer laser systems (Advanced Interventional Systems, Irvine, CA, and Spectranetics, Colorado Springs, CO). Catheters sized of 1.3 to 2.2 mm were used to a maximum catheter-to-artery ratio of 0.66 to 1, followed by adjunctive balloon angioplasty to obtain a residual diameter stenosis of less than 50%.

Balloon Angioplasty

Balloon angioplasty was performed in a standard fashion, using a balloon-to-artery ratio of 1.0 to 1.1. Intention-to-treat analysis was performed primarily, followed by a secondary analysis of the data after accounting for procedural cross-over.

Results

Baseline characteristics

The important baseline clinical and angiographic characteristics of the patients randomly allocated to the three devices are detailed in Table 2-1. In general, the patients were predominantly men and 13% to 18% had unstable angina. One half of the patients had had an MI; three-vessel disease and severe left ventricular dysfunction were uncommon. Half of the lesions were longer than 10 mm, and more than 80% were classified as AHA/ACC class B. Fluoroscopic calcification was noted in 40% of the lesions, and 20% of lesions had less than TIMI (Thrombolysis In Myocardial Infarction) 3 flow prior to the intervention. The left anterior descending artery accounted for half of the treated vessels, and the average reference diameter was 2.9 mm. The three groups were well matched with respect to their baseline characteristics.

Procedural success

As shown in Table 2-2, both laser and rotational atherectomy achieved low rates of "device-alone success," defined as 20% or greater improvement in diameter stenosis (38% and 36%, respectively), and almost all patients had adjunctive balloon angioplasty. The final procedural success rate was significantly greater in the Rotablator group (90%) as compared with laser and balloon angioplasty (77% and 80%, respectively; $P = 0.0016$). Inability to successfully treat the lesion with the assigned device was encountered significantly more frequently in the laser group, with the vast majority receiving balloon angioplasty alone. The procedural success rate, according to the actual device used, was still significantly higher in the Rotablator group compared with laser and balloon angioplasty (91%, 91%, and 83%, respectively; $P = 0.023$). There was no significant difference in the acute gain or resid-

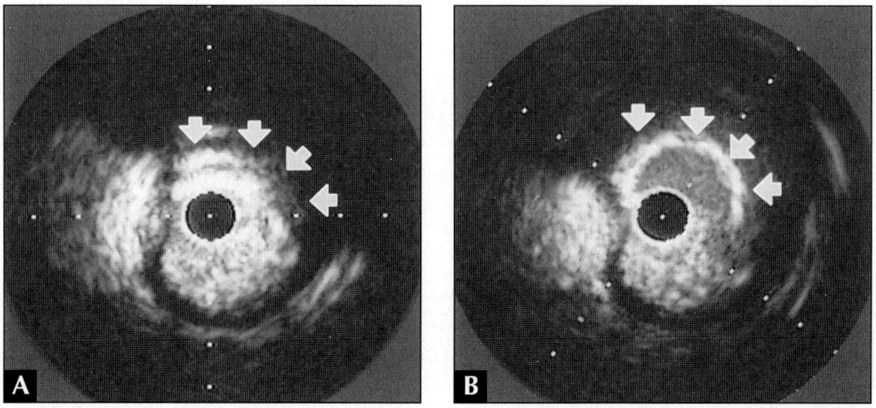

Figure 2-2. Intravascular ultrasound interrogation of the narrowing shown in Figure 2-1, before (**A**) and after (**B**) rotational atherectomy. The *arrows* point to the extensive arc of calcium present in the lesion. The pictures are presented in identical angular orientation to exemplify the preferential cutting ability of the burr. Most of the lumen gain results from plaque ablation in the calcified sector.

ual stenosis among the three groups. The patients treated with rotational atherectomy experienced significantly less severe dissections than those treated with laser or balloon angioplasty (5.3%, 12.3%, and 9.7%, respectively; $P = 0.04$).

In-hospital events

In general, there was no significant difference in the in-hospital outcome of patients treated with any of the three devices tested (Table 2-3). There was a low rate of bail-out stenting, and MI was infrequent, ranging between 2.8% and 4.2%. Despite protocol-mandated CK measurements, the rate of non–Q-wave myocardial infarction (defined as > 2 × upper limit of normal) was extremely low at (1.9% to 2.4%).

Follow-up events at 1 year

As shown in Table 2-3, the three groups differed significantly in the rate of repeat percutaneous intervention to the target vessel, which occurred in 27%, 37%, and 40% of the patients randomly assigned to balloon angioplasty, rotablation, and laser angioplasty, respectively ($P = 0.02$). The majority of repeat revascularization procedures were performed in response to recurrent angina or demonstrable ischemia (73% to 81%), whereas angiographic restenosis alone prompted repeat angioplasty in 20% of patients. There was a strong trend toward more freedom from the composite endpoint of death, MI, and target vessel revascularization in the balloon angioplasty group as compared with Rotablator and laser (63%, 54%, and 52%, respectively; $P = 0.057$). Follow-up angiography was not complete, but was performed in 56%, 68%, and 68% of the groups, respectively ($P = 0.008$). Angiographic restenosis was not different among the three groups, at 47%, 57%, and 59%, respectively ($P = 0.12$).

In summary, this important single center experience demonstrates that for complex lesions in patients with stable angina and preserved left ventricular function, rotational atherectomy achieves superior procedural success rates when compared with balloon angioplasty or laser atherectomy. In ERBAC this advantage was related to the ability of rotational atherectomy, at a burr-to-artery ratio of 0.59 ± 0.14 to 1, to facilitate subsequent balloon angioplasty, rather than to stand-alone success of the Rotablator. In addition, the trial reemphasized the positive association of significant postprocedural residual stenosis with angiographic and clinical restenosis. The increased procedural success with

TABLE 2-1. BASELINE CLINICAL AND ANGIOGRAPHIC CHARACTERISTICS OF PATIENTS RANDOMLY ASSIGNED TO THREE TREATMENTS OF CORONARY STENOSES

	Angioplasty	Laser	Rotablation
Age, y	63 ± 9	62 ± 9	61 ± 10
Diabetes mellitus, %	17	18	15
Unstable angina, %	13	17	18
Previous MI, %	46	43	47
Previous CABG, %	5	6	4
Severe LV dysfunction, %	6	5	6
ACC/AHA B1/B2/C, %	24/65/22	20/68/12	20/66/14
Calcified lesions, %	39	43	40
Lesions longer than 10 mm, %	47	51	49

ACC/AHA—American College of Cardiology/American Heart Association; CABG—coronary artery bypass grafting; LV—left ventricle; MI—myocardial infarction.

rotablation did not translate into an advantage in clinical events or restenosis, as demonstrated by complete clinical follow-up and a reasonable angiographic follow-up. Additional information provided by this study addresses the low incidence of infarction and no-reflow phenomenon observed in the patients treated with rotational atherectomy. The latter is a reflection of the evolution of technique of rotational atherectomy used in this trial (short ablation runs, meticulous attention to burr deceleration, limited burr-to-artery ratio, and addition of vasodilatory substances to the flush solution).

Three important issues were not explored by this trial. The first is the possibility that more aggressive plaque ablation prior to adjunctive balloon angioplasty might reduce restenosis. This hypothesis is based on the observations from intravascular ultrasound that rotational atherectomy reduces the rate of large dissections and lumen irregularities created by balloon angioplasty in complex lesions and that more complete ablation can maximize the postprocedural minimal lumen diameter, thus increasing the likelihood of a durable result [9]. The second remaining dilemma is whether aggressive rotational atherectomy with a large burr-to-artery ratio might provide a sufficiently large lumen to totally obviate the need for adjunctive balloon angioplasty (with its associated deep wall injury), or require only low-pressure inflations (≤ 1 atm) for lumen "smoothing." This strategy may limit the late lumen loss observed after arterial remodeling and intimal reendothelialization. The third unanswered question relates to whether rotational atherectomy should be used only in complex lesions, or if the Rotablator can improve results even in AHA/ACC class A and B1 lesions. Two studies presently underway to clarify these issues are described in the following sections.

The STRATAS Study

STRATAS examines the first two questions mentioned previously, *ie*, what is the optimal ablation strategy as it relates to burr-to-artery ratio and subsequent adjunctive balloon angioplasty?

The objective is to compare an "aggressive" rotablation strategy (burr-to-artery ratio 0.7–0.9 to 1 alone, or with adjunctive ≤ 1 atm balloon angioplasty) with a "conventional" ablation approach (burr-to-artery ratio 0.5–0.7 to 1 followed by routine adjunctive balloon angioplasty at inflation pressures ≥ 4 atm). The two strategies differ significantly in the amount of deep wall injury created with the adjunctive dilatation, thus potentially affecting the reactive hyperplasia and arterial remodeling that ensue. Minimal lumen diameter on 6- to 8-month recatheterization is the primary endpoint of the trial.

Patients and Inclusion Criteria

A multicenter group of experienced operators are now enrolling 500 patients consenting to repeat angiogra-

Table 2-2. Procedural Variables Among Three Treatments of Coronary Stenoses

	Angioplasty	Laser	Rotablation	*P* value
Reference diameter, *mm*	2.91 ± 0.62	2.95 ± 0.55	2.92 ± 0.55	0.84
Preprocedural stenosis, %	74 ± 10	75 ± 10	75 ± 10	0.76
Residual stenosis, %	35 ± 15	34 ± 14	33 ± 14	0.68
Device success, %		38	36	0.40
Procedural success, %	80	77	90	0.002
Cross-over rate, %	5	16	2	< 0.001
Procedural success after crossover, %*	83	91	91	0.023
Bail-out stenting, %	1	1.4	0.5	0.62

**Includes the alternative device.*

phy at 6 to 8 months and undergoing rotablation in native coronary arteries 3.25 mm or smaller in diameter are being enrolled by a multicenter group of experienced operators (Table 2-4). Patients are excluded if there is evidence for intracoronary thrombus, less than TIMI 3 flow in the target vessel, or a suspected MI.

Endpoints

The mechanistic, angiographic endpoint of the trial is the influence of the initial procedural strategy on the 6-month minimal lumen diameter, as assessed by an independent angiographic core laboratory. Multivariate logistic regression analysis will correct for the presence of confounding variables such as diabetes, restenotic lesions, procedural complications, and so on. In addition, procedural success and binary restenosis will be documented and compared between the two strategies.

Clinical endpoints monitored during the trial include death, Q-wave infarction, emergency bypass surgery, and the development of acute vessel closure, slow flow, neurologic deficits, and non–Q-wave infarction. Target vessel revascularization at 9 months will be documented and compared between groups.

A variety of substudies address additional issues related to rotablation, such as intravascular ultrasound interrogation to determine mechanisms of acute lumen gain and late lumen loss (intimal hyperplasia vs arterial remodeling) and use of strip charts to monitor burr deceleration and its relation to adverse outcome [10].

An interim analysis of the first 179 patients enrolled in the trial was presented in November 1995 [11]. The subjects had the typical profile for patients with coronary artery disease. A significantly higher number of burrs was used in the "aggressive" arm as compared with the "routine" approach (2.9 ± 1.1 vs 2.3 ± 0.8, respectively; $P = 0.002$). The burr-to-artery ratio by visual estimates was 0.82 ± 0.08 and 0.70 ± 0.06, respectively ($P = 0.0001$), thus confirming the ability to execute the trial design. The procedural success was 94.2% and there were few major complications (death, 1.5%; Q-wave infarction, none; emergency bypass surgery, 0.8%). The final residual stenosis by QCA was 23 ± 16%. Final data will be available in 1997.

The DART Study (Targeting Restenosis)

The third question unanswered by the ERBAC trial, *ie*, the potential advantage of rotablation over balloon angioplasty in the treatment of less complex lesions, is addressed by the DART study. The objective of DART is to demonstrate that rotational atherectomy (burr-to-artery ratio 0.7–0.85 to 1) followed by adjunctive balloon angioplasty at 1 atm or less

Table 2-3. In-hospital and 1-year Cumulative Events After Treatment for Coronary Stenoses

	Angioplasty		Laser		Rotablation	
	In-hospital	1 year	In-hospital	1 year	In-hospital	1 year
Patients, *n*	195	191	212	211	208	205
Death, %	1.0	3.7	0.9	1.9	0.5	2.4
Q-wave MI, %	2.1	2.6	0.9	2.4	1.0	2.4
Non–Q-wave MI, %	2.1	—	1.9	—	2.4	—
CABG, %	0	6.3	1.9	7.1	1.0	7.3
TLR, %	3.6	27	2.8	40	1.9	37*
Any event, %	3.1	37	3.7	48	2.5	46†

**P = 0.02*
†P = 0.015 angioplasty vs laser; P = 0.04 angioplasty vs rotablation
CABG—coronary artery bypass grafting; MI—myocardial infarction; TLR—target lesion revascularization.

reduces the incidence of target lesion revascularization at 8 months of follow-up compared with balloon angioplasty. The study design incorporates the assessment of clinical restenosis in 1000 patients and angiographic restenosis in a subset of 500 consecutive patients (Table 2-5).

Patients and Inclusion Criteria

A total of 1000 consenting adult patients with stable or unstable angina and class A or B1 lesions in native coronary arteries 2.0 to 2.9 mm in diameter will be enrolled. The lesions have to be amenable to both balloon angioplasty and rotational atherectomy. Patients with recent MI (1 week), recent percutaneous intervention (3 months), or rest angina refractory to medical therapy will be excluded. All patients will have clinical and stress test follow-up, and the first half of the cohort will have repeat angiography at 8 months.

Endpoints

The primary study endpoint is the incidence of target vessel failure at 1 year, which includes periprocedural death, Q-wave MI or bypass surgery, clinical restenosis (target vessel revascularization), or a major adverse event (Q-wave MI or death) that cannot be attributed to a nontarget vessel. This endpoint will be adjudicated by a panel of experts blinded to treatment allocation. In addition, target lesion minimal lumen diameter and binary restenosis will constitute additional prespecified major endpoints for the first 500 patients enrolled in the trial.

A host of secondary endpoints concerning procedure-related complications will be analyzed. Particular emphasis is given to MB-CK elevations(> 8 × normal, 3 to 8 × normal, < 3 × normal), and transfusion requirements; an economic analysis of both strategies will be performed as a separate substudy.

TABLE 2-4. INVESTIGATORS INVOLVED IN THE STRATAS (STUDY TO DETERMINE ROTABLATOR AND TRANSLUMINAL ANGIOPLASTY STRATEGY) TRIAL*†

Clinical site	Site principal investigator
Allegheny General Hospital, Pittsburgh, PA	David M. Lasorda, DO
Arizona Heart Institute, Phoenix, AZ	Richard R. Heuser, MD
Baptist Hospital of Miami, Miami, FL	Michael B. Collins, MD
Baptist Medical Center of Oklahoma City, Oklahoma City, OK	Robert M. Kipperman, MD
Beth Israel Hospital, Boston, MA	Richard E. Kuntz, MD
Cleveland Clinic Foundation, Cleveland, OH	Patrick L. Whitlow, MD
Deborah Heart & Lung Center, Browns Mills, NJ	Marc A. Taylor, MD
Mayo Clinic, Rochester, MN	Kirk N. Garratt, MD
Fairfax Hospital, Falls Church, VA	Bryan D. Raybuck, MD
Lenox Hill Hospital, New York, NY	Jeffrey W. Moses MD
Medical College of Virginia Hospitals, Richmond, VA	Michael J. Cowley, MD
Ochsner Clinic, Baton Rouge, LA	Stephen R. Ramee, MD
Rhode Island Hospital, Providence, RI	David O. Williams, MD
Providence Hospital, Providence, RI	David Warth, MD
Sanger Clinic, Sanger, CA	Robert M. Bersin, MD
University of Chicago Hospital, Chicago, IL	Ted Feldman, MD
University of Florida, Gainesville, FL	Theodore A. Bass, MD

**Principal investigator: Patrick L. Whitlow, MD; coprincipal investigator: Michael J. Cowley, MD*

†Associated investigators: Richard E. Kuntz, MD, MSc (Director, Cardiovascular Data Analysis Center, Harvard University/Beth Israel Hospital, 1295 Boylston Street, Suite 330, Boston, MA 02215); David S. Eccleston, MBBS (Director, STRATAS Strip Chart Core Laboratory, Department of Cardiology, F25, The Cleveland Clinic Foundation, 9500 Euclid Avenue, Cleveland, OH 044195); and David O. Williams, MD, (Director, Angiographic Core Laboratory, Cardiac Projects Office, Rhode Island Hospital, 593 Eddy Street, APC Building, Room 981, Providence, RI 02903).

Conclusions

The field of interventional cardiology is progressing rapidly and new devices are improving on the results of balloon angioplasty. Rotational coronary atherectomy is a unique approach that specifically ablates inelastic atheroma while, theoretically, sparing the normal arterial wall from injury. Rotational atherectomy has shown substantial promise in nonrandomized registries with respect to procedural success, complication rates, and potential to treat lesions otherwise not amenable to balloon angioplasty. Randomized trials (ERBAC, STRATAS, and DART) will answer many unresolved issues regarding this unique coronary interventional strategy. It is expected that the final results of these trials will enable us to define the role and optimal application of rotational coronary atherectomy.

Table 2-5. Investigators and Sites Involved in the DART (Dilation Versus Ablation Revascularization Trial Targeting Restenosis) Trial*†

Clinical site	Site principal investigator
University of Texas Health Science Center, Dallas, TX	Steven Bailey, MD
Beth Israel Hospital, Boston, MA	Donald Baim, MD
Scripps Memorial Hospital, Chula Vista, CA	Maurice Buchbinder, MD
Yale University School of Medicine, New Haven, CT	Michael Cleman, MD
Newark Beth Israel Medical Center, Newark, NJ	Barry Cohen, MD
Hackensack University Medical Center, Hackensack, NJ	Virender Sethi, MD
Kaiser Permanente Medical Center, S.D.	Richard Fortuna, MD
Allegheny General Hospital, Pittsburgh, PA	Robert L. Incorvati, DO
The Christ Hospital, Cincinnati, OH	Dean Kereiakes, MD
St. Luke's Roosevelt Hospital, New York, NY	James Slater, MD
St. Joseph's Hospital of Atlanta, Atlanta, GA	William Knopf, MD
St. Luke's Hospital	Thomas Shimshak, MD
Washington University School of Medicine, Seattle, WA	John Lasala, MD
The Valley Hospital	William K. Lee, MD
Mercy General Hospital, Sacremento, CA	Reginald Low, MD
Washington Hospital Center, Washington, DC	Martin Leon, MD
Milwaukee Heart and Vascular Clinic, Milwaukee, WI	Jack C. Manley, MD
Hahnemann University Hospital, Philadelphia, PA	Dan J. McCormick, DO
Naval Regional Medical Center, Jacksonville, FL	Maurice Buchbinder, MD
Massachusetts General Hospital, Boston, MA	Igor Palacios, MD
Swedish Medical Center, Englewood, CA	Mark Reisman, MD
Scripps Clinic, Chula Vista, CA	Paul Teirstein, MD
St. John Hospital and Medical Center, Detroit, MI	Theodore Schreiber, MD
Maimonides Medical Center, Brooklyn, NY	Jacob Shani, MD
Mount Sinai Hospital, New York, NY	Samin Sharma, MD
Good Samaritan Hospital	Steven Burstein, MD
Loyola University Hospital	Bruce Lewis, MD
Sharp Memorial Hospital, San Diego, CA	Maurice Buchbinder, MD
University of Cincinnati, Cincinnati, OH	Paul Runyan, MD
Virginia Mason Medical Center, Seattle, WA	Mark Reisman, MD
North Shore University Hospital, Manhasset, NY	Chiu Wong, MD
William Beaumont Hospital, Troy, MI	William O'Neill, MD
Houston Veterans Administrative Medical Center, Houston, TX	Nadir Ali, MD
Carle Clinic	Matthew Gibb, MD
Bowman Cray School of Medicine, Winston-Salem, NC	Paul Applegate, MD

**Principal Investigator: Mark Reisman, MD; coprincipal Investigator: Maurice Buchbinder, MD.*

†Associated investigators: Richard E. Kuntz, MD, MSc (Director, Cardiovascular Data Analysis Center, Harvard University/Beth Israel Hospital, 1295 Boylston Street, Suite 330, Boston, MA 02215); and Jeffrey J. Popma, MD (Director, Angiographic Core Laboratory, Washington Cardiology Center, 110 Irving Street NW, Suite 4B14, Washington, DC 20010).

References and Recommended Reading

Recently published papers of particular interest have been highlighted as:

- • Of special interest
- •• Of outstanding interest

1. Hansen DD, Auth DC, Vracko R, Ritchie JL: Rotational atherectomy in atherosclerotic rabbit iliac arteries. *Am Heart J* 1988, 115:160–165.

2.• Ellis SG, Popma JJ, Buchbinder M, Franco I, Leon MB, Kent KM, Pichard AD, Satler LF, Topol EJ, Whitlow PL: Relation of clinical presentation, stenosis morphology, and operator technique to the procedural results of rotational atherectomy-facilitated angioplasty. *Circulation* 1994, 89:882–892.

This article gives a comprehensive review of the clinical and angiographic variables related to rotational atherectomy procedural success and complications.

3. Topol EJ, Ellis SG, Fishman J, Leimgruber P, Myler RK, Stertzer SH, O'Neill WW, Douglas JS, Roubin GS, King SB III: Multicenter study of percutaneous transluminal angioplasty for right coronary artery ostial stenosis. *J Am Coll Cardiol* 1987, 9:1214–1218.

4.•• MacIsaac AI, Bass TA, Buchbinder M, Cowley MJ, Leon MB, Warth DC, Whitlow PL: High speed rotational atherectomy: outcome in calcified and noncalcified artery lesions. *Am Coll Cardiol* 1995, 26:731–736.

This paper compares the outcome of a large cohort of patients, with and without calcified lesions, who were enrolled in the Rotablator registry.

5. Popma JJ, Brogan WC III, Pichard AD, Satler LF, Kent KM, Mintz GS, Leon MB: Rotational coronary atherectomy of ostial stenoses. *Am J Cardiol* 1993, 71:436–438.

6. Mintz GS, Potkin BN, Keren G, Satler LF, Pichard AD, Kent KM, Popma JJ, Leon MB: Intravascular ultrasound evaluation of the effect of rotational atherectomy in obstructive atherosclerotic coronary artery disease. *Circulation* 1992, 86:1383–1393.

7. Warth DC, Leon MB, O'Neill W, Zacca N, Polissar NL, Buchbinder M: Rotational atherectomy multicenter registry: acute results, complications and 6-month angiographic follow-up in 709 patients. *J Am Coll Cardiol* 1994, 24:641–648.

8.• Stertzer SH, Pomerantsev EV, Fitzgerald PJ, Shaw RE, Walton AS, Singer AH, Yeung A, Yock PG, Oesterle SN: Effects of technique modification on immediate results of high speed rotational atherectomy in 710 procedures on 656 patients. *Cathet Cardiovasc Diagn* 1995, 36:304–310.

This article provides an up-to-date review of the advances in rotational atherectomy technique. These modifications have led to a significant reduction in the incidence of periprocedural ischemic complications.

9. Kuntz RE, Gibson CM, Nobuyoshi M, Baim DS: Generalized model of restenosis after conventional balloon angioplasty, stenting and directional atherectomy. *J Am Coll Cardiol* 1993, 21:15–25.

10. Eccleston DS, Horrigan MC, Cowley MJ, Kuntz RE, Williams DO, Whitlow PL, for the STRATAS Investigators: Is there a role for strip chart recording to guide rotational atherectomy? Initial findings from STRATAS [abstract]. *J Am Coll Cardiol* 1996, 27(suppl A):292A.

11. Whitlow PW, Cowley MJ, Kuntz RE, Williams DO, STRATAS Investigators: Study to determine rotablator and transluminal angioplasty strategy [abstract]. *Circulation* 1995, 92(suppl I):I-330.

Chapter 3

Atheroablation Prior to Stents

Mun K. Hong
Gary S. Mintz
Martin B. Leon
Kenneth M. Kent

Conventional angioplasty of calcified, native coronary artery lesions is associated with less than optimal results, higher angiographic complications, reduced procedural success [1], and increased restenosis rate [2]. Rotational atherectomy is particularly effective in the treatment of calcified coronary lesions by preferentially ablating the fibrocalcific plaque [3•] and by changing the lesion compliance [4•]. However, the restenosis rate following rotational atherectomy compared with balloon angioplasty appears to be similar according to the results of a recent randomized study [5••]. Furthermore, in large (> 3 mm) calcified coronary arteries, rotational atherectomy is not a stand-alone device owing to the maximum burr size of 2.5 mm and the recommended burr/artery diameter of 0.8 or less to minimize potential complications.

The Stent Restenosis Study (STRESS) [6••] and the Belgium-Netherlands Stent Trial (BENESTENT) [7••], comparing Palmaz-Schatz tubular slotted stent to balloon angioplasty in large, noncalcified coronary arteries, established the efficacy of stents in reducing restenosis rate. Stents also may reduce restenosis in large, calcified coronary arteries. However, elective use of stents in calcified coronary arteries has not been widespread because of theoretical considerations, such as the inability to fully expand the stent because of lesion rigidity.

Thus, the optimal treatment of calcified lesions in large coronary arteries may be initial rotational atherectomy to change the lesion compliance, followed by immediate stent implantation to maximize the acute gain. Before this procedure can become generalized, it should be proven safe because of the potential complications, such as increased subacute thrombosis from the microvascular disturbance seen with rotational atherectomy [8•] and coronary perforation from stent struts penetrating the vessel wall, especially from high-pressure adjunctive balloon angioplasty.

This chapter illustrates the safety and efficacy of stent implantation after rotational atherectomy in large, calcified native coronary arteries.

Methods

Study Population

The patient cohort included a consecutive series of all patients in the Washington Cardiology Center angioplasty database treated with rotational atherectomy followed by immediate stent implantation. All indications for stent use (*elective use*, to improve acute procedural safety and to reduce late clinical events; *provisional use*, to treat suboptimal primary device results; or *urgent use*, to treat abrupt or threatened closure) were included in this study. Baseline clinical demographics and in-hospital course were confirmed by independent hospital chart review. Clinical outcome data were obtained by serial telephone interviews conducted by research nurses. Late clinical events were adjudicated and corroborated by accompanying documentation.

Device Synergy Procedure

The details of the angioplasty procedures used have been described previously [6••,8•,9]. In brief, an 8-F or 9-F guiding catheter was used depending on the largest burr size anticipated. The dedicated 0.009-inch, 300-cm stainless-steel guidewire (Heart Technology, Bellevue, WA) was advanced beyond the stenosis. Rotational atherectomy was performed using various burr sizes (Heart Technology; 1.5 to 2.5 mm). Unlike other rotational atherectomy procedures (with maximal burr/reference artery diameter of approximately 0.8), the atheroablation during the device synergy procedure was not performed to provide complete ablation of fibrocalcific plaque but to change the lesion compliance. Thus, the maximal burr/reference artery diameter was less than 0.8. After placing the burr tip proximal to the stenosis, the system was activated and the burr tip was advanced slowly through the stenosis, with each run lasting less than 30 seconds. Following the initial ablative procedure, the guidewire was exchanged usually to a 0.014-inch extra-support wire (Advanced Cardiovascular Systems, Inc., Tecumsula, CA) for coronary Palmaz-Schatz stent (Johnson & Johnson Interventional Systems Co., Warren, NJ) implantation or a 0.018-inch extra-support wire for "biliary" Palmaz-Schatz stent or Gianturco-Roubin stent (Cook Inc., Bloomington, IN) implantation. Coronary Palmaz-Schatz stents were used whenever possible; the "biliary" version was reserved for vessels 4 mm or greater in diameter or for ostial lesions because of its improved radioopacity. The Gianturco-Roubin stent was used in smaller (< 3 mm in diameter) vessels or diffuse (> 15 mm) lesions. Coronary or biliary Palmaz-Schatz stents were used in 83% of the patients, and Gianturco-Roubin stents were used in 17% of patients. Following pre-atheroablation, balloon dilatation with 2.5 mm or larger balloon (with balloon/artery diameter close to 1.0 to test for full balloon expansion) was routinely performed in anticipation of subsequent stent placement. Finally, adjunct high-pressure percutaneous transluminal coronary angioplasty (PTCA) was performed after initial stent deployment (routinely to ≥ 16 atm). Angiographic and intravascular ultrasound (IVUS) assessment was performed before and after ablation, after stent implantation, and after adjunct PTCA. Optimal Palmaz-Schatz stent implantation was carefully monitored using an iterative technique with prespecified IVUS endpoints and additional high-pressure inflations as needed. Following Gianturco-Roubin stent implantation, IVUS was not performed to minimize the risk of distorting the stent geometry.

The pre- and poststent anticoagulation regimens varied widely throughout the course of this study. Initially, all patients were treated with aspirin 325 mg daily and postprocedure coumadin for 1 month to keep INR (international normalized ratio) between 2.5 and 3.5 (less than one third of all patients). More recently, all patients were treated with aspirin and ticlopidine 250 mg twice daily for 1 month, and additional low molecular weight heparin 30 mg subcutaneously twice daily (for 2 weeks) in particularly high-risk subsets (*eg*, for treatment of threatened closure). Those patients meeting the prespecified IVUS endpoints were treated with aspirin indefinitely and ticlopidine for 1 month.

Angiographic Analysis

All cineangiograms were reviewed at our Angiographic Core Laboratory by an observer who was unaware of the clinical outcome. Standard morphologic criteria were used for the identification of lesion location, length ("shoulder-to-shoulder"), eccentricity, irregularity, fluoroscopic calcification, and ulceration. These criteria were used to grade the American College of Cardiology/American Heart Association lesion criteria [1] as modified by Ellis [10]. Abrupt closure was defined as transient or permanent occlusion of the artery during the procedure. Dissection was graded using the National Heart, Lung, and Blood Institute classification [11]. Perforation was defined as extravasation of contrast agent outside the arterial lumen. Distal embolization was defined as thrombolysis in myocardial infarction flow less than 2 [12] or complete occlusion of a major distal branch at any point during the procedure. No reflow was defined as delayed clearance of contrast agent despite no obstructive epicardial lesion.

Quantitative angiographic analysis was performed using selected end-diastolic cineframes demonstrating the stenosis in its most severe and unforeshortened projection. Cineframes were optically magnified (2.4:1) and digitized using a cine-video converter. Using the contrast-filled guiding catheter as the calibration standard, reference and minimal lumen diameters were determined before and after rotational atherectomy, after stent implantation, and after final adjunct balloon inflation using a validated, automated edge-detection algorithm (Cardiovascular Measurement Systems, Medis, Leiden, the Netherlands). Based on these measurements, percent diameter stenoses were determined.

Intravascular Ultrasound Technique

Intravascular ultrasound studies were performed using one of two systems available commercially. The first system (InterTherapy Inc., Sunnyvale, CA) incorporated a single-element 25-MHz transducer and an angled mirror mounted on the tip of a flexible shaft, which was rotated at 1800 rpm within a 3.9-F short monorail polyethylene imaging sheath to form planar cross-sectional images in real time. With this system, the transducer was withdrawn automatically at 0.5 mm/s to perform the imaging sequence. The second system (Cardiovascular Imaging Systems, Inc., Sunnyvale, CA) used a single-element 30-MHz beveled transducer mounted on the end of a flexible shaft and rotated at 1800 rpm within a 2.9-F long monorail/common distal lumen imaging sheath or within a 3.2-F short monorail polyethylene imaging sheath. With this system, the transducer also was withdrawn automatically at 0.5 mm/s to perform the imaging sequence. Intravascular ultrasound measurements were performed on-line during the procedure and also were recorded on half-inch high resolution s-VHS videotapes for off-line analysis. Measurements at the same anatomic image slice were made before and after rotational atherectomy, after stent implantation, and after adjunct balloon angioplasty and included length, location, and arcs of calcium, areas of external elastic membrane, and lumen at lesion and reference sites.

Table 3-1. Baseline Characteristics of the Study Population*

Mean age, *y*	65 ± 11[†]
Male gender, %	66
Unstable angina, %	81
Hypertension, %	8.1
Diabetes mellitus, %	30
Prior myocardial infarction, %	36
Prior coronary artery bypass surgery, %	29
Left ventricular ejection fraction, %	48 ± 13

*Total number of patients, 178.
[†]Continuous variables are presented as mean±SD.*

Results

Clinical Demographics

Data regarding demographics of the study population are shown in Table 3-1. The baseline characteristics are representative of patients undergoing angioplasty, except that the mean age (65 ± 11 years) is slightly higher than our usual patient population (62 ± 11 years) and that no patients had experienced an acute myocardial infarction (AMI), because intraluminal thrombus is a contraindication for rotational atherectomy.

Angiographic and Intravascular Ultrasound Findings

Findings of angiography and IVUS are presented in Table 3-2. The majority of the lesions were de novo, nonostial lesions in heavily calcified coronary arteries. A few lesions were suggestive of intraluminal throm-

Table 3-2. Angiographic and Intravascular Ultrasound Findings*

Quantitative and qualitative coronary angiography	
Target artery, %	
Right coronary	36
Left main	4.5
Left anterior descending	38
Left circumflex	17
Lesion location, %	
Ostial	13
Proximal	41
Mid	39
Distal	6.3
Calcium, %	70
Restenotic lesion, %	22
Length, *mm*	9 ± 7[†]
Eccentricity, %	43
Ulceration, %	7.3
Thrombus, %	4.4
Total occlusion, %	2.2
Reference vessel, *mm*	2.81 ± 0.43
Minimal lumen diameter, *mm*	
Preintervention	1.05 ± 0.44
Post–rotational atherectomy	1.76 ± 0.61
Post-stent	2.57 ± 0.69
Final	2.81 ± 0.69
Intravascular ultrasound	
Lesion calcification, %	85
Superficial calcium, %	65
Superficial and deep calcium, %	25
Preintervention arc of calcium,°	209 ± 115

*Total number of patients, 224.
[†]Continuous variables are presented as mean ± SD.*

bus, although these also could have represented calcification [13••].

Reference vessel size was 2.81 ± 0.43 mm, and preintervention lesion had 62.4% ± 14.4% diameter stenosis. Incremental gains were obtained with each device use, and the final minimal lumen diameter closely matched that of the reference diameter (Fig. 3-1). Angiographic complications were rare: no incidence of no-reflow, one incidence of distal embolization, three episodes of abrupt closure, and one incidence of coronary perforation successfully sealed by the end of the procedure. Four patients were found to have at least type C dissection at the end of the procedure. These patients were treated with continued anticoagulation.

Preintervention IVUS confirmed the presence of extensive lesion calcification (Fig. 3-2). The majority (85%) of the patients had lesion calcification, and the remainder of patients had fibrotic component. There were both superficial (65%), and combined superficial and deep wall calcifications (25%) in these lesions, with 209 ± 115° arcs of superficial calcium. Off-line IVUS analysis showed that 19% of the stents were not fully apposed at the end of the procedure and that 6% of the stents did not expand fully (minor/major axis < 0.7).

Procedural results

Data regarding procedural effectiveness and long-term outcome are provided in Table 3-3. Angiographic success (final diameter stenosis < 50%) was obtained in 98% of patients. Procedural success (final diameter stenosis < 50% and no in-hospital death, Q-wave myocardial infarction [MI], or emergency coronary artery bypass surgery) was obtained in 92% of patients. The major ischemic complications included 4.1% death, 2.7% Q-wave MI, and 2.8% emergency coronary artery bypass surgery. There was one incidence of in-hospital stent thrombosis. Conversely non–Q-wave MI (creatine phosphokinase > 5 × normal) was seen in 24% of the patients. Vascular complications occurred in 3.9% of patients.

Subsequent Cardiac Events

During the first 30 days after the procedure, there was no incidence of subacute thrombosis in patients undergoing elective stent placement. However, in the

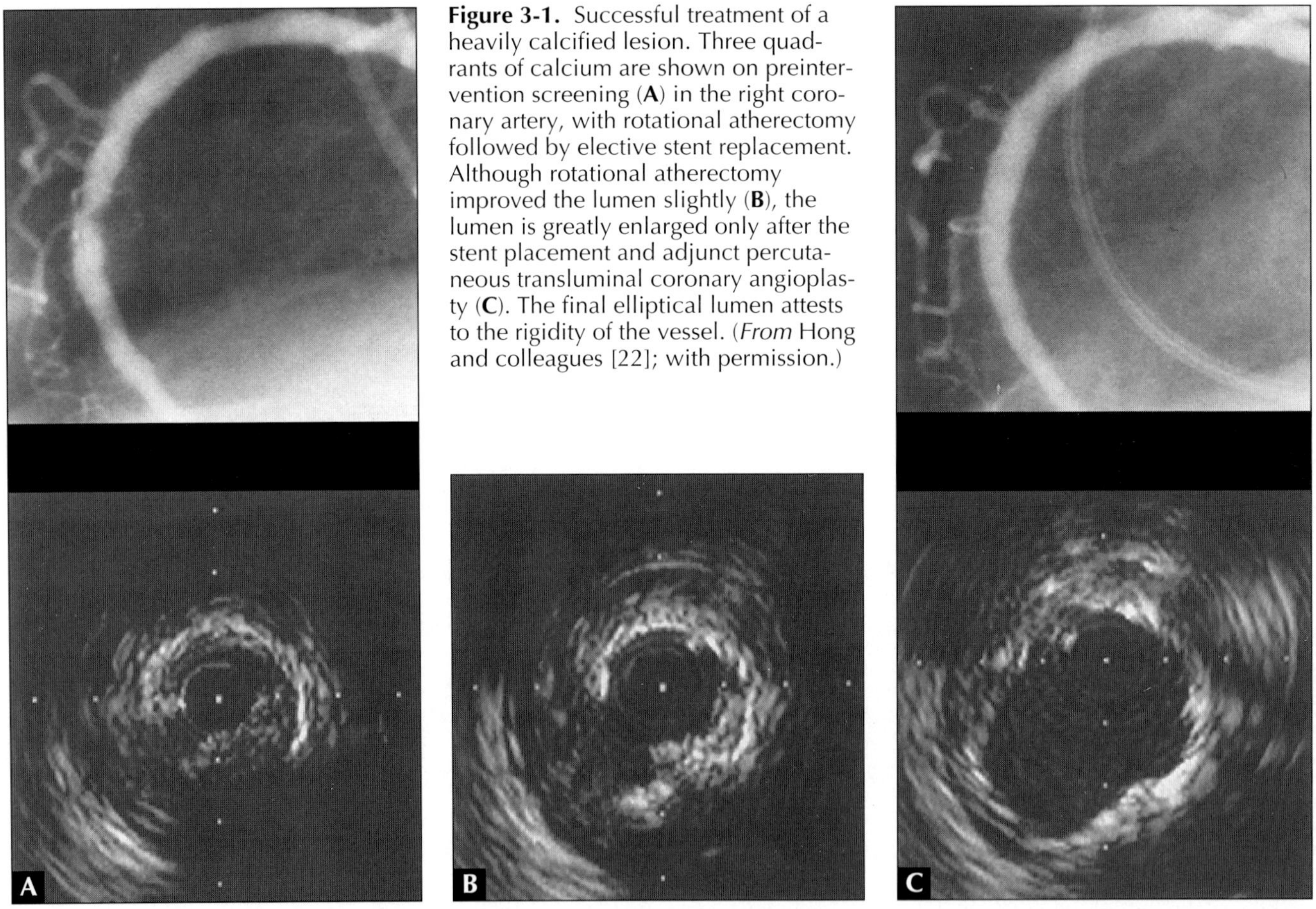

Figure 3-1. Successful treatment of a heavily calcified lesion. Three quadrants of calcium are shown on preintervention screening (**A**) in the right coronary artery, with rotational atherectomy followed by elective stent replacement. Although rotational atherectomy improved the lumen slightly (**B**), the lumen is greatly enlarged only after the stent placement and adjunct percutaneous transluminal coronary angioplasty (**C**). The final elliptical lumen attests to the rigidity of the vessel. (*From* Hong and colleagues [22]; with permission.)

other groups, four patients experienced subacute thrombosis. Including the one patient with in-hospital subacute thrombosis, the overall incidence of subacute thrombosis in this mixed patient population was 2.7%, although the incidence in the elective group was zero.

Long-Term Outcome

With complete clinical follow-up on those patients with successful initial procedure and 80% of patients with greater than 4-month follow-up, the overall target lesion revascularization was 13%. Death occurred in 2.7% of patients, and Q-wave MI occurred in 0.5% of patients.

Discussion

This review of stent placement following rotational atherectomy in large, calcified coronary arteries shows that this approach appears to be safe and effective. Overall procedural success was achieved in 92% of patients with 8.1% major ischemic complications. After the successful procedure, 2.7% incidence of subacute thrombosis was found up to 30 days of follow-up. Clinical follow-up suggests relatively low (13%) target-lesion revascularization.

Previous Reports

There are only a few reports of immediate stent placement following rotational atherectomy [14,15], both of which describe emergency stenting for treatment of coronary dissection complicating rotational atherectomy. In the larger series of 10 patients, three patients experienced major ischemic complications (one death and two Q-wave MI) and three patients had non–Q-wave MI with one stent thrombosis [15]. Thus, emergency bail-out stenting after complicated rotational atherectomy is associated with a high complication rate (30%) as well as an equally high incidence of non–Q-wave MI. The complications from rotational atherectomy were probably responsible for subsequent major ischemic sequelae, rather than the bail-out stent procedure.

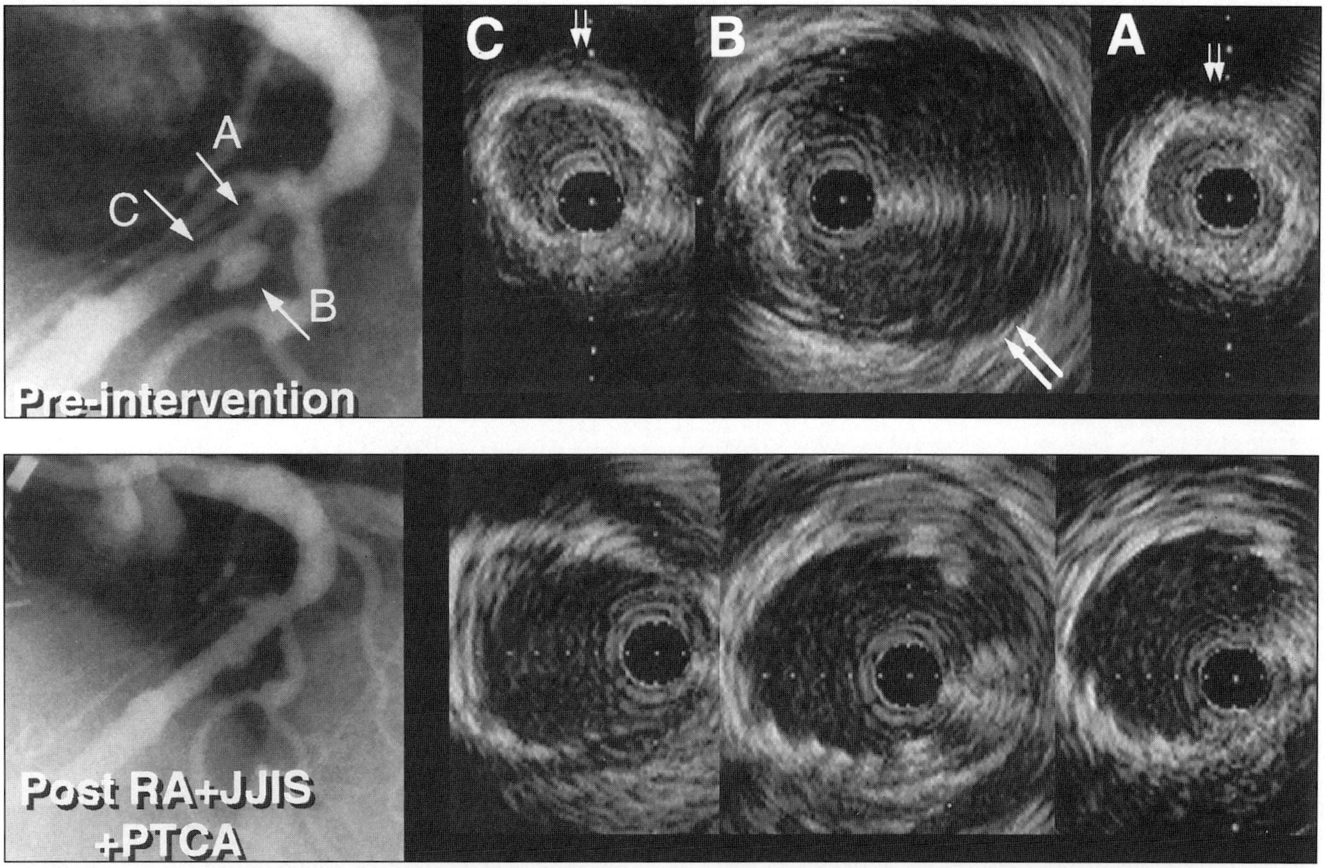

Figure 3-2. Successful device synergy treatment of a heavily calcified, ulcerated lesion (360° superficial calcium). Excellent circumferential lumen throughout the lesion. **A** and **C** show calcified lesion; **B** illustrates the ulcerated lesion. *Small double arrows* in top right hand panel point out the calcified intima; *large double arrows* illustrate the ulcerated area. JJIS—Johnson and Johnson Interventional Systems Co. (Warren, NJ); PTCA—percutaneous transluminal coronary angioplasty; RA—rotational atherectomy. (*From* Hong and colleagues [23]; with permission.)

Rationale

There are several reasons for stent placement after rotational atherectomy, especially in large, calcified coronary arteries. The first reason is the treatment of dissections following rotational atherectomy. Although the incidence of dissection is related to the lesion complexity, the Rotational Atherectomy Multicenter Registry found 11% angiographic evidence of dissection [16]. The incidence may be higher if IVUS is routinely employed [17••]. Thus, immediate stent implantation should reduce the abrupt closure rate following rotational atherectomy. The second reason is the high restenosis rate seen in a recent randomized study for comparable lesion subsets [5••]. The predominant mechanism of restenosis after rotational atherectomy is chronic geometric remodeling [18••]. Because the stents have been found to resist geometric remodeling [19••] and reduce restenosis in noncalcified coronary lesions [6••,7••], stent implantation after rotational atherectomy also may provide the optimal long-term benefit in large, calcified coronary arteries. Finally, stent implantation following rotational atherectomy should improve the coronary blood flow and normalize the coronary flow reserve, which may be abnormal after rotational atherectomy with or without adjunct balloon angioplasty (Fig. 3-3).

Results

The positive findings of this preliminary study confirm the safety of this approach. Despite theoretical concerns regarding the microcirculatory disturbance from rotational atherectomy, the potential inability to fully expand the stent in calcified vessels, the ill effects from high-pressure adjunct angioplasty after rotational atherectomy, and the subacute stent thrombosis, this study shows that in selected patients, the procedure can be successful without procedural or subacute complications.

However, the high incidence of non–Q-wave MI is still of concern and will require careful follow-up. Recent studies of atherectomy suggest that periprocedural non–Q-wave MI may not portend benign long-term results [20••,21••].

Future Directions

The safety and the long-term efficacy of this combined device procedure need to be confirmed in a larger patient cohort. To address these issues, the SPORT (Stent Implantation Post Rotational Atherectomy Trial) study, a multicenter registry of 100 consecutive patients with calcified native vessel coronary artery disease undergoing planned rotational atherectomy and adjunct IVUS-guided stent placement, will begin in the near future. This study will include angiographic follow-up to address the long-term efficacy of the approach.

Limitations of the Study

This consecutive series included only those patients who did not have complications during the rotational atherectomy, such as no-reflow phenomenon or coronary perforation, that would have precluded stent placement. Thus, the percentage of the patients with planned device synergy approach who actually received the combined procedure is unknown. In addition, it is difficult to clearly separate the three groups (elective vs provisional vs urgent use) from retrospective analysis of the registry data and the corresponding in-hospital and long-term sequelae. There has been no previous study or attempt on our part to implant stents without initial atheroablation in calcified vessels. This precludes comparison of our results to primary stenting in calcified coronary lesions. Furthermore, the restenosis rate needs to be determined, because these patients do not undergo routine follow-up angiography. Finally, the equipment cost of the procedure is much higher than balloon angioplasty or either device alone. Therefore, the cost-effectiveness of this approach needs to be confirmed in future studies evaluating the overall cost of the initial procedure and subsequent need for target-lesion revascularization.

Table 3-3. Procedural Long-Term Outcome*

Acute results	Percent
Angiographic success	98
Procedural success	92
Major complications	8.1
Death	4.1
Q-wave MI	2.7
Emergency CABG	2.8
Non–Q-wave MI	24
Subacute thrombosis	2.7
Vascular complication	3.9
Long-term results	
No event	84
Death	2.7
Q-wave MI	0.5
TLR-CABG	4.0
TLR-PTCA	8.5

**Total number of patients, 178.*

MI—myocardial infarction; CABG—coronary artery bypass surgery; TLR—target-lesion revascularization; PTCA—percutaneous transluminal coronary angioplasty.

Conclusions

This study demonstrates that stent implantation after rotational atherectomy in large, calcified coronary arteries appears to be a safe and effective approach. Despite theoretical concerns with this approach mentioned previously, the results of this study confirm that, in this patient cohort with unfavorable clinical (older age) and lesion (heavy calcification) characteristics, this device synergy results in high procedural success and acceptable periprocedural complications, with low subacute stent thrombosis. The long-term safety and benefit need to be confirmed in a larger, prospective patient cohort.

References and Recommended Reading

Recently published papers of particular interest have been highlighted as follows:

- • Of special interest
- •• Of outstanding interest

1. Ryan TJ, Subcommittee on Percutaneous Transluminal Coronary Angioplasty: Guidelines for percutaneous transluminal coronary angioplasty: a report of the American College of Cardiology/American Heart Association Task Force on assessment of diagnostic and therapeutic cardiovascular procedures. *J Am Coll Cardiol* 1988, 12:529–545.

2. Mintz GS, Pichard AD, Kent KM, *et al.*: Intravascular ultrasound comparison of restenotic and de novo coronary artery narrowings. *Am J Cardiol* 1994, 74:1278–1280.

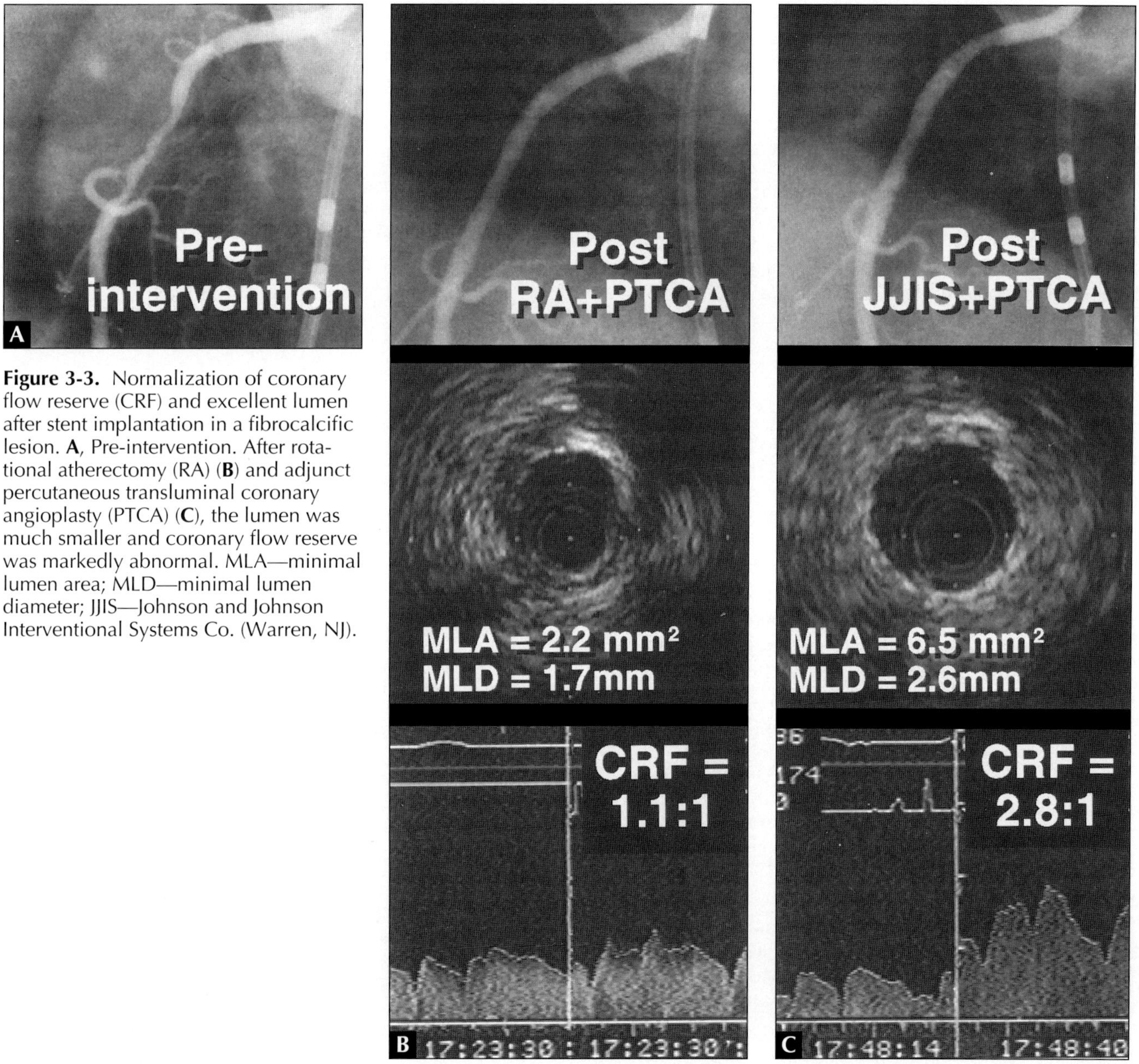

Figure 3-3. Normalization of coronary flow reserve (CRF) and excellent lumen after stent implantation in a fibrocalcific lesion. **A**, Pre-intervention. After rotational atherectomy (RA) (**B**) and adjunct percutaneous transluminal coronary angioplasty (PTCA) (**C**), the lumen was much smaller and coronary flow reserve was markedly abnormal. MLA—minimal lumen area; MLD—minimal lumen diameter; JJIS—Johnson and Johnson Interventional Systems Co. (Warren, NJ).

3.• Kovach JA, Mintz GS, Pichard AD, *et al.*: Sequential intravascular ultrasound characterization of the mechanisms of rotational atherectomy and adjunct balloon angioplasty. *J Am Coll Cardiol* 1993, 22:1024–1032.

Intravascular ultrasound study documenting the selective ablation of fibrocalcific atherosclerotic plaque by rotational atherectomy.

4.• Brogan WC, Popma JJ, Pichard AD, *et al.*: Rotational coronary atherectomy after unsuccessful coronary balloon angioplasty. *Am J Cardiol* 1993, 71:794–798.

Rotational atherectomy may change lesion compliance in "undilatable" lesions.

5.•• Vandormael M, Reifart N, Preusler W, *et al.*: Six months follow-up results following excimer laser angioplasty, rotational atherectomy and balloon angioplasty for complex lesions: ERBAC study [abstract]. *Circulation* 1994, 90:I-213.

First randomized study in comparable lesion subsets among balloon angioplasty, rotational atherectomy, and excimer laser angioplasty. Six-month follow-up shows no difference in restenosis rates, although the initial success rate was higher in the rotational atherectomy group.

6.•• Fischman DL, Leon MB, Baim DS, *et al.*: A randomized comparison of coronary-stent placement and balloon angioplasty in the treatment of coronary artery disease. *N Engl J Med* 1994, 331:496–501.

One of two randomized studies documenting the efficacy of Palmaz-Schatz stents in reducing restenosis compared with balloon angioplasty.

7.•• Serruys PW, de Jaegere P, Kiemeneij F, *et al.*: A comparison of balloon-expandable-stent implantation with balloon angioplasty in patients with coronary artery disease. *N Engl J Med* 1994, 331:489–495.

The other randomized study documenting the efficacy of Palmaz-Schatz stents in reducing restenosis compared with balloon angioplasty.

8.• Ellis SG, Popma JJ, Buchbinder M, *et al.*: Relation of clinical presentation, stenosis morphology, and operator technique to the procedural results of rotational atherectomy and rotational atherectomy–facilitated angioplasty. *Circulation* 1994, 89:882–892.

Careful analysis of success and complications during rotational atherectomy in three high-volume centers.

9. Roubin GS, Cannon AD, Agrawal SK, *et al.*: Intracoronary stenting for acute and threatened closure complicating percutaneous transluminal coronary angioplasty. *Circulation* 1992, 85:916–927.

10. Ellis S, Vandormael M, Cowley M, *et al.*: Coronary morphologic and clinical determinants of procedural outcome with angioplasty for multivessel coronary disease. *Circulation* 1990, 82:1193–1202.

11. Huber MS, Mooney JF, Madison J, *et al.*: Use of a morphologic classification to predict clinical outcome after dissection from coronary angioplasty. *Am J Cardiol* 1991, 68:467–471.

12. Chesebro J, Knatterud G, Roberts R, *et al.*: Thrombolysis in Myocardial Infarction (TIMI) Trial, Phase I: a comparison between intravenous tissue plasminogen activator and intravenous streptokinase. Clinical findings through hospital discharge. *Circulation* 1987, 76:142–154.

13.•• Duissaillant GD, Mintz GS, Pichard AD, *et al.*: Intravascular ultrasound identification of calcified intraluminal lesions misdiagnosed as thrombi by coronary angiography. *Am Heart J*, in press.

Intravascular ultrasound study showing calcified lesions masquerading as intraluminal thrombi.

14. McKenna CJ, McCann HA, Sugrue DD: Emergency bail-out stenting for major coronary dissection complicating rotational atherectomy. *Irish Med J* 1995, 88:32.

15. Levin TN, Carroll JD, Feldman T: Bail-out stenting for flow limiting dissections after rotational atherectomy in complex coronary lesions. *Cathet Cardiovasc Diagn* 1996, 37:300–304.

16. Warth DC, Leon MB, O'Neill W, *et al.*: Rotational atherectomy multicenter registry: acute results, complications and 6-month angiographic follow-up in 709 patients. *J Am Coll Cardiol* 1994, 24:641–648.

17.•• Fitzgerald PJ, Ports TA, Yock PG: Contribution of localized calcium deposits to dissection after angioplasty: an observational study using intravascular ultrasound. *Circulation* 1992, 86:64–70.

Intravascular ultrasound study showing high incidence of dissection following angioplasty.

18.•• Mintz GS, Popma JJ, Pichard AD, *et al.*: Arterial remodeling after coronary angioplasty: a serial intravascular ultrasound study. *Circulation*, 1996, 94:35–43.

Serial intravascular ultrasound study in patients undergoing angioplasty, including rotational atherectomy, which shows that geometric remodeling is the major mechanism of restenosis in these lesions.

19.•• Painter JA, Mintz GS, Wong SC, *et al.*: Serial intravascular ultrasound studies fail to show evidence of chronic Palmaz-Schatz stent recoil. *Am J Cardiol* 1995, 75:398–400.

Serial intravascular ultrasound study showing no chronic stent recoil.

20.•• Elliot JM, Berdan LG, Holmes DR, *et al.*: One-year follow-up in the coronary angioplasty versus excisional atherectomy trial (CAVEAT I). *Circulation* 1995, 91:2158–2166.

Long-term follow-up study in patients undergoing directional atherectomy, showing the unfavorable late outcome in patients with periprocedural enzyme elevations.

21.•• Redwood SR, Popma JJ, Kent KM, *et al.*: "Minor" CPK-MB elevations are associated with increased late mortality following ablative new-device angioplasty in native coronary arteries [abstract]. *Circulation* 1995, 92(suppl I):544.

Another study documenting the unfavorable late outcome of patients undergoing new-device angioplasty, including rotational atherectomy, and periprocedural enzyme elevation.

22. Hong MK, Mintz GS, Popma JJ, *et al.*: Safety and efficacy of elective stent implantation following rotational atherectomy in large, calcified coronary arteries. *Cathet Cardiovasc Diagn*, 1996, (suppl 3):50–54.

23. Hong MK, Mintz GS, Popma JJ, *et al.*: Angiographic results and late clinical outcomes utilizing a stent synergy (pre-stent atheroablation) approach in complex lesion subsets. *J Invas Cardiol* 1996, 8:15–22.

Chapter 4

Minimally Traumatic Recanalization of Atherosclerotic Arteries

David C. Auth
Mark Reisman

The Rotablator® (Boston Scientific Corporation, Northwest Technology Center [formerly Heart Technology], Redmond, WA) atherectomy device has been described previously [1–4] as a high-speed rotary sander that selectively ablates inelastic tissue without damaging elastic tissue. Serendipitously, all forms of atherosclerotic tissue are relatively inelastic, whereas healthy tissue is elastic. Thus, the Rotablator is able to convert atheromatous mass automatically whether fatty or calcified into a collection of microparticles that under ideal conditions pass through the capillary bed and ultimately meet their end by phagocytic ingestion in the reticuloendothelial system [5]. As such, the device should be able to remove all forms of plaque without damaging adjacent healthy tissue structures, including those found in even the most eccentric lesion morphologies, and do so without causing damage to the arterial wall, which is known to lead to restenosis [6–8].

The foregoing description of the Rotablator makes it sound like the perfect instrument for trauma-free removal of plaque, which should predict low restenosis. The question is, *"What has limited its acceptance in many clinics around the world?"* Although it is being used frequently by some interventionalists and, on occasion, pulled off the shelf for the really "tough" cases by others, there still exists a widespread opinion that the device is largely a product for the nondilatable or grossly calcified lesions and, furthermore, that its restenosis rate is essentially the same as conventional percutaneous transluminal coronary angioplasty (PTCA). One thing has become increasingly clear: *The results obtainable with the Rotablator are unique and are closely tied up with the particular technique with which it is applied.*

This chapter discusses the best technique for the use of the Rotablator to maximize acute and long-term success for the Rotablator-treated patient. In particular, the specific recommendations for avoiding heat damage, for avoiding stretch damage, and for removing large amounts of plaque mass safely and effectively are dealt with from a basic science as well as a practical application point of view.

Chemistry of Ablation: Heat as a Byproduct or as a Prime Mover

The word *ablation* has taken on a variety of interpretations in the medical literature, including necrosis of neural pathways and laser evaporation of tissue mass. In this chapter, the interpretation is one of physical removal of tissue mass by way of surface sanding. Lasers have been characterized as ablative devices that evaporate tissue mass by physically converting a solid into an atomic or molecular gas, consisting of the elemental components of the original structure. Actually, this is inaccurate, in that laser ablation occurs by the fragmentation of mass resulting from microbubbles of evolving steam in the tissue depth. As such, it is similar to conventional radiofrequency electrosurgery (BOVIE). The size of the fragments that evolve from laser ebullition depend upon the wavelength of electromagnetic energy used—excimer lasers produce fragments of about 20 μm. Longer wavelength lasers produce larger fragments because the size of the steam vesicle is generally larger and deeper before an eruption can break the surface. This type of ablation takes place by way of a thermal pathway: Energy is absorbed as photons and converted to thermal phonons, which, in turn, produce steam, which then erupts and fragments the tissue. When these eruptions occur in small time frames of the order of hundreds of nanoseconds, they can produce secondary shock waves, which can also destroy tissue mass at greater depths than would be expected simply on the basis of normal radiative penetration depth.

In contrast, sanding machines produce fragments that vary in size according to the depth to which the sanding crystals penetrate the surface being treated. Obviously, fine sandpaper can provide crystal penetration of only limited depth and thus produces particles or fragments that are generally quite small. An additional important factor that controls the depth of the crystalline invagination within the mass to be sanded is the pressure with which the sanding element is pushed into the mass. For this reason, light pressure produces generally smaller sanding dust fragments than does heavy pressure for the same grit size of the sanding surface. In the Rotablator device, the sanding crystals are natural diamonds with protuberant pyramids of approximately 5 μm. With light pressure, the Rotablator produces particles of approximately 1 μm [9]. The sanding process is able to cleave chemical bonds directly by forceful shearing of the molecular structure. This is direct mechanical shear rather than shear induced by expanding vesicles of steam as with laser surgery or electrosurgery. As such, ablation occurs by way of a direct mechanical pathway rather than a thermal pathway. Thermal energy, however, can and will generally be liberated as a byproduct of the sanding action because the cutting action of the sanding crystals is not without some level of friction, which necessarily produces heat. (Although a sharp saw produces less heat than a dull one, it still inevitably produces some heating.) The challenge with the Rotablator is to have a sanding tip that is sharp yet delicate; thus, the use of fine, sharp diamond crystals. Some heat, however, is generated when the Rotablator is used to sand atheroma or when it slips over normal tissue. The heat is dissipated in the blood and saline flush, which is in contact with the diamond burr tip. Some heat can be directly transmitted to the arterial wall and may result in an unacceptable temperature rise if too much sanding pressure is applied. Such pressure is controllable by the clinician noting the drop in revolutions per minute (rpm) of the Rotablator (Delta decrement) and by controlling the baseline (platform) operating rpm. We have now performed a number of experiments to determine safe operation parameters for use of the Rotablator.

Using an experimental model that included 12-mm cylinders derived from bovine femurs with 0.35-mm cored lumens to permit passage of the Rotablator guidewire, four thermal probes were placed at intervals of 3 mm to assess temperature changes as the burr engaged that segment of bone (Fig. 4-1*A*). With continuous saline infusion at normal body temperature, 2.0-mm burrs were advanced through the model, and simultaneous data acquisition included rpm and temperature. Two methods of advancement of the burr were applied, either a continuous ablation through the entire segment or an oscillating technique, which consisted of 2 seconds of engagement of the bone followed by 2 seconds of withdrawal to permit reestablishment of antegrade flow. Both methods were tested using an aggressive ablation technique that permitted significant decelerations (14,000 to 18,000 rpm) or a gentle advancement technique that limited the rpm deceleration to a range of 4000 to 6000. The results are shown in Figure 4-1*B* [10••]. Subsequent experimentation to assess the impact of heat generation using various techniques was accomplished using an in vivo miniswine model. The femoral artery was exposed and cradled in a constricting sheath containing thermal probes (Fig. 4-2*A*). The probes were in contact with the adventitia of the artery, and simultaneous recording of rpm and temperature were acquired as the burr was advanced through the cradled segment. The burr was activated proximal to the sheath and was advanced either aggressively with significant decelerations of 10,000 to 15,000 rpm or gently with decelerations ranging between 5000 to 9000 rpm with corresponding temperature elevations of 11.3 ± 6.2°C and 4.1 ± 1.2°C, respectively. The results are shown in Figure 4-2*B*.

Previous studies have demonstrated evidence of thermal injury [11•] by studying specimens that have undergone rotational atherectomy followed by directional atherectomy as well as work in animal models. The literature is replete with studies demonstrating the association of thermal injury with smooth muscle proliferation, high restenosis rates, erythrocyte aggregation, and platelet activation [12–17]. Interestingly, the benchmark studies of rotational atherectomy [18••,19••,20] applied the old recommendations, which included activating all burr sizes at 190,000 to 200,000 rpm with a 10% deceleration as the burr crosses the lesion (19,000 to 20,000 rpm) as acceptable.

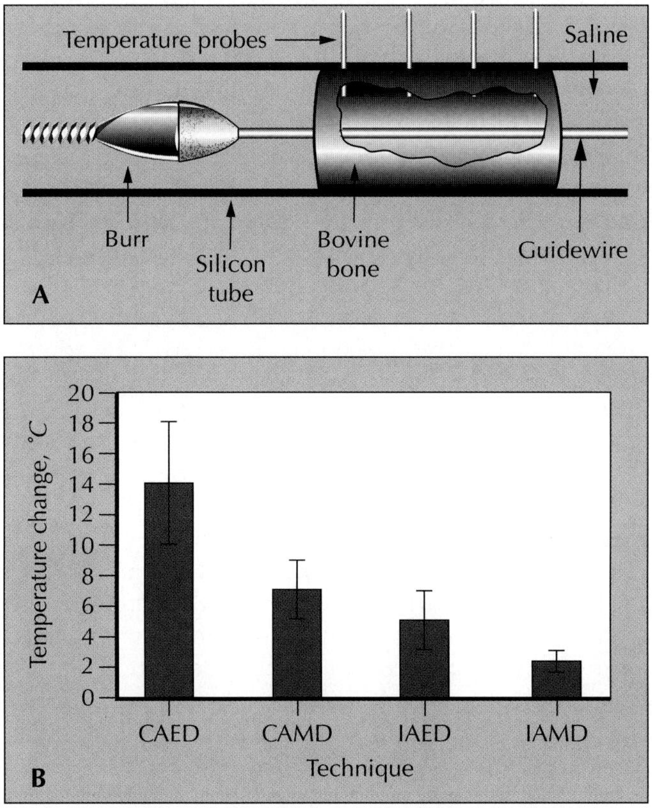

Figure 4-1. Experimental design to assess temperature changes as burr engages bone. **A**, Temperatures were measured by four thermal probes as the 2.0-mm burr advanced through the 0.35-mm lumen in the bone. **B**, Comparison of two methods of burr advancement in a bovine bone model. The difference in heat generation depends on the technique and degree of decelerations used. Nine bovine bones were used in each test; $P < 0.05$ between IAMD and all other tests. *T-bars* indicate ± SD.

The studies described strongly suggest that the optimal technique to minimize heat generation is to apply an oscillating technique with minimal (< 5000 rpm) decelerations. The acute and long-term implications for rotational atherectomy [18••,19••,20] are only speculative at present. Data derived from the STRATAS (Study to Determine Rotablator and Transluminal Angioplasty Strategy) trial, however, suggest creatine phosphokinase elevations with significant drops in rpm [21]. Several trials are ongoing, exploring the outcomes of various lesion subsets using these technique modifications.

Stretch Damage, Restenosis, and Technique

The previous section dealt with the generation of heat when the Rotablator is applied suboptimally. In this section, the issues related to stretch trauma are discussed. The most important of these relate to the adjunctive use of balloon angioplasty following a Rotablator procedure. For the past 8 years of clinical use, most investigators have used adjunctive balloon angioplasty following the Rotablator to maximize angiographic lumen. Different strategies of debulking before adjunctive therapy have been used:

1. Minimal debulking: a single burr with a burr-to-artery ratio of 0.3 to 0.6.
2. Moderate debulking with burr-to-artery ratio of 0.6 to 0.75.
3. Ideal debulking with a burr-to-artery ratio of 0.75 to 0.9.

Strategies 2 and 3 frequently require the use of two or more burrs in a stepwise fashion of about 0.5 mm per step and, for most economy-minded users, is an approach with reluctant acceptance, unless the cost of complications is included in the overall cost analysis.

There has been widespread failure to achieve lumen diameters of a size approximately equal to the burr diameter because of the problem of "watermelon seeding" or the burr "slipping" past the lesion. Because of the absence [22] of longitudinal friction when the burr is spinning at high rpm (orthogonal displacement of friction), it is frequently difficult for the interventionalist to judge the amount of time necessary to debulk a lesion unless careful surveillance of the rpm decrement is taken. Many early trials of the Rotablator were flawed because care was not taken to ensure that full debulking had, in fact, taken place. Ideally the first pass across the lesion is taken at a sufficiently slow pace so as not to drop the rpm more than 5000 to avoid heat production and to avoid "skipping" across the lesion. In the final pass when there is no drop in rpm as the burr crosses the lesion, the operator can be certain that full debulking has occurred. In many of the early trials of the Rotablator, either the lesion was not adequately debulked because of watermelon seeding, or the final burr size was simply too small and the operator felt compelled to use a balloon to achieve an angiographically satisfying lumen. Unfortunately, for many of these cases in which angiographic lumen was improved after balloon angioplasty, the flow was not significantly improved because the actual useful flow channel was not changed much, but rather a crack was induced in the plaque so as to provide space for angiographic contrast media, which provided the seeming improvement in lumen, as seen by angiography. Intravascular ultrasound (IVUS) studies have shown repeatedly that angiographic lumens can be misleading because of the crack-full-of-contrast shadowgram [23]. Thus, although the angiographic shadowgram provides a more satisfying picture of the arterial therapy, most of the time the actual improvement in flow capacity resulting from post-Rotablator barotrauma when measured at 24 hours is minimal and the price paid is high: *deep wall stretch trauma*. The use of stents may be justified for some anatomic situations, particularly for large arteries in the range of 4.0 mm. With stenting, deep wall damage certainly happens, but obviously the larger initial lumen may provide more margin for neointimal growth, allowing for a good long-term outcome [24–26]. It is more important to note that long-term minimal lumen diameter (MLD) in various stent trials averages out to approximately 1.8 mm [24,26]. It is worthwhile to consider what flow capacity is provided by a 1.8-mm MLD. Figure 4-3 illustrates the flow capacity for a series of narrowed arterial segments. These segments are each 15 mm long, varying in lumen diameter from 0.5 to 2.5 mm. The pressure drop across each segment is 7.5 mm Hg, or about 10% of diastolic pressure. Poiseuille's law [27] states that:

eq. 1. $\Delta P = 8\,L\,F\,V/\pi\,R^4$
thus, eq. 2. $F = \Delta P\,\pi\,R^4/8\,LV$ flow rate
Where ΔP is pressure drop; R = radius;
L = length; V = viscosity; and F = flow rate.

Thus, the flow rate, F, is proportional to R^4. Figure 4-3 illustrates dramatically the rise in flow capacity with relatively modest increases in R or D (diameter). The flow rate is obviously somewhat reduced during systole when the arteries are compressed. Nonetheless, equation 2 provides a good reference point for flow capacity. It is clear why a *long-term stent result* of only 1.8 mm MLD can be quite satisfactory, in that the flow capacity would be (with ΔP of only 7.5 mm Hg) nearly 200 mL/min. Obviously the flow that occurs is modulated by the autoregulatory system of the distal circulation, including precapillary sphincters. The goal of revascularization should be one of achieving a long-term result that allows for as much flow as the myocardium needs. Under maximal exertion, the blood flow requirements are 400 mL/min per 100 g of myocardium, or 70 mL/min per 100 g of myocardium

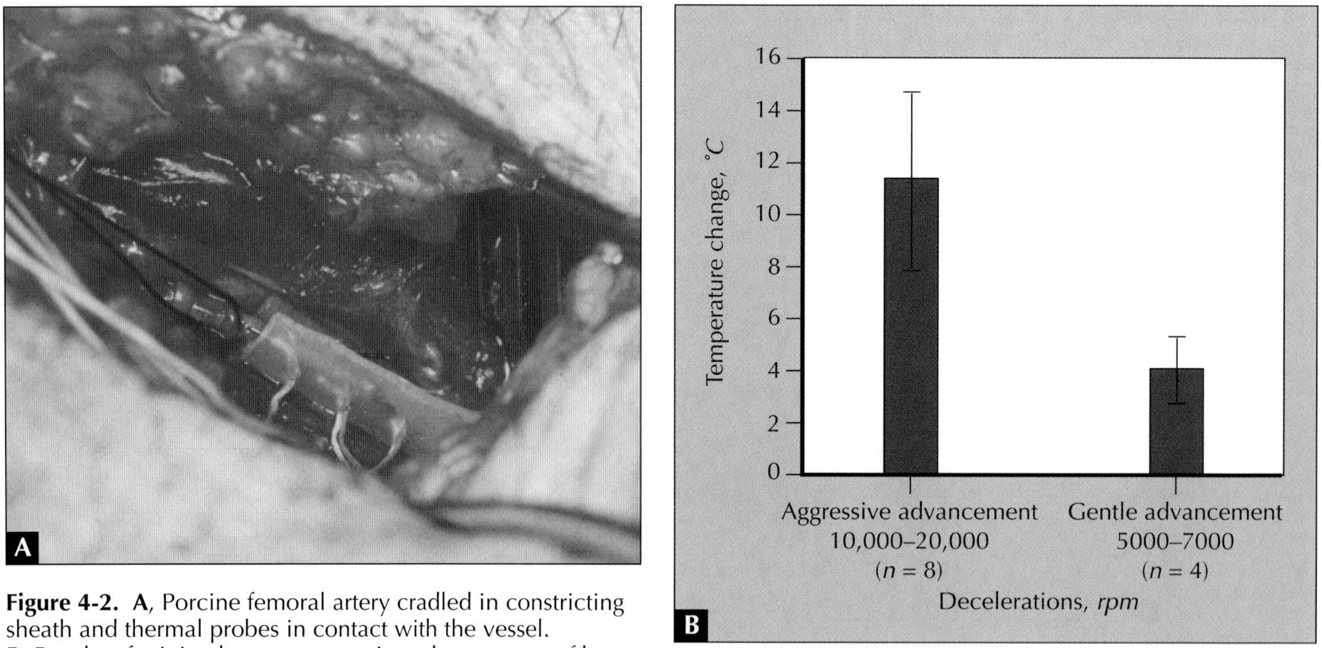

Figure 4-2. **A**, Porcine femoral artery cradled in constricting sheath and thermal probes in contact with the vessel. **B**, Results of minimal versus aggressive advancement of burr in porcine femoral artery. *T-bars* indicate ± SD.

at rest [27]. Realizing that a ΔP of more than 7.5 mm Hg is normally readily available to drive blood through the revascularized segment, it becomes clear why a 2-mm diameter internal mammary artery (IMA) can be quite serviceable, even though several centimeters in length, and why a surgical probe of 1.5 mm in diameter is adequate to check for patency of the distal (IMA) anastomosis.

Figure 4-3 and the fact that modest long-term MLDs [24–26] provide satisfactory clinical outcome suggest that balloon-trauma–induced neointimal formation, elastic recoil, and adventitial remodeling may well be a disadvantage after a Rotablator atherectomy, in which adequate, deep, trauma-free debulking was achieved and in which a final MLD of 2.25 mm or larger is achieved by ablation alone without deep wall damage when good technique is employed. Two randomized clinical trials are currently underway to attempt to determine the long-term outcome for angiographic, sonographic, and clinical restenosis after Rotablator ablation as a stand-alone method of revascularization (with or without a 1 atm adjunctive balloon [oversize] postablation tamponade) versus Rotablator with high (normal) pressure adjunctive angioplasty (STRATAS) or conventional angioplasty (DART [Dilation versus Ablation Revascularization Trial]). In the STRATAS trial, the pure ablation arm strives for a burr to artery ratio of 0.7 to 0.9 mm. More aggressive debulking to a diameter of approximately 0.8 mm of the reference vessel diameter has in three separate nonrandomized clinical trials resulted in clinical restenosis rates of 6% to 20% [28,29,30•]. The ability for a balloon to break the internal elastic lamina (IEL) when used at nominal diameters comparable to the reference vessel diameter is reduced as the stenosis diameter is increased. Thus, for a nondiseased vessel with no plaque bulk, inflating a balloon to a diameter equal to the normal arterial diameter does not break

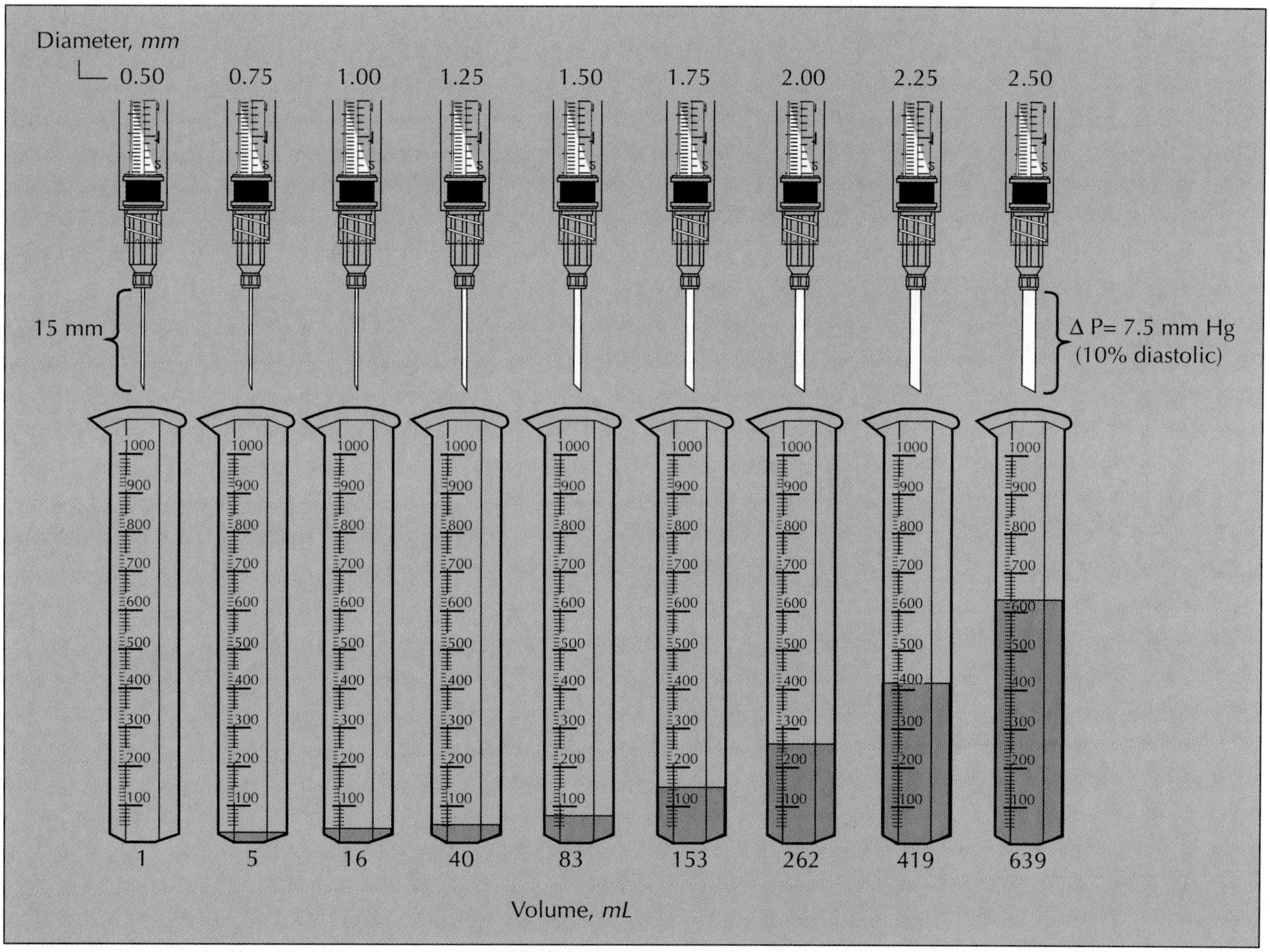

Figure 4-3. Flow rate capabilities for true cylindrical lesions as a function of recanalized lumen diameter. The pressure drop (lesion gradient) across lesion equals 10% of diastolic pressure (7.5 mm Hg).

the IEL. As the plaque mass becomes larger, the effective diameter of the angioplasty stretch is the balloon diameter plus the plaque mass. Thus, for total occlusions, the effective angioplasty stretch diameter is the worst case, because the plaque contribution to stretch diameter is at its largest dimension. When ablation is truly successful at reducing plaque mass to the point at which only 20% of the mass remains relative to the reference diameter, adjunctive balloon angioplasty may not provide stretching to the point of breaking the IEL.

The CARAT (Coronary Angioplasty vs Rotational Atherectomy Trial) [30•] provides insight into the issue of restenosis and the role of dilatational trauma in exciting neointimal proliferation and adventitial remodeling. It was found that when inadvertently *undersized* balloons were used in conjunction with aggressive debulking with the Rotablator, the target vessel revascularization rate was 9%. Consistent with the previous discussion, undersized balloons used in lumens in which most of the plaque mass has been removed result in little stretching of the artery (if any) and, thus, greatly diminish the possibility for breaking of the IEL and significant stretching of the adventitia. The elastic recoil component of restenosis is inherently eliminated with aggressive debulking because with good technique, stretching was *never* a part of the lumen enlargement. The fact that the restenosis rate associated with the Rotablator is considered by many to be nearly identical to conventional PTCA is the result of trials in which adjunctive use of balloon angioplasty after modest size ablated lumens essentially produced massive dilatational trauma [18••,19••]. This is easily explained by Lamé's equation (Fig. 4-4), which states that the tension in the wall of an artery is proportional to the diameter of the lumen and inversely proportional to the thickness of the wall. Coupling Lamé's equation with the reduction in wall strength that accompanies debulking, it comes as no surprise that angioplasty with a pressurized balloon after minimal or modest atherectomy delivers a much graver insult to the arterial wall in the form of stretch injury than if no debulking were present. Figure 4-4 provides an example of an artery in which arterial wall tension is calculated with (*right side*) and without (*left side*) preballoon debulking. In this example, the wall tension is shown to increase by a *factor of 10* after debulking for the same amount of balloon inflation pressure. Thus, although some of the contribution to elastic recoil can be expected to be reduced by modest debulking, one must necessarily expect that the contribution of neointimal proliferation and adventitial remodeling will be major for balloon-stretched arteries after primary debulking, unless, in fact, the stretch injury is avoided by aggressive debulking and undersize ballooning.

An alternative to undersized balloons is the use of *oversize balloons at a maximum of 1 atm pressure*. Figure 4-5 illustrates the results of controlled pressure on healthy porcine coronary arteries; on the two histologic sections at the left, one can see a control segment of artery that has adjacently received a true applied pressure of 1 atm. Clearly, minimal damage and stretch trauma is in evidence. By contrast, the right side of Figure 4-5 illustrates the stretch trauma associated with only 2 atm of controlled pressure. The left upper quadrant of the artery is massively stretched, and one can certainly predict that severe restenosis would be the result. In these experiments, an oversize balloon was used so as to ensure that all of the indeflator pres-

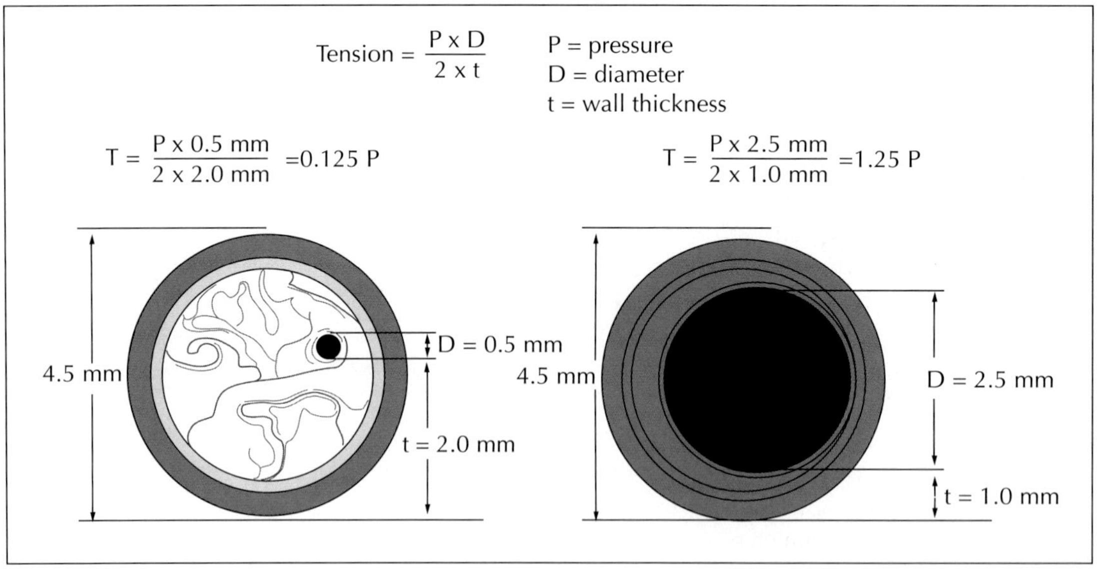

Figure 4-4. Comparative wall tension in artery computed by Lamé's equation (*top*) in artery with and without debulking. Ten atm of balloon pressure before Rotablator system debulking produces a tension on the vessel wall that is equal to 1 atm after primary Rotablator debulking.

sure was reaching the artery wall without containment by the hoop strength of the balloon material. In other words, to define the mechanical strength and resistance of the healthy artery to stretch tension trauma, a known amount of pressure was applied. In an actual PTCA procedure or in a balloon-delivered stent procedure, the tension delivered to the arterial wall is typically ambiguous because the pressure inside the balloon is contained by the cumulative hoop strength of the balloon *and* the artery *and* the stent, if one is used. The lesson that comes from Figure 4-5 is simply that pressures of 1 atm are manageable by healthy porcine arteries, whereas pressures as low as 2 atm are not. From an evolutionary point of view, this is quite reasonable in that 1 atm = 6 × systolic pressure and 2 atm = 12 × systolic pressure. It stands to reason that nature would not unduly overdesign a fluid pipe for pressures grossly exceeding normal operating parameters.

The question arises as to what benefit a 1-atm pressure tamponade can supply after primary Rotablator debulking. Three useful benefits can occur:

1. Immediate relief of spasm and a glimpse of what the result would look like 24 hours later [31••], when it is known that typically, after moderate to aggressive debulking with the Rotablator, the luminal dimensions are actually improved 1 day later.
2. Immediate smoothing of luminal irregularities, which may occur as a result of sanding across inhomogeneous plaque boundary planes.
3. Immediate clarification of haziness, which may be intraluminal thrombus.

Clinical use of 1-atm balloon inflations after Rotablator atherectomy have now routinely provided the benefits cited previously. By confining the pressure to 1 atm (and no more), the likelihood for balloon-induced dissection and deep wall trauma is minimized. One question that frequently is posed is what size balloon to use when operating at a maximum of 1 atm. Most balloons will not have achieved nominal size at 1 atm. Furthermore, for the plastic membrane of the balloon to appose itself uniformly throughout all of the varying dimensions of the lumen, including the reference segment, it is important that the sausage shape of the balloon never manifest itself because it then imposes high-pressure and low-pressure points on a nonuniform lumen. Thus, when used adjunctively with the Rotablator, where it is desirable to apply

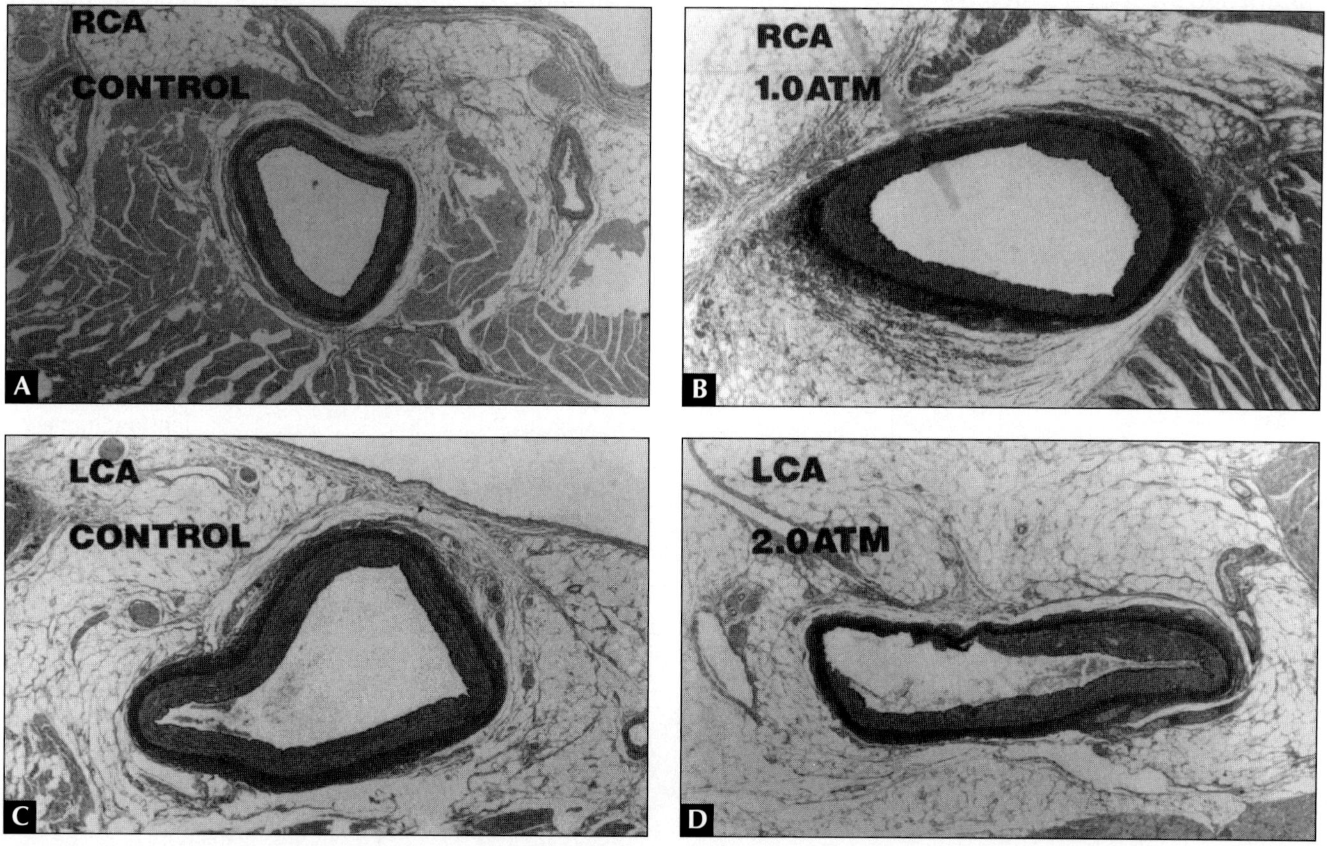

Figure 4-5. Histology of normal porcine arteries subjected to 1 atm (**A** and **B**) or 2 atm (**C** and **D**) of indeflation pressure. Note that as little as 2 atm of pressure delivered to the arterial wall causes deep trauma to a healthy artery, with severe medial and adventitial distention.

gentle and uniform tamponade pressure by way of a slick plastic membrane to the inner surface of the artery, including the atherectomized segment, it is best to use a grossly oversized (at least 1.5 mm larger than final Rotablator burr diameter) balloon, so that the sphincter of the sausage never manifests itself and the balloon functions as a flaccid plastic sock, which conveys uniform pressure at a nondestructive level to the inside of the artery, enabling one or more of the therapeutic benefits described previously and at the same time not causing deep wall trauma. Figure 4-6 illustrates schematically the appearance of an oversize balloon in an artery that is not subjected to pressures at a level which would cause mechanically traumatic stretching. In the *left side* of Figure 4-6, the pleats of the balloon membrane are depicted. As long as the balloon contains pleats, it cannot provide hoop strength. All of the pressure containment of hoop retention is provided by the arterial structure itself. In the *right side* of Figure 4-6, the sausage shape (in cross section) of the balloon is in evidence, and the tension in the wall of the artery is shared with the tension in the wall of the balloon to contain the pressure within the balloon, as shown by the accompanying equation. When using balloons in this way, not only is wall damage minimized, but also the balloon is capable of conforming to noncircular lumens and providing a continuous, constant, and well-defined pressure transition into the nontreated segments of the artery. Experience has now shown this to be a highly effective, safe adjunct to primary Rotablator therapy. Even though some residual "waist" may be evident on the balloon, the flow capacity is more than adequate.

Stertzer and colleagues [29] and Kaplan and coworkers [30•] both speak to the "sweet spot" (*ie*, the best range) of burr-to-artery ratio, wherein too little debulking or too much debulking leads to more restenosis, and targeting a burr-to-artery ratio of about 0.8 appears to be ideal. It is important to note that at 0.8 burr-to-artery ratio with good debulking technique, only about 20% to 30% of the plaque diameter is left relative to the reference segment. For a typical 3.00-mm artery, this implies the use of a 2.38-mm final burr size with a true lumen (as measured by IVUS) of approximately 2.3 mm. As can be seen in Figure 4-3, this has the capacity to deliver more than 400 mL of blood per minute (more than an IMA graft). If such a lumen is achieved without causing deep wall trauma, the prognosis for long-term patency should be improved. Although randomized clinical trials are currently underway, registry data for restenosis with the Rotablator when used in the "sweet spot" regimen of burr-to-artery ratio and without significant balloon-induced deep wall trauma [30•] are compelling. Another registry of Rotablator stand-alone treated patients was accumulated in the early 1990s as part of the Food and Drug Administration clinical trial on the Rotablator [31••]. These data are presented in Figure 4-7. These data were compiled by Petersen at the University of California. Figure 4-7 depicts a population average of 43 patients who were treated with Rotablator stand-alone therapy and followed at 24 hours and 6 months with quantitative coronary angiography.

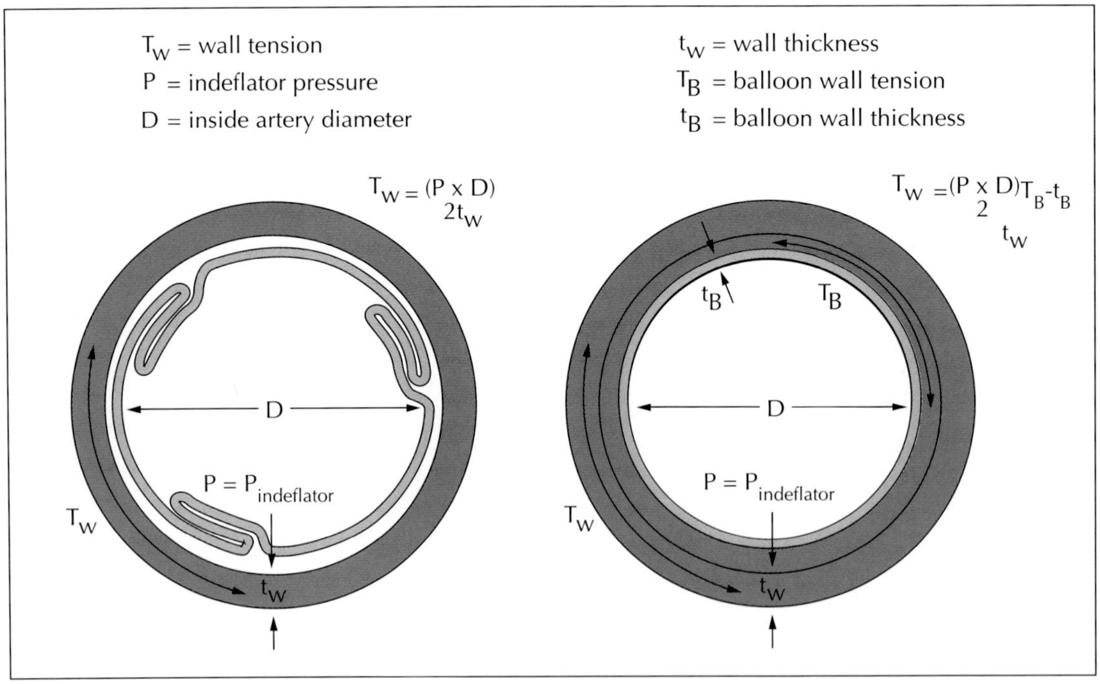

Figure 4-6. A pleated (oversized) balloon inside a resistant lumen. The *left side* illustrates folds (pleats) of balloon before lumen expands or cracks to the point of tightening the skin of the balloon. The *right side* illustrates balloon with pleats completely unfolded and the skin of the balloon taking up a portion of the indeflator pressure.

Surprisingly the late loss in MLD compared with the acute MLD was only 0.03 mm. These data have been criticized because final MLD was so low to begin with, partly because of the watermelon seeding effect discussed earlier and partly because of the use of relatively smaller sized burrs, which could fit through the lumens of the guide catheters that were available at that period of time (however, it is especially noteworthy that the 6-month MLD of the stent population average in the STRESS trial for arteries of less than 3.00 mm was only 1.55 mm [32], not significantly different than that for patients in Figure 4-7 at 6 months, which was 1.39 mm even with guide catheter limitations of 1989). With the advent of large lumen guide catheters, it is now possible to pass a 2.38-mm burr through some 9-F catheters and a 2.5-mm burr through most 10-F catheters. Thus, if similar late loss accompanies the use of larger burrs more in keeping with a burr-to-artery ratio of 0.75 to 0.90 mm and if thermal damage is avoided by paying close attention to drops in rpm while engaging the lesion, long-term success in the range found in the CARAT trial [30•] should be reproducible for other interventionalists.

Considerable discussion has taken place about the safety of using larger burrs in rotary ablation. The STRATAS trial early report [33] has provided encouraging new information on maximal debulking without causing unduly high complication rates. In the STRATAS trial, investigators are using strip chart recorders to monitor in real time the drops in rpm. Careful attention to gentle advancement of the burr avoids heat production and torsional dissection. (It may also reduce the incidence of spasm.)

A further confounding factor in comparing restenosis of the Rotablator with balloons and stents in the absence of complete randomized trials rests in the incomparability of Rotablator populations to those treated with stents and balloons as reported in the literature. In the registry data [19••], Warth and colleagues report a restenosis rate of 37.7% for the Rotablator, with 64% angiographic follow-up and 73% B and C lesions. Furthermore, many of the lesions were in smaller arteries and in long diffuse disease. In arteries less than 3 mm in diameter, the restenosis rate reported [32] for the PTCA arm of the STRESS trial was 54% in a population of much less complex disease. It appears that in a head-to-head randomized trial of Rotablator versus PTCA in arteries less than 3 mm based on historical comparisons, the Rotablator fares much better even with the antiquated techniques that were practiced during the late 1980s and early 1990s.

Preferred Technique of Rotary Ablation: Ablation Technique

The most recent modification of Rotablator technique has focused on the slow, gentle advancement through the lesion based on rpm surveillance. The rotational speed should be maintained within 5000 rpm of the platform speed (setting proximal to the lesion). Aggressive forward burr advancement, indicated by excessive deceleration, could result in heat generation [10••] and formation of large particles. In addition to monitoring the rotational speed, contrast material should be injected intermittently to provide visual

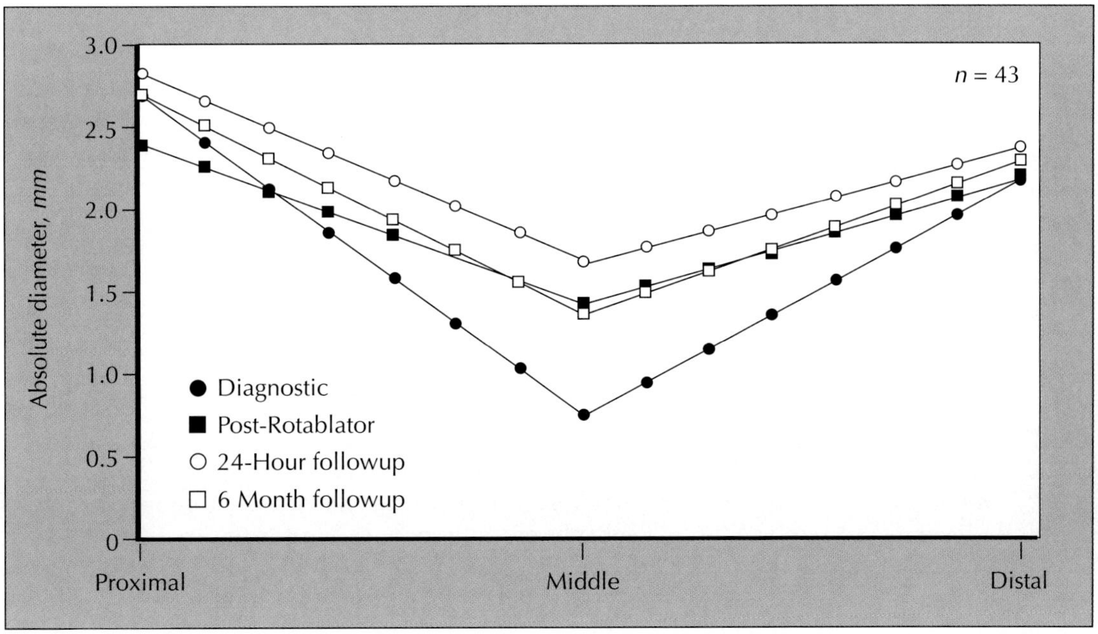

Figure 4-7. Pre-, post-, 24-hour, and 6-month lumen dimensions by quantitative coronary angiography (QCA) for Rotablator treatment as stand-alone therapy. Note minimal late loss (0.03). These data depict an average of 43 patients not treated with adjunctive percutaneous transluminal coronary angioplasty (Rotablator stand-alone).

assessment of burr advancement; these injections identify the borders of the lesion, the orientation of the device in tortuous segments, and the burr-to-artery relationship. If egress of contrast material is not observed, the burr should be withdrawn slightly to reestablish antegrade flow and allow particle clearance during ablation; contrast material injections may provide secondary benefit by inducing reactive hyperemia. The optimal duration of ablation is based on lesion morphology, distal runoff, and hemodynamic and clinical parameters. In general, 15 to 30 seconds is recommended, with a time interval between runs to allow for particle clearance and administration of vasodilators. In the cases in which there are electrocardiogram changes, significant chest discomfort, or hemodynamic compromise, the interval between ablations should be increased until the patient is clinically stable. Several ablation runs may be performed until the lesion is completely treated; the final "polishing run" is distinguished by smooth tracking of the burr through the treated segment as seen on fluoroscopy and no drop in rpm during advancement.

Plugging the Drain

How Much Debris Is Tolerable

Slow-flow and no-reflow remain significant complications of rotational atherectomy. Although the exact cause has yet to be clarified, there are two possible mechanisms defined as primary or secondary. The primary mechanism implies that the debris is the culprit and mechanically clogs the microcirculation. The fine particle mist that is generated by the Rotablator's ablative attrition of plaque and conversion into mechanically subdivided pieces of the original mass has been assumed to be the direct cause of slow-flow by sludging of the distal capillary bed. Even though a number of studies have been published attesting to the particle size being less than the diameter of red blood cells, the disturbances to the distal bed have been largely assumed to be related to the actual particles plugging the drain. Two clinically observed features have led us to suspect that there is much more to the story:

1. Rotablator treatment of restenotic tissue mass rarely is compromised by slow-flow.
2. Sometimes even a small amount of liberated tissue in the range of 1 mg of microparticles of plaque leads to chest pain and electrocardiogram changes, particularly when the plaque is highly calcified (aorto-ostial lesions). When normal flow occurs in a larger coronary artery, approximately 25,000 mg of red blood cell solids are sent to the distal bed per minute; in other words, four orders of magnitude more particulate mass than has been observed to cause flow disturbance in certain cases with ablated plaque particles.

Items 1 and 2 strongly suggest that another chemically magnified effect is taking place in the distal bed. Perhaps the bed responds to the chemical insult of effluent by shutting down the flow, by way of the precapillary sphincters. Perhaps the ground-up tissue factors stimulate activation of platelets, which, in turn, plug up the distal bed. Several empiric methods for reducing or, according to some clinicians, essentially eliminating flow disturbance have now evolved. These include maintaining an adequate diastolic blood pressure to achieve the optimal hydrostatic force for particle clearance [34•]. In addition, administering vasodilators through the Rotablator infusate port (Rotaflush) reduces the incidence of vasospasm and should improve coronary flow characteristics [35,36]. Technique modifications include minimizing the individual ablation times to 15 to 30 seconds and waiting between ablation treatments for baseline hemodynamic, electrocardiogram, and clinical parameters to be reestablished. The oscillating ablation (Fig. 4-8) is beneficial because it minimizes the bolus effect by generating a small amount of debris that is cleared by the antegrade blood flow and the effluent from the Rotablator infusate.

Chemical Adjuvants

Dilators and blockers

The ubiquitous nature of vasospasm during rotational atherectomy varies from minimal to severe. The opportunity to administer vasodilators in a subselective manner is a fortuitous design benefit of the Rotablator system. Taking advantage of the infusate port that is primarily responsible for cooling the driveshaft, the majority of Rotablator users "spike" the infusate with vasodilators. Several reports have documented the safety and efficacy of this technique [35–37]. The use of heparinized saline with 4 mg of nitroglycerin in a liter bag as the Rotaflush is recommended and has precluded the need for additional vasodilator treatment during the procedure in the majority of cases.

Platelet inhibitors

Excitement has been generated by a new class of compounds that inhibit platelet activation, specifically the glycoprotein IIb/IIIa inhibitors. The Rotablator can, by way of several mechanisms, induce platelet activation and subsequent aggregation. They include shear forces from the spinning burr, heat generation, and possibly the release of tissue factors from the ablated tissue. Several operators with extensive Rotablator experience have used ReoPro (Centocor B.V., Leiden, the Netherlands) in selected patients that would be considered at a higher risk for slow-flow and no-reflow. These include lesions greater than 20 mm, heavily calcified lesions, and patients presenting within several days of an acute myocardial infarction or unstable angina. The initial results are encouraging with an ongoing registry and a formal multicenter randomized trial (RotaPro) to be initiated in the near future.

ROTASTENTING

Stenting has taken a prominent position in percutaneous revascularization as a result of the improved long-term results compared to balloon angioplasty reported in the BENESTENT (Belgium Netherlands Stent Trial) and STRESS trials [24,26]. These trials targeted lesions in larger vessels (> 3 mm) with minimal complexity. The question becomes whether stenting can achieve comparable outcomes in lesions with less favorable characteristics. To determine the viability of broadening the indications for stenting, two strategies can be applied. One strategy is to "push the envelope" of stenting (*ie,* to test whether the clinical trials can be replicated in a less favorable lesion subset). This approach may have little justification considering the existing experience attesting to the difficulty of stent delivery and optimal deployment in calcified and diffusely diseased vessels. The second approach raises the specter of "lesion modification," that is, to transform the lesion to a less complex morphology by debulking (Fig. 4-9). Rotational atherectomy can affect stenting by facilitating delivery of the stent and increasing compliance in calcified or diffusely diseased vessels [38,39]. Increased compliance may enable greater stretch of the vessel with high balloon pressures or permit optimal stent deployment at lower pressures. Rotational atherectomy generally creates a smooth, round lumen, as shown with IVUS, which may provide greater opportunity for concentric stent apposition. A randomized clinical trial to determine significant benefits of rotational atherectomy debulking before stenting in complex lesions is presently being designed.

SPECIAL ISSUES

Guidewire Bias

Rotational atherectomy of coronary lesions is predicated on the principle of differential cutting. The high-speed sander is directed through the vessel and is oriented to the lesion based on the position of the guidewire. Because the architecture of the coronary anatomy is often tortuous and lesions often located on bends or in angulated segments, the stiff guidewire used in the Rotablator system may not lie centrally in the vessel. The final orientation or resultant vector of the guidewire is the balance between the guidewire "attempting" to be straight (lowest energy state) and the vessel opposing these forces while "attempting" to maintain its native configuration. In the case of a highly elastic tortuous vessel, the Rotablator guidewire produces a straightening effect on the vessel, and the result, angiographically, is *pseudolesions* (Fig. 4-10). Advancing the burr through such segments may result in the device, by virtue of the

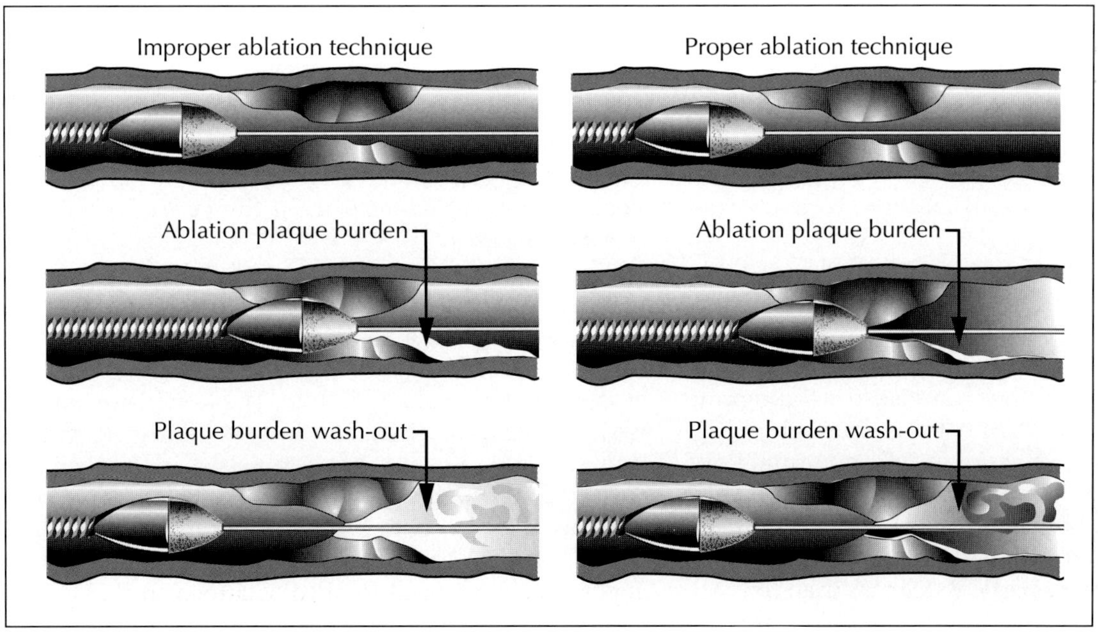

Figure 4-8. Demonstrates the proper versus improper technique of ablation. Using an oscillating technique (proper) reduces the "bolus" of microparticles and allows smaller quantities to be delivered as a function of time and provides for better dilution of the particles and their chemical toxicity in each milliliter of blood reaching the microcirculation.

guidewire, being directed toward the vessel wall and potentially results in tangential cutting. The impact of tangential cutting can be reduced by using smaller burrs and spinning the device at lower speeds (< 130,000 rpm) to minimize the cutting of the vessel. Conversely, guidewire bias may have a favorable impact on the treatment. In the case in which the burr is directed toward an eccentric lesion based on the guidewire position, the result now referred to as directional rotational atherectomy may generate a lumen greater than the selected burr size (Fig. 4-11). Finally, severely angulated lesions require close scrutiny and are treated with trepidation with the Rotablator system. Lesions situated at branch ostial locations (obtuse marginal off the circumflex) can be severely angulated with the guidewire oriented off-axis and placing significant stress on the arterial wall. A burr presented into this anatomy may ablate tangentially and in some cases result in perforation. Therefore, it is strongly recommended that in these cases the burr-to-artery ratio be low (< 0.5), with the goal to perform lesion modification (improve vessel compliance) for an adjunctive therapy such as PTCA.

With the now recognized importance of guidewire placement, several operators are manipulating the guidewire for improved positioning. Use of guide catheters that remove angulation is one technique. An example is treatment of an ostial circumflex lesion from the left main. An Amplatz guide catheter can be telescoped into the direction of the circumflex, with the guidewire then having a coaxial alignment into the vessel. Additional techniques such as placing the guidewire just beyond the lesion, as opposed to anchoring it in the distal vessel, may allow the guidewire to have less preference to lay along a wall and result in central cutting of concentric lesions.

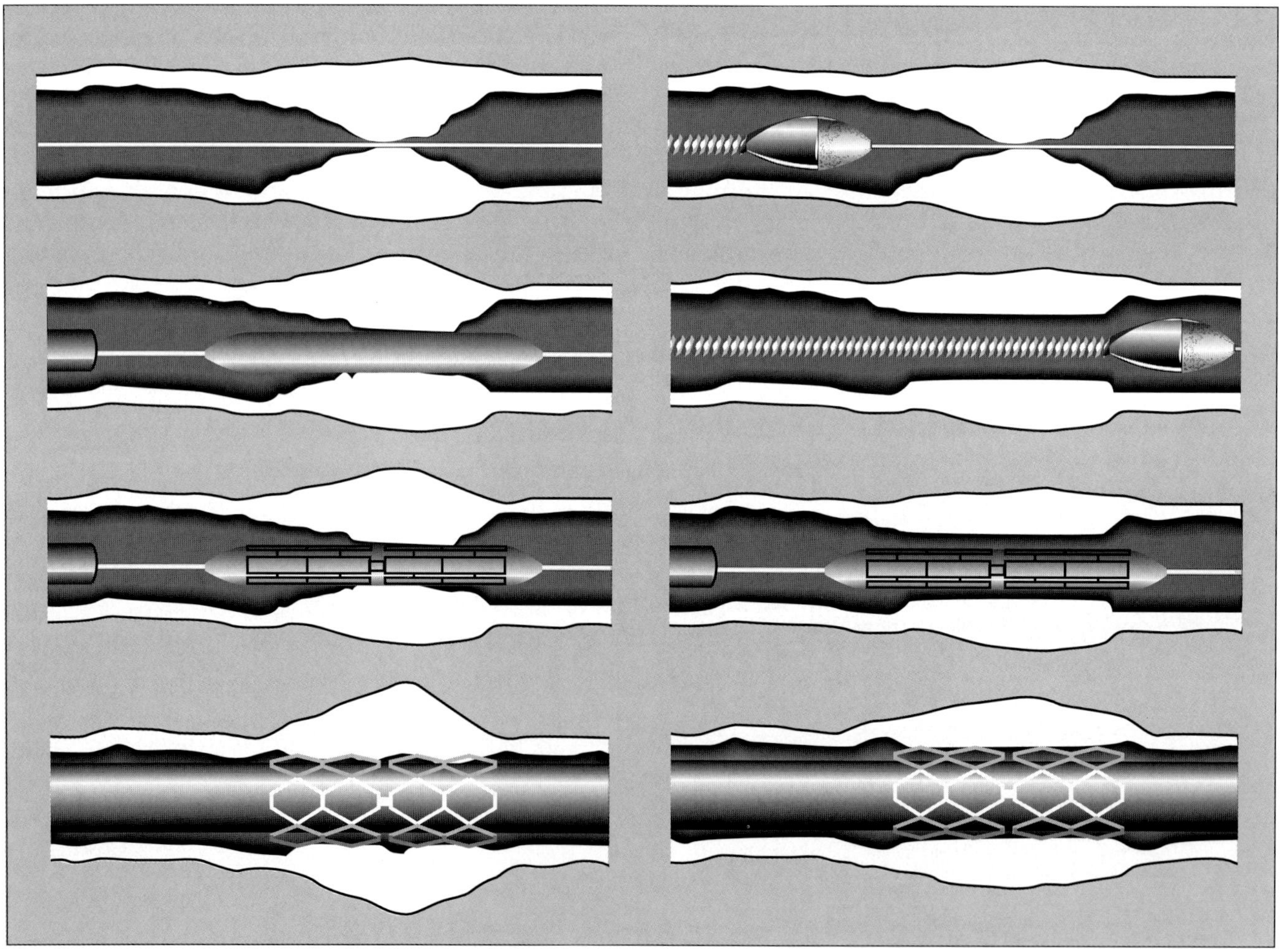

Figure 4-9. Demonstrates the advantage of debulking (*right*) versus not debulking (*left*) prior to stent implantation. The reduction of plaque by debulking potentially may improve deployment and, by increasing vessel compliance, may translate into a larger and more cylindrical final lumen.

Prebending the Guidewire

As discussed previously, because of the tendency for the guidewire to be straight, it lies along that side of the arterial lumen that allows it to be as straight as possible. To get a desirable trajectory for the burr in the artery, it can be beneficial to prebend the wire to follow the natural pathway of the artery. Thus, after noticing the way in which the wire lays in a vessel, the wire can be withdrawn using an exchange catheter or balloon (that could be used later) and bent using a forming tool, such as a needle to contour gently (by stroking) the wire to mimic the curve in the artery. Longitudinal location can be controlled by placing the curve a known distance from the platinum spring tip, which ideally is relatively close to the region of ablation as discussed previously (in other words, do not place the platinum tip distally during the ablative run because it tends to anchor the wire adversely). When the wire is reinserted into the artery, the bend location can be adjusted according to the reference length of the platinum spring tip as displayed on x-ray film. The plane of the bend automatically aligns itself with the plane of the curve in the vessel because nature insists on minimizing the elastic potential energy of the system. Even if the bend of the wire is not perfectly congruent with the bend of the artery, an approximate congruency makes a major difference in the magnitude of wire bias effect. For some cases in which an eccentric plaque is on the opposite side of the lumen from the natural "lay" of the wire, prebending can nicely redirect the burr to the eccentric plaque location. In all of this discussion, the goal of wire bias control and override is to allow the burr to behave in its true differential cutting fashion without prejudice based on extraneous mechanical vector forces.

New Technology Developments

To provide less intrinsic wire-bias, a new wire called the RotaWire (Boston Scientific Corp., Northwest Technology Center, Redmond, WA) has now been developed and approved by the Food and Drug Administration. This wire has a distal section of about 30 cm, which is tapered so as to provide a nearly ideal "bullwhip" mechanical characteristic that provides for a relatively high level of torsional rigidity in the body of the wire, while providing for distal zone flexibility and tractability. Distal zone flexibility implies more transverse compliance, which, in turn, implies less radial vector force or "bias" when the wire is insinuated into tortuous anatomy. To take full advantage of this more limber wire characteristic, a new Rotablator driveshaft has been approved by the Food and Drug Administration which, in turn, is much more flexible and capable of conforming to the tortuous trajectory of the wire and vessel without imposing excessive radial force ("driveshaft bias"). This new driveshaft, when

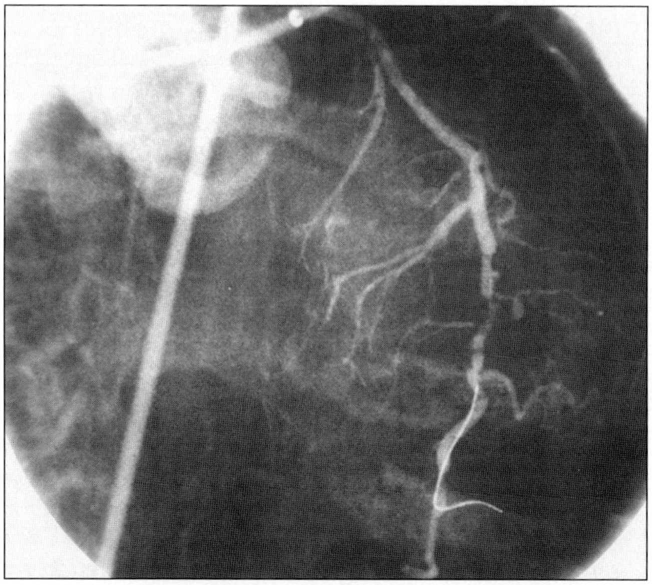

Figure 4-10. Demonstrates the significant straightening of the vessel caused by the stiff Rotablator guidewire. As clearly shown, there is significant deformity of the vessel (pseudolesions).

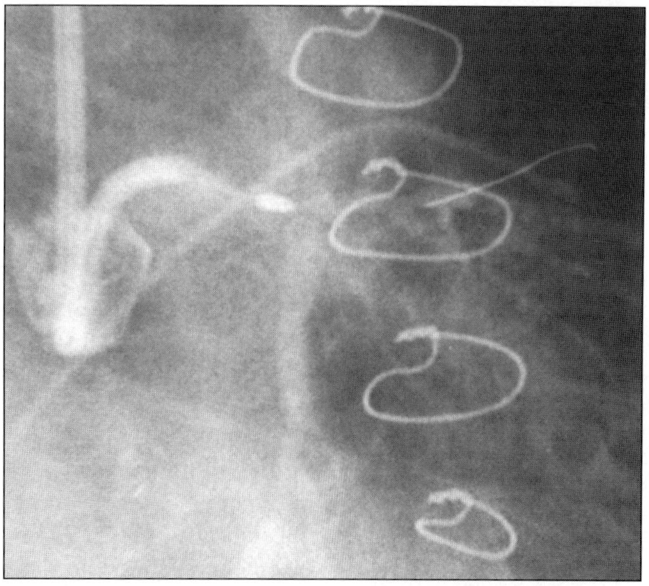

Figure 4-11. Placing the guidewire into a small diagonal branch allows the burr to be directed superiorly into the plaque mass of this eccentric lesion. By performing rotational atherectomy using this technique, a favorable guidewire bias ("directional") rotational atherectomy can be performed.

combined with the RotaWire, enables Rotablator operation around tortuous anatomy with a significant reduction in guidewire and driveshaft bias, although not totally eliminating the issue and the need for the interventionalist always to consider how the force vectors are directed within the lumen.

Soft Plaque and Compliant Substrates

The concept of differential cutting has often been misunderstood to mean preferential cutting of hard versus soft material. The proper concept is one of inelastic versus elastic. The Rotablator is relatively unable to ablate or sand material that is compliant and able to deflect out of the path of the diamond crystals. Atheromatous plaque exhibits marked inelasticity (as opposed to thrombus) and is effectively sanded by the Rotablator, provided that sanding pressure can be applied. One study [40] showed with intracoronary ultrasound surveillance that the Rotablator was capable of debulking fatty plaque. It is a little bit like asking the question: Can one sand butter or cheese? Of course the answer is "yes," but the sand paper will fill up with butter or cheese and lose its ablative efficiency. The Rotablator does not fill up with fat in the diamond crystals because it is spinning at a high rate of speed, which automatically sheds the particles by centrifugal force. What does become a serious clinical problem in association with Rotablator debulking of fatty plaque is the issue of vessel substrate compliance. When the fatty plaques rest on a normally compliant vessel wall, it becomes increasingly difficult to achieve effective purchase of the diamond sanding surface on the fatty plaque because the underlying tissue gives way. Thus, what may appear as a situation in which fatty plaque is not effectively ablated is usually a situation in which the underlying tissue does not provide adequate support for the sanding process. Some investigators report that using the Rotablator for removing neointima from restenotic (but well deployed) stents is the easiest procedure they do because the soft neointimal is rapidly ablated by the Rotablator, and the stent scaffolding ensures a firm foundation against which to sand and remove the restenotic mass. When a clinical situation presents itself in a soft plaque resting on a compliant substrate, it is important to recognize why the ablative effectiveness is reduced. Several anatomic situations manifest this condition: ostial lesions, eccentric lesions, and noticeably noncalcified lesions. (It is important to note that even calcified lesions sometimes rest on compliant substrates and resist rapid sanding.) When these situations present themselves, there is no substitute for patience. Although the sanding pressure that can be applied is noticeably reduced, it is never equal to zero. Thus, sanding still occurs, although at a much reduced rate. It simply takes more time to finish the atherectomy. At times, favorable guidewire bias or guide catheter bias improves the sanding pressure and speeds up the ablation. Prebending the wire as mentioned earlier can also speed up the process by getting better purchase.

Some might argue that soft plaque is easily pushed aside by conventional PTCA or stenting, and therefore debulking is unnecessary or useless. It is always important to remember that pushing aside plaque, whether it is soft or hard, implies stretching and perhaps rupturing the IEL, media, and adventitia.

Conclusions

Rotablator removal of obstructive atheroma without causing damage to healthy tissue structures and most particularly to the wall of the artery is not only possible, but also in many clinics is routine, as verified by IVUS. Randomized trials are underway to measure clinically the magnitude of the impact of restenosis. Using the Rotablator in such a manner so as not to cause stretch or ablative trauma or thermal damage requires adherence to a specific technique that is now well understood. For the more skillful user, it is now possible for many lesions to be treated with high-speed rotary ablation without seeing any damage to the arterial wall beneath the intimal level; the IEL, media, and adventitia are completely free of any histologic changes. In many stand-alone Rotablator treatments, the lesion residual can actually function as its own native stent possessing significant radial strength (sometimes more than stainless steel). To intervene in such a case with PTCA actually reduces the radial strength of the artery. Angiographic determinants of procedure conclusion can be misleading. IVUS has shown repeatedly that Rotablator treatment leaves a clean, round, untraumatized cylindrical hole. Attempting to improve on the angiogram with vessel rupturing adjunctive PTCA will assuredly lead to high levels of restenosis, as shown in the ERBAC (Excimer Rotational Ballon Angioplasty Comparison) trial. Blood flow capacity in cylinders of greater than 2.0 mm diameter is nearly always adequate. When a 2.0-mm waist "pops" with adjunctive PTCA as the balloon pressure is increased from 1 to 2 atm of indeflation pressure, it is a sure sign that the arterial wall has given way and that high levels of restenosis are likely. The temptation to balloon to an angiographic endpoint will lead to frequent episodes of wall damage and subsequent restenosis. The recent clinical experience with platelet aggregation inhibitors in conjunction with Rotablator attrition of plaque suggests that slow-flow or no-flow issues after rotary ablation are the result of the release of ground-up tissue factors, which can lead to platelet aggregation in the microcirculation. The clinical experience with ReoPro, in the setting of unstable syndromes, long, diffuse, and calcified plaques, has provided significant encouragement for the rotary ablation of these lesion subsets with reduced fear of severely restricted outflow.

The Rotablator is a surgical instrument operated at the end of a 2-m catheter instrument. It has more accuracy than a scalpel and requires even more attention to detail to avoid complications and enjoy the surgical precision implicit within.

Acknowledgment

In preparation of this text, special thanks are extended to Verna Harms, PhD, RN, Cindy Ogden, and Maria Fulton.

References and Recommended Reading

Recently published papers of particular interest have been highlighted as:

- • Of special interest
- •• Of outstanding interest

1. Hansen DD, Auth DC, Vrocko R, *et al.*: Rotational atherectomy in atherosclerotic rabbit iliac arteries. *Am Heart J* 1988, 115:160–165.
2. Hansen DD, Auth DC, Hall M, *et al.*: Rotational endarterectomy in normal canine coronary arteries. *J Am Coll Cardiol* 1988, 11:1073–1077.
3. O'Neill WW, Bates RE, Kirsch M, *et al.*: Mechanical transluminal coronary endarterectomy: initial clinical experience with the Auth mechanical rotary catheter [abstract]. *J Am Coll Cardiol* 1989, 13:227A.
4. Erbel R, O'Neill W, Auth D, *et al.*: Hochfrequenz-Rotationsatherektomie bei koronarer Herzkrankheit (High frequency rotational atherectomy in coronary heart disease). *Deutsche Medizinische Wochenschrift* 1989, 114:487–495.
5. Ahn S, Auth DC, Marcus D, *et al.*: Removal of focal atheromatous lesions by angioscopically guided high-speed rotary atherectomy. *J Vasc Surg* 1988, 7:292–300.
6. Schwartz R, Huber K, Murphy J, *et al.*: Restenosis and the proportional neointimal response to coronary artery injury: results in a porcine model. *J Am Coll Cardiol* 1992, 19:267–274.
7. Schwartz RS: Models of human coronary restenosis. In *Textbook of Interventional Cardiology*, edn 2, vol 1. Edited by Topol EJ. Philadelphia: WB Saunders, 1994: 365.
8. Nobuyoshi M, Kimura T, Ohishi H, *et al.*: Restenosis after percutaneous transluminal coronary angioplasty: pathologic observations in 20 patients. *J Am Coll Cardiol* 1991, 17:433–439.
9. Villa AE, Whitlow PL: Rotational coronary atherectomy. In *Textbook of Interventional Cardiology*, update 9. Edited by Topol EJ. Philadelphia: WB Saunders, 1994:135–146.
10. •• Reisman M, DeVore LJ, Ferguson M, *et al.*: Analysis of heat generation during high-speed rotational ablation: Technical implications [abstract]. *J Am Coll Cardiol* 1996, 27:292A.

Gentle ablation with deceleration of less than 7000 rpm and an oscillating technique were shown in an animal model to result in minimal heat generation, whereas more aggressive technique resulted in significant heat.

11. • Hong MK, Tjurmin A, Haudenschild CC, *et al.*: Historical findings in directional atherectomy specimens after rotational atherectomy in calcified coronary arteries [abstract]. *Circulation* 1994, 90:I-213.

Histologic specimens taken by DCA after rotational atherectomy in human coronary arteries demonstrated heat damage to the tissue, which may impact restenosis.

12. Douek PC, Correa R, Neville R, Unger EF: Dose dependent smooth muscle cell proliferation induced by thermal injury. *Circulation* 1992, 86:1249–1256.
13. Yamashita K, Satake S, Ohira H, *et al.*: Radiofrequency thermal balloon coronary angioplasty: A new device for successful percutaneous transluminal coronary angioplasty. *J Am Coll Cardiol* 1994, 23:336–340.
14. Reis GJ, Pomerantz M, Jenkins RD, *et al.*: Laser balloon angioplasty: clinical, angiographic and histologic results. *J Am Coll Cardiol* 1991, 18:193–202.
15. Snabre P, Braumler H, Mills P, *et al.*: Aggregation of human red blood cells after moderate heat treatment. *Biorheology* 1985, 22:185–195.
16. Lapshina EA, Biokizika IB: Thermal stability of erythrocyte membrane proteins at varying ionic strength and media composition. *Biofizika* 1994, 396:1015–1020.
17. Gader AM, al-Mashhadani SA, al-Harthy SS, *et al.*: Direct activation of platelets by heat is the possible trigger of the coagulopathy of heat stroke. *Br J Haematol* 1990, 74:86–92.
18. •• Vandormael M, Reifart N, Preusler W, *et al.*: Comparison of excimer laser, rotablator and balloon angioplasty for the treatment of complex lesions: ERBAC study final results [abstract]. *J Am Coll Cardiol* 1994, 23:57A.

Patients with complex lesions were randomized to treatment with balloon angioplasty or laser or rotational atherectomy (about 100 patients in each group). For rotational atherectomy major complications were lower and procedural success was higher. Restenosis rates for all procedures were greater than 50%, and target vessel revascularization was higher for laser and rotational atherectomy.

19. •• Warth DC, Leon MB, O'Neill W, *et al.*: Rotational atherectomy multicenter registry: Acute results, complications and 6-

month angiographic follow-up in 709 patients. *J Am Coll Cardiol* 1994, 24:641–648.

This report on the results of the first 709 patients in the Rotablator multicenter registry documents patient and lesion characteristics, procedural success, complications, and 6-month follow-up.

20. Stertzer SH, Rosenblum J, Shaw RE, *et al.*: Coronary rotational ablation: initial experience in 302 procedures [see comments]. *J Am Coll Cardiol* 1993, 21:287–295.

21. Eccleston DS, Horrigan MC, Cowley MJ, *et al.*: Is there a role for strip chart recording to guide rotational atherectomy? Initial findings from STRATAS [abstract]. *J Am Coll Cardiol* 1996, 27:292A.

22. Auth DC: Introduction: Angioplasty with high speed rotary ablation. In *Restenosis after Intervention with New Mechanical Devices.* Edited by Serruys PW, Strauss BH, King SB III. Boston: Kluwer Academic Publishers, 1992:282.

23. Nissen SE, Gurley JC: Intervascular ultrasound imaging following mechanical coronary interventions: theoretic advantages and initial clinical experience. In *Restenosis after Intervention with New Mechanical Devices.* Edited by Serruys PW, Strauss BH, King SB III . Boston: Kluwer Academic Publishers, 1992:75.

24. Fischman DL, Leon MB, Baim DS, *et al.*: A randomized comparison of coronary-stent placement and balloon angioplasty in the treatment of coronary artery disease. *N Engl J Med* 1994, 331:496–501.

25. Kuntz RE, Gibson MC, Nobuyoshi M, *et al.*: Generalized model of restenosis after conventional balloon angioplasty, stenting and directional atherectomy. *J Am Coll Cardiol* 1993, 21:15–25.

26. Serruys PW, Jaegere P, Kiemeneij F, *et al.*: A comparison of balloon-expandable-stent implantation with balloon angioplasty in patients with coronary artery disease. *N Engl J Med* 1994, 331:489–495.

27. Rushmer RF: *Cardiovascular Dynamics*: edn 4. Philadelphia: WB Saunders, 1976.

28. Leguizamon JH, Chambre DF, Torresani EM, *et al.*: High-speed coronary rotational atherectomy. Are angiographic factors predictive of failure, major complications or restenosis? A multivariate analysis [abstract]. *J Am Coll Cardiol* 1995, 25:95A.

29. Stertzer SH, Rosenblum J, Shaw RE, *et al.*: Restenosis following successful rotational ablation of de novo coronary stenosis. *J Invas Cardiol* 1993, 5:295–301.

30.• Kaplan BM, Mojares JJ, Safian RD, *et al.*: Optimal burr and adjunctive balloon sizing alters the need for target vessel revascularization after rotablator atherectomy [abstract]. *J Am Coll Cardiol* 1996, 27:291A.

Restenosis rates appear lower if the burr-to-artery ratio for debulking was optimal (0.75–0.95). Higher rates of restenosis occurred with too little debulking or with excessive debulking, which may have induced medial damage.

31.•• Peterson KL, Rivera I, McDaniel M, *et al.*: Percutaneous transluminal coronary rotational ablation: serial follow-up by quantitative angiography. In *Restenosis after Intervention with New Mechanical Devices.* Edited by Serruys PW, Strauss BH, King SB III. Boston: Kluwer Academic Publishers, 1992:319.

Angiographic films from patients in the Rotablator multicenter registry who had procedural, 24-hour, and 6-month follow-up angiograms were analyzed by quantitative coronary angiography. At 24 hours the minimum luminal diameter had increased in size from the postprocedural film; at 6 months it had decreased by 0.3 mm.

32. Savage M, Fischman D, Rake R, *et al.*: Elective coronary stenting versus balloon angioplasty in smaller native coronary arteries: results from STRESS [abstract]. *J Am Coll Cardiol* 1996, 27:253A.

33. Whitlow PL, Cowley M, Kuntz R, *et al.*: Study to determine rotablator and transluminal angioplasty strategy [abstract]. *Circulation* 1995, 92:I-330.

34.• O'Murchu B, Foreman RD, Shaw RE, *et al.*: Role of the intraaortic balloon pump counterpulsation in high risk coronary atherectomy. *J Am Coll Cardiol* 1995, 26:1270–1275.

In 159 patients at high risk due to low ejection fraction, myocardium at risk, and complexity of lesion site, prophylactic preprocedure insertion of an intra-aortic balloon pump in 28 patients resulted in higher procedural success without hypotension than in the remaining patients who did not receive a balloon pump or an intraprocedural pump in response to hypotension.

35. Cohen BM, Weber V, Cohen D, *et al.*: Intracoronary cocktail infusion during rotational ablation: safety and efficacy [abstract]. *J Invas Cardiol* 1995, 7:3A.

36. Coletti RH, Haik BJ, Wiedermann JG: Marked reduction in slow-reflow after rotational atherectomy through the use of a novel flushing solution [abstract]. *J Invas Cardiol* 1996, 8:32A.

37. Stertzer SH, Pomerants EV, Fitzgerald PJ, *et al.*: Effects of technique modification on immediate results of high speed rotational atherectomy in 710 procedures on 656 patients. *Cathet Cardiovasc Diag* 1995, 36:304–310.

38. Mintz GS, Dussaillant G, Wong S, *et al.*: Rotational atherectomy followed by adjunct stents: the preferred therapy for calcified lesions in large vessels? *Circulation* 1995, 92:I-329.

39. Guarneri EM, Norman SL, Stevens KM, *et al.*: Rotational atherectomy prior to stent implantation [abstract]. *J Am Coll Cardiol* 1996, 27:252A.

40. Dussaillant G, Mintz GS, Walsh C, *et al.*: Volumetric intravascular ultrasound analysis shows that rotational atherectomy effectively ablates soft atherosclerotic plaque [abstract]. *Circulation* 1995, 92:I-17.

Chapter 5

The Current Status of Laser Angioplasty Technology

David R. Holmes, Jr.

During the development of laser angioplasty in the late 1980s, there was great enthusiasm for the technology and its potential role in solving the problems of interventional cardiology. The dominant problems for interventional cardiology then, as today, include 1) chronic total occlusion, which is associated with decreased success rates with conventional percutaneous transluminal coronary angioplasty (PTCA), mainly related to inability to cross the occlusion with a guidewire; 2) specific adverse lesion morphology including diffuse disease, the presence of intracoronary thrombus, lesion calcification, eccentricity, and ostial location, all of which are associated with decreased success rates and often increased restenosis with conventional PTCA technology; 3) the unpredictable nature of barotrauma on the vessel wall after balloon angioplasty with the potential for dissection and acute closure; and 4) restenosis, which was believed at that time to be primarily the result of neointimal hyperplasia. Although our understanding of restenosis has advanced, it remains a problem.

Laser technology had the potential to address many of these problems. The concept of ablating atheromatous tissue with an excimer laser to produce a smooth surface without eschar remains attractive [1]. Such a device could either be used as a stand-alone procedure or would facilitate subsequent adjunctive PTCA. Early animal and in vitro studies documented the potential for "clean cutting" of even calcified diffuse disease. In addition, there was interest in developing a system that could be used to create a pilot channel through a chronic total occlusion.

With these goals in mind, laser therapy was developed with initial evaluation of continuous wave lasers; these lasers ablated by inducing intense localized heating, resulting in concentric zones of carbonized material, eosinophilic coagulum, and vacuolization. These lasers were subsequently abandoned for pulsed excimer laser technology with a 308-nm xenon chloride (XeCl) laser, which was believed to produce relatively few thermal effects and only small zones of thermal or blast injury. This laser has dominated the field, although solid-state lasers including holmium:YAG systems operating in the mid-infrared zone at 1.94- to 2.09-μm wavelengths have also been used [2]. These latter lasers have some potential advantages in that they operate close to the water absorption peak and may provide excellent ablation with minimal thermal damage to the arterial wall. After these systems were developed, patient treatment cohorts were accrued and multicenter registries were developed that resulted in Food and Drug Administration (FDA) approval of excimer laser coronary angioplasty (ELCA) in the United States in 1991.

Since FDA approval and more widespread experience, the role of ELCA has changed dramatically. Initial pilot studies documented improved outcome in complex lesion subsets compared with historical cohort comparisons of patients treated with conventional PTCA [3]. In the first 3000 patients with 3592 lesions treated reported by the industry-sponsored Advanced Interventional Systems (AIS) registry [4], only 7% of the lesions were type A; the remainder were either type B (61%) or type C (32%). In these higher risk lesion subsets, laser success was achieved in 84% and procedural success in 90%. Major complications were infrequent and included death (0.5%), Q-wave myocardial infarction (MI) (2.1%), and coronary bypass graft surgery (CABG) (3.8%).

Similarly, the other industry-sponsored study (percutaneous excimer laser coronary angioplasty [PELCA]) of 1521 patients with 1592 treated lesions also included predominantly type B and C lesions. In this registry, the laser success rate was 81.1% and procedural success was 89.3% [5]. As with the AIS registry, the PELCA registry documented a low incidence of major complications (death, 0.7%; Q-wave MI, 1.0%; and in-hospital CABG, 3.1%). A striking finding was the fact that there was no difference in success rates or in-hospital complications between any of the major lesion subtypes. This finding played a major role in the approval process because it was in contrast to the widely held belief that, with conventional dilatation, increasing lesion complexity was associated with decreased success rates. These findings led to an increasing interest in ELCA, with special emphasis on high-risk patients with ostial lesions, diffuse disease, and chronic total occlusion.

Against this backdrop, several events occurred that greatly ameliorated the increase in enthusiasm. These include 1) continued concern over the cost of the devices (approximately $250,000) and need for adjunctive PTCA, 2) lack of significant effect on the incidence of restenosis [6], 3) inability of excimer laser to successfully ablate calcified lesions, 4) development of Rotablator (Boston Scientific Corporation, Northwest Technology Center [formerly Heart Technology]; Redmond, WA) and long balloon technology, and 5) the problem of dissection. The last factors have been most important in retarding a significant increase in laser angioplasty.

Lack of Impact on Restenosis

One goal of new technology is to improve the long-term outcome in patients by reducing restenosis. There was initial considerable interest in stand-alone laser therapy to avoid the barotrauma of balloon inflation as a means to decrease restenosis. Unfortunately, such a strategy with the device sizes available left a substantial residual stenosis and was associated with restenosis rates of approximately 50% [6]. Randomized trials have now documented that restenosis rates with this procedure are not improved compared with rates for conventional PTCA [7••,8]. It must be remembered that small vessels with more diffuse disease have markedly increased restenosis rates with any technology, even with stents. In addition, these early randomized trials did not incorporate what is now believed to be optimal laser technique [8].

Inability of Excimer Laser to Treat Lesion Calcification

Although excimer laser was initially documented in in vitro models to result in clean tissue ablation without charring or vessel damage, in actual practice calcified lesions often could not be treated successfully. In such heavily calcified lesions, even increasing the fluence or frequency was often not successful, and vessel trauma would result. In addition, the introduction of ultrasound allowed the observation that calcification was very frequent, even if not seen on angiography, particularly in longer, diffuse disease. Therefore, when calcium was identified, operators often tended to avoid selecting the laser for use. Another factor was the introduction of rotational atherectomy, which was found to be very effective for lesion calcification and soon became the treatment of choice. For the treatment of other diffusely diseased vessels, long balloons were also introduced that were found to result in excellent initial success rates. These long balloons, 40 to 80 mm in length, were less expensive and easier to use than excimer laser.

Laser-Induced Dissection and Vessel Injury

The most problematic area of ELCA was that of unpredictable laser-induced dissection. Dissection occurred in 13% of the AIS registry [4] and 22% of the PELCA registry [5] and was associated with acute vessel closure in 6.5% and 6.1%, respectively. The increased incidence of dissection was unexpected based on the initial in vitro testing. Subsequent studies documented intense effects with cavitation and expansion, particularly when lasing in the presence of contrast media. This has led to recent efforts with saline flushing to minimize vessel damage, which has been reported to decrease dissection [9].

In addition to dissection, perforation has been a potential concern with ELCA [10]. Perforation is extremely uncommon with conventional PTCA but is increased with ablative devices. In the ELCA registry of 2759 patients, 36 (1.3%) developed a perforation [10]. The frequency of perforation declined over time with increasing operator experience, from 1.6% in the first 1888 patients to only 0.4% in the final 1000 patients. Although perforation is relatively uncommon, it is associated with increased morbidity and even mortality. In the ELCA Registry, among patients with perforation, 36.1% required emergency CABG, 16.7% experienced an MI, and 5.6% died. Recent advances with covered stents may alleviate the need for urgent surgery. Although factors associated with increased perforation rates have been identified, they are relatively weak predictors, and the event remains unpredictable.

All of these factors led to the dramatic decrease in ELCA, with many laboratories either abandoning the technique, never starting it, or limiting it to a very small percentage of cases. More recently, however, there has been a rebirth of interest in the technique. This is the result of two major factors: 1) the increasing number of patients with instent restenosis [11••], and 2) the development of the laser total occlusion wire system [12••,13]. An additional factor is continued interest in laser for diffuse vein graft disease [14••].

Instent Restenosis

The incidence of restenosis has decreased in selected patients undergoing stent implantation; even in these selected patients, however, restenosis rates may occur in 15% to 20%. In the larger group of patients currently undergoing stent implantation who do not meet the STRESS (Stent Restenosis Study)/BENESTENT (Belgium Netherland's Stent Trial) criteria, the restenosis rates have been found to be increased to 20% to 40%. In these patients with "instent" restenosis, neointimal hyperplasia is the dominant or perhaps sole mechanism. Several patterns of restenosis have been documented, including focal (either occurring at the site of articulation or at either end of the stent) and diffuse. In the former, conventional PTCA is very effective. In the latter, conventional dilatation is associated with very high recurrent restenosis rates. In this latter group, laser angioplasty is being performed with increasing frequency to debulk the mass of neointima followed then by dilatation. Although attractive, there are only limited longer-term efficacy data on this approach.

Laser Total Occlusion Wire System

Chronic total occlusion is a relatively frequent finding in patients with symptomatic coronary artery disease and is one of the most common reasons for surgical referral. Although conventional PTCA has been used (in some series of conventional PTCA patients, treatment of a chronic total occlusion accounts for 10% of case volumes), it is characterized by decreased success rates of approximately 60% due to inability to cross the lesion with a guidewire.

Recently, a laser wire consisting of optical fibers encased in a 0.018-inch hypodermic tube shaft has been evaluated [12••,13]. This device is steerable with a movable torque device mounted on the proximal shaft and is delivered with a sheath to the point of occlusion. By visualizing the course of the distal vessel via either ipsilateral or contralateral injections and collateral vessels and by using biplane imaging, the laser wire is activated and slowly advanced with frequent test injections until it penetrates the chronic total occlusion into the distal vessel. In selected case series, even with lesions that have been refractory to attempts at conventional guidewire recanalization, success rates of approximately 80% can be achieved. Complications have been found to be infrequent. Single "laser wire exits" are common, occurring in approximately 20% of cases, but clinical sequelae are extremely uncommon. The procedure of lasing for chronic total occlusion is often long and involves substantial contrast volume and radiation exposure. Continued documentation of these results in larger patient series with an expanded group of operators will allow further growth in ELCA. If the procedure is found to greatly improve the ability to access chronic occlusions, there will be a marked increase in the use of excimer laser angioplasty.

Conclusions

There has been a definite rebirth of interest in ELCA based on application of the technique for the treatment of diffuse instent restenosis and for the treatment of chronic total occlusion. Other future developments, including multiplexing approaches and saline flushing techniques, will also have the potential to increase the utility and the outcome of this procedure.

References and Recommended Reading

Recently published papers of particular interest have been highlighted as:

- • Of special interest
- •• Of outstanding interest

1. Grundfest WS, Litvack F, Forrester JS, *et al.*: Laser ablation of human atherosclerotic plaque without adjacent tissue injury. *J Am Coll Cardiol* 1985, 5:929–933.

2. Topaz O: Solid-state Laser: The Holmium:YAG System. In *Strategic Approaches in Coronary Intervention.* Edited by Ellis SG, Holmes DR Jr. Baltimore: Williams & Wilkins; 1996:50–62.

3. Eigler NL, Weinstock B, Douglas JS Jr, *et al.*: Excimer laser coronary angioplasty of aorto-ostial stenoses: results of the Excimer Laser Coronary Angioplasty (ELCA) Registry in the first 200 patients. *Circulation* 1993, 88(part I):2049–2057.

4. Litvack F, Eigler N, Margolis J, *et al.*: Percutaneous excimer laser angioplasty: results of the first consecutive 3000 patients. *J Am Coll Cardiol* 1994, 23:323–329.

5. Baumbach A, Bittl JA, Fleck E, *et al.*: Acute complications of excimer laser coronary angioplasty: a detailed analysis of multicenter results. *J Am Coll Cardiol* 1994, 23:1305–1313.

6. Bittl JA, Kuntz RE, Estella P: Analysis of late lumen narrowing after excimer laser facilitated coronary angioplasty. *J Am Coll Cardiol* 1994, 23:1314–1320.

7.•• Appelman YEA, Piek JJ, Strikwerda S, *et al.*: Randomized trial of excimer laser angioplasty versus balloon angioplasty for treatment of obstructive coronary artery disease. *Lancet* 1996, 347:79–84.

The first fully repeated randomized study of excimer laser versus conventional PTCA.

8. Vandormael M, Reifart N, Preusler W, *et al.*: Six-month follow-up results following excimer laser angioplasty, rotational atherectomy and balloon angioplasty for complex lesions: ERBAC study [abstract]. *Circulation* 1994, 90:1143.

9. Deckelbaum LI, Strauss BH, Bittl JA, *et al.* and the PELCA Investigators: Effect of intracoronary saline infusion on dissection during excimer laser coronary angioplasty: a randomized trial [abstract]. *Circulation* 1994, 90:1774.

10. Holmes DR Jr, Reeder GS, Ghazzal ZMB, *et al.*: Coronary perforation after excimer laser coronary angioplasty: the Excimer Laser Coronary Angioplasty Registry experience. *J Am Coll Cardiol* 1994, 23:330–335.

11.•• Mehran R, Mintz GS, Popma JJ, *et al.*: Excimer laser angioplasty in the treatment of instent restenosis: an intravascular ultrasound study [abstract]. *J Am Coll Cardiol* 1996, 27 (2, suppl A):362A.

An early experience dealing with the problem of instent restenosis. This will be one of the major indications for laser angioplasty.

12.•• Serruys PW, Leon M, Hamburger JN, *et al.*: Recanalization of chronic total coronary occlusions using a laser guide wire: the Eu and US Total experience [abstract]. *J Am Coll Cardiol* 1996, 27(2, suppl A):152A.

The future of laser angioplasty rests in major part on its utility and effectiveness for treating chronic total occlusions.

13. Popma JJ, Leon MB, O'Neill W, *et al.*: Angiographic outcomes after arterial recanalization of refractory occlusions with the PRIMA excimer laser wire [abstract]. *J Am Coll Cardiol* 1996, 27(2, suppl A):152A.

14.•• Hong MK, Wong SC, Popma JJ, *et al.*: Favorable results of debulking followed by immediate adjunct stent therapy for high risk saphenous vein graft lesions [abstract]. *J Am Coll Cardiol* 1996, 27(2, suppl A):179A.

Although in abstract form, this study documents one of the reasons for the increase in laser use.

Chapter 6

The Role of Saline Flush in Reducing Collateral Damage During Excimer Laser Angioplasty

Raj Makkar
Neal Eigler
Frank Litvack

Excimer laser coronary angioplasty (ELCA) has retained its place in the interventional cardiology armamentarium. In the 1980s, when new interventional devices were emerging with great promise, none generated more excitement than ELCA. Expectations for the technology were high, but the complexity of the in vivo laser tissue interaction was incompletely understood. This technology, more so than any of the other second-generation interventional devices, has experienced the classic pendular shift in favor. ELCA was expected by some to solve the deficiencies, including restenosis, of balloon angioplasty. However, the occurrence of unpredictable and sometimes extensive dissections remained an enigmatic problem. Currently, there is a resurgence in acceptance of the technology, in part due to an improved understanding of the laser tissue interaction as well as better delineation of its appropriate applications [1••,2,3].

Originally, the idea of using the excimer laser in angioplasty procedures was derived from observations by physical scientists that precise etching of polymer films was possible using ultraviolet light [4]. Early biologic researchers were encouraged by their findings and research was extended to in vitro studies of vascular tissue [5]. It was demonstrated that a 308-nm excimer laser was capable of cutting precise channels in atherosclerotic material without causing the collateral thermal or blast injury that was commonly seen with the continuous-wave lasers then in use. However, there were no commercially available medical excimer laser systems, and the tasks required to transform the available excimer laser technology to a viable angioplasty system were formidable. It was said that transmission of excimer laser light through fiberoptics was impossible because of the short wavelength and the high-peak instantaneous power of the pulses. In addition, catheter systems had to be designed that were compatible with existing angioplasty technique.

The Problem of Dissection

Many thousands of patients underwent ELCA, and it has emerged as a useful therapy for selected patients with complex coronary disease. Several registries from the early clinical experience demonstrated that the procedure could be safely applied, even in a variety of complex lesions that are not well suited for conventional percutaneous transluminal coronary angioplasty (PTCA). These include aorto-ostial, long lesions, total occlusions crossable with the wire, diffuse disease, and vein grafts [6,7]. Currently, this procedure is being used in patients with in-stent restenosis, and the laser wire that has been developed has the potential to be used in the treatment of chronic total occlusions [8]. Major ischemic complications in the early registries were in keeping with standards at that time [6,7]. This notwithstanding, coronary dissection was a persistent, perplexing, and vexing problem. This led to an unpredictability of the procedure and was in part responsible for the dampening of enthusiasm for ELCA. In a detailed analysis of multicenter results from Europe and the United States, dissection was noted in 22%, vasospasm in 6.1%, filling defects in 4.8%, and abrupt closure in 6.1% of patients [7]. In another large registry of 3000 patients, angiographic dissection occurred in 13% of lesions, transient occlusion in 3.4%, and sustained occlusion in 3.1% [6]. Although at first glance the incidence of dissection would not appear to be substantially greater than that seen with conventional balloon angioplasty, it was the nature, severity, and unpredictability of these dissections that was so troubling. Specifically, lesions that would typically yield good results with conventional balloon angioplasty could, following laser angioplasty, become complicated with long spiral or deep dissections. The incidence and severity of dissections varied from investigator to investigator and no clear delineation of causality was obvious. These findings were particularly troublesome in view of the clear demonstration that excimer energy was capable of ablating atherosclerotic plaque with minimal collateral damage in vitro.

Mechanism of Dissection After ELCA

The clue to the dissection problem lay in the literature that existed from the 1960s and in a series of experiments that resulted in papers in the late 1980s and early 1990s. It was first demonstrated that pulsed laser energy produces cavitation or bubbles in a fluid medium when a pulsed 694-nm ruby laser produced acoustic transients, probably as a result of the development of dielectric fields [9]. This observation was repeated with different pulsed lasers [10]. In 1988 Isner and colleagues, using myocardial tissue in a blood medium, demonstrated a sequence of cavity formation, growth, collapse, and rebound [11]. Van Leeuwen and colleagues demonstrated that intraluminal vapor bubbles induced by excimer laser pulses cause microsecond arterial dilatation and invagination leading to extensive wall damage in the rabbit model [12]. These authors concluded that in a blood field, each excimer laser pulse generated a fast expanding and imploding vapor bubble that induced dissections and extensive wall damage far beyond the penetration depth of a 308-nm laser light (Fig. 6-1). They postulated that this unique pattern of extensive wall damage observed in the rabbit may explain the mechanism of

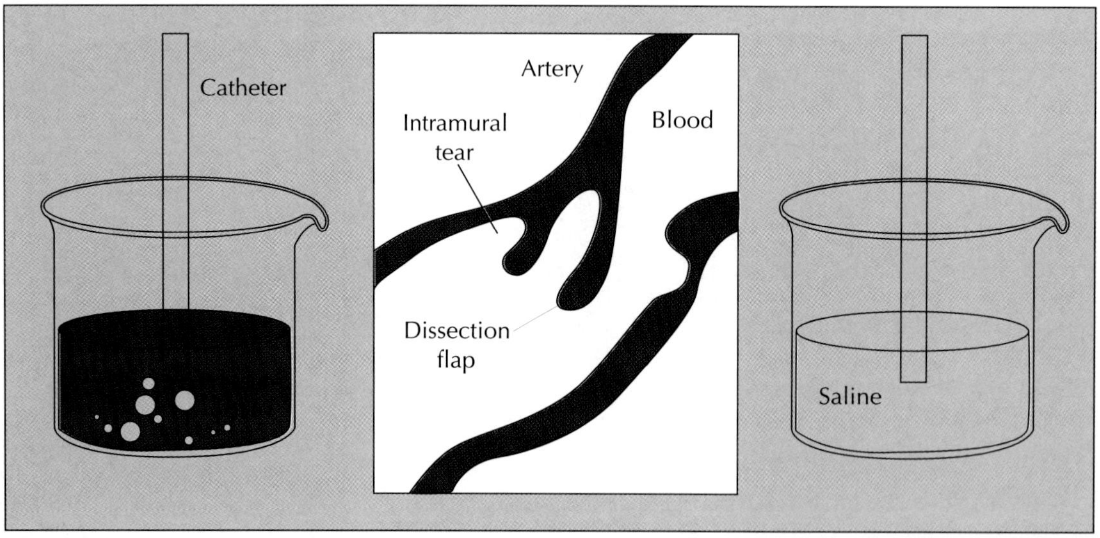

Figure 6-1. Laser-induced tearing of the arterial wall. Excimer laser energy, absorbed by blood (*left*), causes rapidly expanding bubbles that disrupt the arterial wall. Such coronary dissection (*middle*) is avoided by clearing the artery of blood and infusing saline through the guiding catheter. The light beam transmits through the saline and is not absorbed (*right*).

dissection observed in humans during the clinical procedure [12].

Baumbach and colleagues [13•] further theorized that pressure transmitted during excimer laser ablation of vascular tissue may be the culprit in the clinically observed dissections. They conducted an experiment in which pressure waves were measured during excimer laser radiation in blood and contrast media using a sensitive hydrophone. At 4-mm distance from the tip of a 1.7-mm multifiber catheter excimer irradiation in blood resulted in a linear increase of peak pressures. When the experiments were repeated in radiographic contrast media, peak pressure increased two- to threefold over that which was observed in the blood media (Fig. 6-2*A*). They then diluted the blood with either contrast media or saline. At a concentration of 60% contrast in blood, a 3.4-fold increase of peak pressures was documented, as compared with pure blood. Concentrations of saline in blood of 90% reduced the peak pressures by 16%, and concentrations of saline in blood of 96% reduced the peak pressures by more than 50%, as compared with pure blood (Fig. 6-2*B*).

These experiments provided the important series of clues necessary to solve the excimer laser angioplasty dissection problem. It appeared that excimer laser energy was negatively interacting with blood or, even worse, radiographic contrast and causing rapidly expanding and imploding bubbles that yielded the damaging forces responsible for the unpredictable dissections. This explained the interoperator variation and the commonly observed finding that diffuse, tubular lesions were less prone to dissection. The dissection-prone operators would be heavy footed and provide a great deal of energy in a confined space. On the other hand, some operators held their pulse trains to just a couple of seconds, limiting the amount of energy that was input. The simple, type A lesions that yield good results with balloon angioplasty were those commonly associated with unpredictable and frustrating dissections. This is probably because these lesions did not allow the catheter to be buried deep within them and, as such, were exposed to flowing blood. Finally, some operators, in a futile attempt to limit dissections, would be very "careful." They would precisely position the laser catheter with the aid of frequent injections of radiographic contrast. This resulted in excimer irradiation within a contrast medium—the worst possible scenario for dissection.

Role of Saline Flush Technique

Tcheng and colleagues [14••] proposed a new technique for reducing pressure pulse generation during 308-nm excimer laser coronary angioplasty. They observed that in vitro ablation of porcine aorta in the presence of blood or contrast resulted in tissue dissection, whereas ablation and pure crystalloid did not (Fig. 6-3). The crystalloid did not absorb the 308-nm radiation. Therefore, vapor bubbles were not created. Next, they developed a "flush and bathe" technique designed to replace all blood and contrast with crystal-

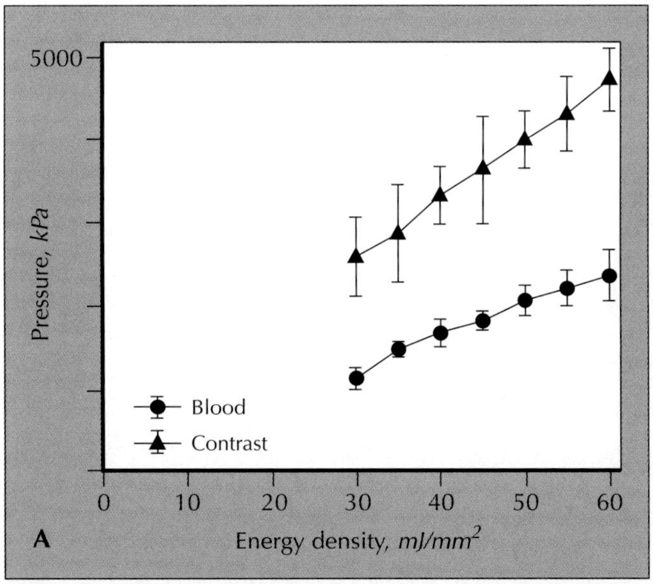

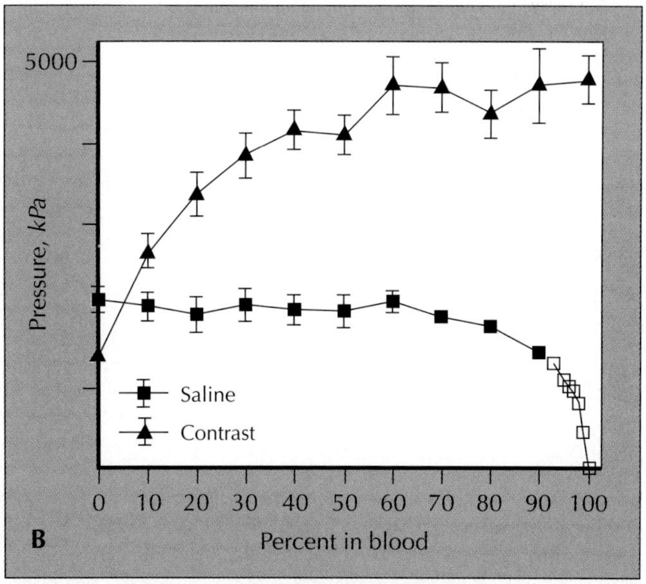

Figure 6-2. A, Peak pressures (mean ± SD) at a distance of 4 mm to the catheter tip during excimer laser irradiation with different energy densities in blood and contrast media. **B**, Peak pressures (mean ± SD) in a distance of 4 mm to the catheter tip during excimer laser irradiation with 45 mJ/mm^2 in solutions of saline or contrast media in blood. (*From* Baumbach and colleagues [7]; with permission.)

loid. As demonstrated in the experimental models, there would need to be sufficient dilution of blood to reduce the concentration by more than 90%. They reported a pilot study of safety and feasibility involving the treatment of 57 consecutive excimer laser angioplasty patients. No patients developed complications from the infusion. The procedure success rate was 95%, and there were no acute ischemic complications. Dissections following laser ablation were seen in 14%. However, all were classified as Grade I dissections and judged to be clinically inconsequential. This was in contradistinction to prior experience, in which the frequency of dissections would be the same but the severity of dissections would be far worse than with PTCA [14••].

This early experience led to the design and execution of a small, randomized trial of conventional and saline technique. Moderately severe or worse dissections occurred in 21% of conventionally treated lesions but in only 4% of saline-treated lesions [15••]. Based on these data and the anecdotal experience of many operators, the saline infusion technique is now the standard for excimer angioplasty. This simple technique has changed the complexion of the procedure. Excimer laser angioplasty has now become a predictable procedure with a low incidence of clinically significant dissections and acute occlusion.

Saline Flush Protocol

The following protocol for saline infusion during excimer laser angioplasty is recommended:

1. Position a laser catheter within the coronary artery in contact with the target lesion.
2. Remove the contrast syringe from the manifold.
3. Attach a 20-cm^3 syringe for saline infusion.
4. Very carefully flush the manifold and the guiding catheter of all contrast.
5. Tighten the Y-adapter so the laser catheter can move forward without leaking saline during the infusion.
6. Inject a 10-mL bolus of saline via the guide catheter.
7. Immediately, slow the injection rate to 1 to 3 mL/s.
8. Activate the laser immediately after the 10-mL bolus infusion and during the 1- to 3-mL saline slow infusion.
9. Repeat the procedure for each pulse train and do not apply laser energy for more than 3 seconds at a time.

Conclusions

In summary, excimer laser angioplasty has been an evolving procedure both technically and clinically. At present, the technology appears to be best applied to the debulking of selected complex lesion types as a prelude to stenting or in vessels that cannot be stented and for the treatment of in-stent restenosis. Unpredictable and severe coronary dissections were a persistent problem in the early years of this technology, although the incidence and severity tended to be somewhat operator-dependent. Recognition that laser irradiation within a blood or contrast medium would result in rapidly expanding and imploding vapor bubbles capable of generating sufficient energy to induce

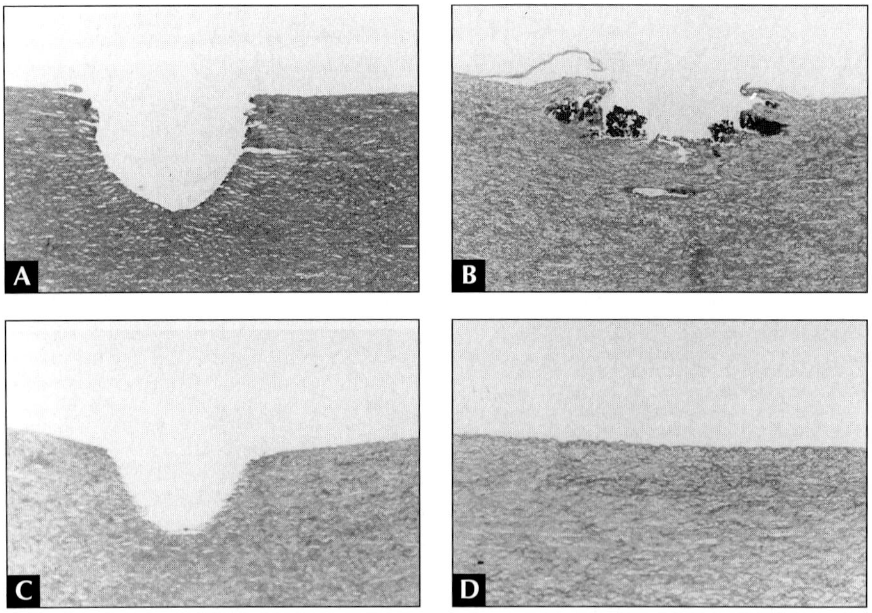

Figure 6-3. Histology of porcine aorta following excimer laser irradiation. One thousand pulses of 308-nm radiation were delivered via an 800 μm optical fiber, with the fiber maintained in a stationary position oriented vertically to the surface of the specimen during the ablation. **A** and **C** were obtained with the specimen and fiber in normal saline, whereas **B** and **D** were obtained with the specimen and fiber in a blood field. **A** and **B** were obtained with the tip of the laser catheter initially in contact with the specimen. **C** and **D** were obtained with the tip of the laser fiber 1 mm from the tissue. Note the tissue disruption shown with contact ablation in a blood field (**B**), whereas attempted ablation at a distance of 1 mm in a blood field (**D**) shows no ablation of tissue. Trichrome stain, ×15. (*From* Tcheng and colleagues [14]; with permission.)

vascular dissection yielded critical information suggesting a simple technical change that improved the procedure. In contemporary practice, all excimer angioplasty procedures are performed using the saline infusion technique via the coronary guide catheter. A small, randomized trial demonstrated significant diminution in the incidence of serious dissections [15••]. This simple modification of technique has vastly improved the predictability of the procedure and the comfort level of the operators.

REFERENCES AND RECOMMENDED READING

Recently published papers of particular interest have been highlighted as:

- • Of special interest
- •• Of outstanding interest

1.•• Litvack F, Eigler NL, Forrester JS: Excimer laser coronary angioplasty. *Scientific American Sci Med* 1996, 3:42–51.

A comprehensive review of laser angioplasty.

2. Deckelbaum IL: Coronary laser angioplasty. *Lasers Surg Med* 1994, 14:101–110.

3. Litvack F, Eigler NL, Forrester JS: In search of the optimized excimer laser angioplasty system. *Circulation* 1993, 87:1421–1422.

4. Srinivasan R, Mayne-Banton V: Self developing photoetching of poly(ethylene terephthalate) laser radiation. *Appl Phys Lett* 1982, 41:576–578.

5. Grundfest WS, Litvack F, Forrester JS, *et al.*: Laser ablation of human atherosclerotic plaque without adjacent tissue injury. *J Am Coll Cardiol* 1985, 5:929–933.

6. Litvack F, Eigler N, Margolis J, *et al.* for the ELCA investigators: Percutaneous excimer laser coronary angioplasty: results in the first consecutive 3,000 patients. *J Am Coll Cardiol* 1994, 23:323–329.

7. Baumbach A, Haas KK, Carsten R, *et al.*: Formation of pressure waves during in vitro excimer laser irradiation in whole blood and the effect of dilution with contrast media and saline. *Lasers Surg Med* 1994, 14:3–6.

8. Serruys PW, *et al.*: Use of laser guidewire on total occlusions. *Circulation* 1994, 90:I–331.

9. Carome EF, Mueller CE, Clark NA: Intense ruby-laser-induced acoustic impulses in liquids. *J Acoust Soc Am* 1966, 40:1462–1466.

10. Bell CE, Landt JA: Laser-induced high-pressure shock waves in water. *Appl Phys Lett* 1967, 10:46–51.

11. Isner JM, DeJesus SR, Clarke RH, *et al.*: Mechanism of laser ablation in an absorbing fluid field. *Lasers Surg Med* 1988, 8:543–554.

12. van Leeuwen TG, Meertens JH, Velema E, *et al.*: Intraluminal vapor bubble induced by excimer laser pulse causes microsecond arterial dilation and invagination leading to extensive wall damage in the rabbit. *Circulation* 1993, 87:1258–1263.

13.• Baumbach A, Haase KK, Rose C, *et al.*: Formation of pressure waves during in vitro excimer laser irradiation in whole blood and the effect of dilution with contrast media and saline. *Lasers Surg Med* 1994, 14:3–6.

This review reports that collateral tissue damage is more extensive when lasing is performed in contrast medium than when it is performed in saline.

14.•• Tcheng JE, Wells LD, Phillips HR, *et al.*: Development of a new technique for reducing pressure pulse generation during 308-nm excimer laser coronary angioplasty. *Cathet and Cardiovasc Diagn* 1995, 34:15–22.

Excellent article dedicated to describing the mechanism of dissection after ELCA and the role of saline flushing.

15.•• Deckelbaum LI, *et al.*: Trial examining effects of saline infusion. *Circulation* 1994, 90:I–331.

Randomized trial comparing saline flush technique with standard technique of ELCA. The saline flush technique was effective in reducing significant dissections (4% vs 21% for standard technique).

Chapter 7

The Multiplex Approach as a Means of Reducing Collateral Damage

Andreas Baumbach
Karl K. Haase
Karl R. Karsch

With the rapid development of catheter and system technology during the past 10 years, excimer lasers have evolved from benchwork setups to clinically applicable systems for coronary angioplasty [1•]. The basic concept of laser angioplasty is very attractive: removal of the atherosclerotic plaque by controlled application of light without the extensive trauma to surrounding vessel wall structures that characterizes balloon dilatation. After initial experimental and clinical trials, the potential benefits of using excimer lasers as compared with standard balloon dilatation were thought to be as follows: increased success in complicated lesions due to debulking as a different mechanism of action, successful angioplasty of former nondilatable lesions, reduced acute vessel complications, and reduced incidence of restenosis as a result of the less traumatic procedure.

However, these expectations were not met in clinical practice [1•,2••]. With increasing knowledge of the process, which leads to tissue removal in vitro and in vivo, it becomes apparent that excimer laser ablation is invariably associated with side effects. Research has now focused on systems that provide equal ablation efficacy with reduced trauma to adjacent vessel wall structures.

Excimer Lasers

Laser is the acronym for "light amplification by stimulated emission of radiation." Regardless of what type of amplification medium (solid, liquid, or gas) is used for the generation of coherent and monochromatic laser light, all laser systems operate by the same physical process of stimulated emission of radiation. The laser resonator consists of an active or gain medium enclosed in a set of reflection mirrors. The medium of excimer lasers is a mixture of xenon and chloride gases, which forms a dimer in the excited state. The acronym excimer stands for "excited dimer." The gain medium is pumped by an external energy source controlled by an electronic circuit, which is responsible for the duration of the pump pulse to the active medium. Within the resonator, light bounces back and forth between two mirrors, stimulating more light emission from the active medium. One of the mirrors is only partially reflective, allowing some of the laser light to exit the resonator. An optical switch inside or outside the laser cavity can further reduce the pulse duration of the laser output. The laser light exiting the laser cavity is characterized by wavelength, pulse duration, fluence, and repetition rate. Xenon chloride excimer lasers for angioplasty emit light at a wavelength of 308 nm, which is in the ultraviolet part of the spectrum, at pulse durations of 120 to more than 180 ns, fluences between 40 to 55 mJ/mm^2, and repetition rates of 10 to 25 Hz.

Tissue Ablation and Side Effects

The process of tissue ablation is complex. In contrast to holmium and neodymium:yttrium-aluminum-garnet (Nd:YAG) lasers, excimer laser light is not absorbed in water. At 308 nm, the light is absorbed by tissue proteins, which leads to the breaking of molecular bonds and then results in the transformation of tissue from the solid into the gas phase [3].

The removal of tissue is associated with little or no thermal damage to adjacent tissue [4]. However, this ablation of tissue is associated with at least two important side effects. First, van Leeuwen and colleagues demonstrated that a vapor bubble expands and collapses within 300 µs following the laser pulse [5]. The bubble size is determined by the irradiation area (or tip size) and the energy per pulse. With larger catheters working at higher energy densities, the bubble size can exceed the vessel size significantly, leading to dilation and invagination of the vessel wall. Furthermore, the bubble can cause severe damage when forced to expand into the tissue, leading to dissection. The second side effect represents a basic mechanism of tissue removal by laser light. Acoustic pressure waves result from absorption of laser light in tissue and blood. These pressure waves can exceed 50 bars at the lateral side of the catheter tip, therefore leading to acoustic damage of adjacent tissue. The peak pressures are determined by the energy per pulse. Compared with tissue absorption, the irradiation of blood and the irradiation of contrast media potentiate the extent of pressure-wave formation [6] (*see* Chapter 6, Fig. 6-2*A*). No absorption of excimer laser light occurs in saline, and therefore, no pressure waves result from irradiation of saline (*see* Chapter 6; Fig. 6-2*B*).

This clinical relevance of the correlation between catheter size, fluence, and the extent of trauma can be demonstrated in an analysis of multicenter results. Data regarding 1595 interventions of coronary excimer laser angioplasty in 1521 patients were analyzed using a merged database from the United States Spectranetics and European Percutaneous Coronary Excimer Laser Angioplasty Registries [7]. Complications included dissection (22.0%), vasospasm (6.1%), filling defects (4.8%), abrupt reclosure (6.1%), embolization (2.3%), perforation (2.4%), arrhythmia (0.7%), and aneurysm formation (0.3%). Major complications were non–Q-wave myocardial infarction (MI) (2.3%), Q-wave MI (1.0%), coronary artery bypass graft (3.1%), and death (0.7%). Logistic regression analysis revealed a correlation between dissections and the use of larger catheter size ($P = 0.0005$), high energy per pulselevels ($P = 0.0001$ for native vessels), as well as lesion length >10 mm ($P = 0.001$), and presence of a side branch ($P = 0.01$).

Thus, the primary approach to reduce side effects is to decrease the catheter size and to reduce the fluence. However, this will further reduce the ablation efficacy of the system. Tissue ablation with excimer lasers is a slow and stepwise process. The maximum ablation depth in atherosclerotic tissue is 2 to 40 µm per pulse, depending on tissue characteristics, catheter size, fluence, and force applied to the tip [8]. For calcified tissue, the etch rate (tissue removal per pulse) is lower. Assuming a high ablation depth of 20 µm per pulse, ablation of a noncalcified 1-cm lesion will still require 500 pulses. At a standard repetition rate of 20 Hz, this will need 25 seconds of irradiation.

Reduction of Side Effects

Options for reducing bubble size and extent of pressure-wave formation include the prevention of unnecessary absorption of laser light in blood and the reduction of side effects during tissue ablation. First, irradiation in the presence of contrast media should be avoided, and irradiation of blood should be reduced to a minimum. Saline infusion [9•] may decrease blood irradiation and lead to a reduction of complications. While still under development, characterization of tissue by spectroscopic analysis may be a means for optimizing tissue irradiation. Second, homogenized light distribution may result in a better ablation efficiency with reduced side effects.

Smooth Excimer Laser Coronary Angioplasty

A different principle is realized in the multiplex approach or smooth excimer laser coronary angioplasty (SELCA). An innovative excimer laser system (MAX Fiberscan; Medolas, Gräfelfing, Germany) couples the laser beam sequentially into one of eight or 12 fiber sectors of the catheter device, thus reducing the area irradiated and the amount of mass explosion per each shot (Fig. 7-1). Thus, instead of reducing the catheter size, the size of the effective area at a given time is reduced. A Fiberscan tip with one of eight sectors illuminated is shown in Figure 7-2. The repetition rate of the system is 150 Hz. With eight sectors, this results in 18.75 Hz for the whole tip area.

Experimental results demonstrated a reduction of pressure-wave formation and bubble size. For ablation of blood, contrast agent, and normal vessel wall, the maximum pressure pulse is found to be five times lower, and for calcified plaque the peak pressure is reduced by a factor of 8. The efficacy in vitro is similar to conventional excimer laser irradiation: at a fluence of 50 mJ/mm^2 the etch rate per 8 pulses is > 2.0 μm [10].

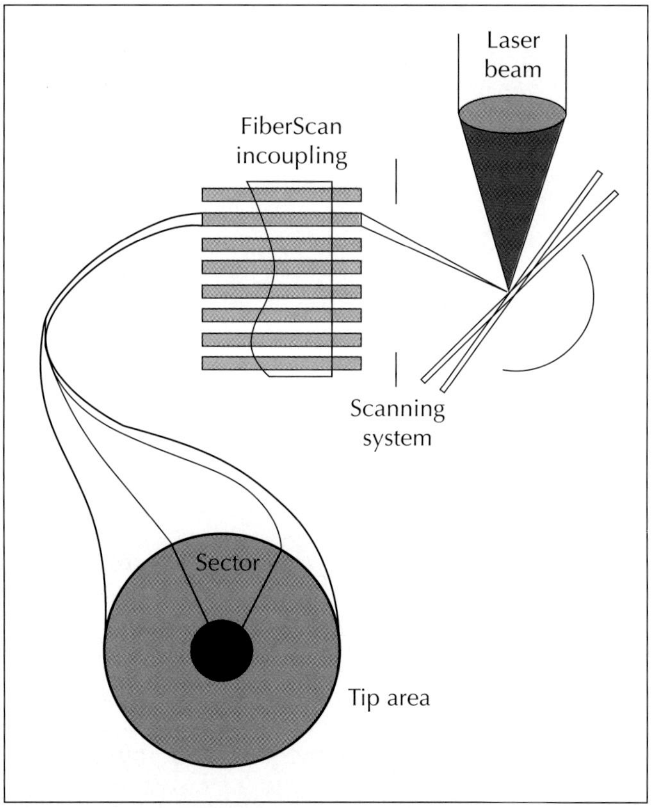

Figure 7-1. Principle of the multiplex or smooth excimer laser coronary angioplasty (SELCA) system. The laser beam is sequentially coupled to one of eight fiber segments of the catheter tip.

Initial results of the human application were promising; however, only a limited number of patients have been treated with this technology. At our institution, a total of 51 patients were treated. The baseline characteristics are illustrated in Table 7-1. Acute success was achieved in all patients. Balloon angioplasty was performed in 33 patients because of insufficient results or haziness and closure of the vessel. The results and complications are listed in Table 7-2. Quantitative analysis of the angiographic results is presented for the initial 32 cases and is compared with 37 cases performed using conventional excimer laser angioplasty in Figure 7-3. Lumen achievement by SELCA was lower than with the standard system, because only 1.5-mm catheters were available for the majority of SELCA cases. For 24 patients, a 6-month follow-up was available. There was no reduction in the incidence of restenosis (diameter stenosis > 50%) in this small series (n = 14 of 24).

The incidence of severe acute clinical complications is low, although extravasation of dye occurred in two patients. These minor perforations had no clinical sequelae and were sealed with balloon angioplasty. When laser angioplasty is not immediately followed by balloon dilatation, serial angiographic controls may demonstrate a higher rate of laser-related phenomena. The incidence of major dissections in the present series is low, but the occurrence of dissection membranes, hazy appearance of the vessel after laser angioplasty, and delayed closure within 10 minutes is still present and compares to conventional excimer laser angioplasty performed with the same protocol at our institution. Future approaches require additional saline flushing to further reduce unnecessary side effects.

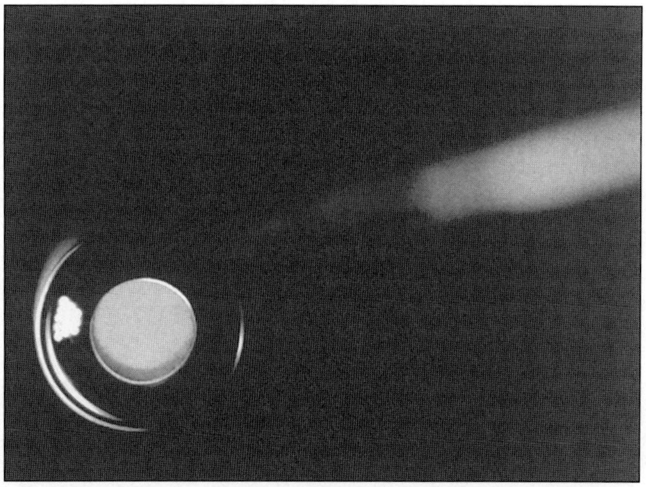

Figure 7-2. Photograph of a catheter tip with one illuminated segment.

Although SELCA represents an interesting and effective development of excimer laser technology, the general limitations of laser angioplasty still apply. In theory, SELCA is equally efficient as standard excimer laser systems, but the passage of a high-grade stenosis seems to take even more time. Additional removal or scattering of tissue by shock waves and bubble propagation, which both facilitate the advancement of the catheter in conventional excimer laser coronary angioplasty, is reduced considerably. Thus, the system is effective in limiting the side effects, but as a consequence, advancement of the catheter is restricted to the slow ablation rates known from experimental investigations.

Another drawback is the restriction to small catheter sizes. It has recently been shown with intravascular ultrasound that only a small lumen is achieved by the passage of an excimer laser catheter [11]. Catheters of 2.5 to 3.0 mm would be required to achieve a sufficient lumen and to allow for comparison of stand-alone laser angioplasty with balloon angioplasty. However, catheters of this size are far too bulky and represent no realistic option in coronary angioplasty. In clinical practice, laser angioplasty is used as an adjunct to balloon angioplasty. In recent trials, laser irradiation was almost invariably followed by balloon dilatation. Apart from economic considerations, this approach clearly differs from the initial idea of atraumatic tissue removal. Thus, an effect on the incidence of restenosis cannot be expected after the combined trauma of laser and balloon angioplasty. However, initial laser passage may facilitate balloon dilatation of otherwise difficult lesions and may increase the acute success rates for a subgroup of target lesions.

Table 7-1. Baseline Characteristics of 50 Patients (51 Lesions) Treated with Smooth Excimer Laser Coronary Angioplasty

Male/female	41/9
Age	58 ± 7
Angina pectoris	
CCS I	0
CCS II	10
CCS III	22
CCS IV	6
Unstable angina	2
Acute MI	0
Extent of CAD	
One vessel	18
Two vessels	25
Three vessels	6
Prior MI	19
Prior PTCA (target vessel)	5
Prior CABG	0
Hypertension	16
Diabetes mellitus	5
Current smoker	9
Target vessel	
LAD (including one diagonal branch)	31
LCX	6
RCA	14

CABG—coronary artery bypass graft; CAD—coronary artery disease; CCS—Canadian Cardiovascular Society Score; LAD—left anterior descending artery; LCX—left circumflex artery; MI—myocardial infarction; RCA—right coronary artery.

Conclusions

The multiplex approach or SELCA represents an improved technology for excimer laser angioplasty. Compared with the standard system, side effects are reduced, but are not eliminated. The suppression of shock waves and bubbles is achieved at the cost of a decreased efficacy in the clinical practice. Further research on laser technology is mandatory to achieve the goal of highly efficient tissue removal without collateral damage.

Table 7-2. Results of Smooth Excimer Laser Coronary Angioplasty

	Patients, *n*(%)
Reduction of stenosis severity	51(100)
Stand-alone laser angioplasty	18(35)
Angiographic success	51(100)
Dissection minor	15(29)
with reduction of flow	2(3.9)
Spasm	5(10)
Perforation	2(3.9)
Acute closure	7(14)
MI/CABG/death	0(0)

CABG—coronary artery bypass graft; MI—myocardial infarction.

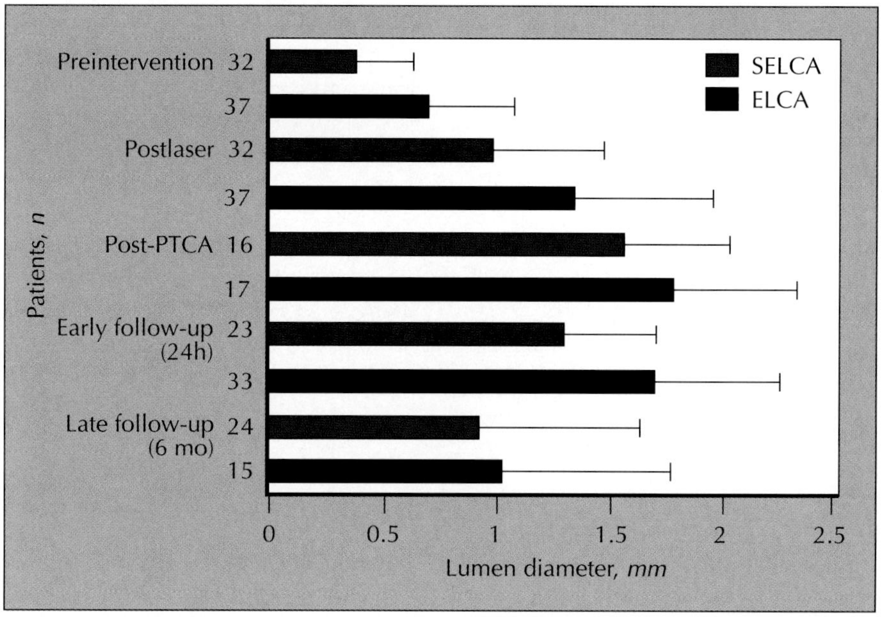

Figure 7-3. Minimal lumen diameter following SELCA and conventional excimer laser irradiation. Acute results, early (24 hours), and late follow-up. ELCA—excimer laser coronary angioplasty; SELCA—smooth excimer laser coronary angioplasty.

References and Recommended Reading

Recently published papers of particular interest have been highlighted as:

- • Of special interest
- •• Of outstanding interest

1.• Litvack F, Eigler NL, Margolis JR, *et al.*: Percutaneous excimer laser coronary angioplasty: results of the first consecutive 3000 patients. *J Am Coll Cardiol* 1994, 23:323–329.

Data of the US Excimer Laser Registry, representing the largest single database on excimer laser angioplasty.

2.•• Appelmann YEA, Piek JJ, Strikwerda S, *et al.*: Randomised trial of excimer laser angioplasty versus balloon angioplasty for treatment of obstructive coronary artery disease. *Lancet* 1996, 347:79–84.

First randomized trial on laser angioplasty, showing no difference in the incidence of restenosis following conventional excimer laser angioplasty and balloon dilatation for long (> 10 mm) lesions.

3. Srinivasan R: Ablation of polymers and biological tissue by ultraviolet lasers. *Science* 1986, 234:559–565.

4. Grundfest WS, Litvack F, Forrester JS, *et al.*: Laser ablation of human atherosclerotic plaque without adjacent tissue injury. *J Am Coll Cardiol* 1985, 5:929–933.

5. Van Leeuwen TG, Van Erven L, Meertens JH, et al.: Origin of arterial wall dissections induced by pulsed excimer and mid-infrared laser ablation in the pig. J Am Coll Cardiol 1992, 19:1610–1618.

6. Baumbach A, Haase KK, Rose C, *et al.*: Formation of pressure waves during in-vitro excimer laser irradiation in whole blood and the effect of dilution with contrast media and saline. *Lasers Surg Med* 1994, 14:3–6.

7. Baumbach A, Bittl JA, Fleck E, *et al.*: Acute complications of coronary excimer laser angioplasty: a detailed analysis of multicenter results. *J Am Coll Cardiol* 1994, 23:1305–1313.

8. Kvasnicka J, Nakamura F, Lange F, Geschwind JH: Tissue ablation with excimer laser and multifiber catheter: effects of optical fiber density and fluence. *J Intervent Cardiol* 1992, 5:263–273.

9.• Tcheng JE, Wells LD, Phillips HR, *et al.*: Development of a new technique for reducing pressure pulse generation during 308-nm excimer laser coronary angioplasty. *Cathet Cardiovasc Diagn* 1995, 34:15–22.

Study relevant for clinical practice presenting the effect of saline infusion during excimer laser angioplasty on the incidence of dissections.

10. Xie DY, Hassenstein S, Oberhoff M, *et al.*: In vitro evaluation of ablation parameters of normal and fibrous aorta using smooth excimer laser coronary angioplasty. *Lasers Surg Med* 1993, 13:618–624.

11. Honye J, Mahon DJ, Nakamura S, *et al.*: Intravascular ultrasound imaging after excimer laser angioplasty. *Cathet Cardiovasc Diagn* 1994, 32:213–222.

Chapter 8

Recanalization of Chronic Total Coronary Occlusions Using a Laser Guidewire: A Single-Institution Experience With the Initial 100 Cases

Jaap N. Hamburger
Sergei Airiian
Geert H.M. Gijsbers
Pim J. de Feyter
Patrick W. Serruys

Total coronary occlusion is estimated to be present in approximately one third of the patient population undergoing diagnostic angiography for symptomatic coronary artery disease [1]. Despite a steady improvement in the quality of devices available for percutaneous transluminal coronary angioplasty (PTCA), success rates of recanalization of total occlusions have failed to keep pace with the increasing success rates of dilation of coronary stenoses [2–13]. However, a number of studies have shown long-term clinical benefit of successful recanalization. For this reason, we decided to evaluate the potential of a recently developed laser guidewire to recanalize chronically occluded coronary arteries. The initial experience with this laser guidewire, which combines the mechanical properties of a conventional coronary guidewire with the ablative energy of a xenon chloride (XeCl) excimer laser, has been favorable (Hamburger and colleagues, unpublished data). Here we report on the continued experience and describe the results in the first 100 patients treated in our institution.

Methods

In August 1993 a pilot study was initiated at the Thoraxcenter of the University Hospital of Rotterdam to evaluate the performance of the Spectranetics Prima Total Occlusion System (Spectranetics; Colorado

Springs, CO). The study protocol had the approval of the University Hospital of Rotterdam Medical Ethics Committee. Informed consent was obtained from all patients. Inclusion criteria for the study were a TIMI (Thrombolysis In Myocardial Infarction) class 0 flow [14] coronary occlusion on diagnostic angiography, with a documented minimum age of occlusion of 2 weeks. Initially a mechanical attempt to cross the total occlusion was required and, in the case of failure, an additional attempt was made with the laser guidewire. In order to evaluate the true potential of this new device, those lesions that are considered to be unfavorable for a mechanical attempt at recanalization were intentionally not excluded. Therefore, with the exception of acute myocardial infarction (AMI) within 2 weeks prior to the intervention, there were no exclusion criteria. The age of occlusion was assessed by angiographic data and, whenever possible, estimated from clinical history. The stump morphology was evaluated on the preprocedural angiogram. Routinely, the distal vessel lumen was visualized through a contrast medium injection in the contralateral coronary artery. The length of occlusion was measured by quantitative coronary angiography (QCA) after visualization of both the occluded stump and the distal lumen by means of a simultaneous bilateral coronary injection at the start of the procedure (Fig. 8-1). Fluoroscopic time, total procedure time, and the amount of contrast medium used were recorded. Blood samples for creatine phosphokinase (CPK) analysis were taken 6 and 12 hours after the procedure.

Laser guidewire success was defined as angiographic evidence of reaching the true lumen of any branch distal to the occlusion. Procedural success was defined as an average diameter stenosis of less than 50% in at least two orthogonal views by visual assessment at completion of the procedure. Clinical success was defined as procedural success without death, Q-wave myocardial infarction (MI), coronary bypass surgery, or repeat angioplasty during the index hospital stay.

The Laser Guidewire

The design of the Spectranetics laser guidewire, the technique of the laser guidewire procedure [15•], and the mechanism of excimer laser tissue interaction [16,17], have been described in detail elsewhere. In short, the laser guidewire consists of an 0.018-in wire containing 12 silica fibers with a 45 μm diameter. The supplied support catheter has a 2.5-F tapered tip providing additional backup support. The Model 018-001 (Generation 1) had a nonshapeable nonsteerable tip, which consequently could only be advanced in straight coronary segments. The Model 018-003, which is the model currently being used, was introduced in April 1994. The laser guidewire was designed to function as an exchange wire with a working length of 175 cm, which can be lengthened to 300 cm by removing the proximal coupler. The distal section of the wire has

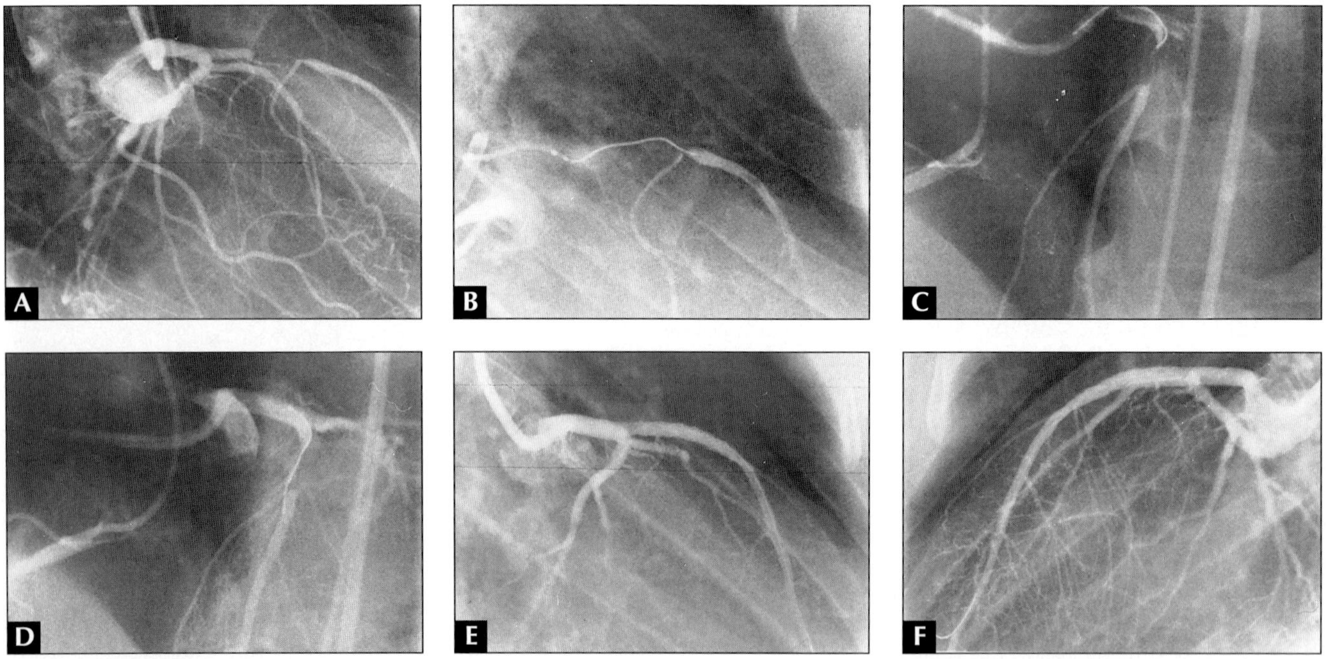

Figure 8-1. A total occlusion of the proximal left coronary artery (LAD). **A**, Simultaneous cannulation of the LAD with an 8-F guiding catheter and a 7-F diagnostic catheter in the ostium of the right coronary artery. Bilateral simultaneous injection showing the occlusion and the distal lumen. **B–D**, Advancing the laser guidewire during a contralateral injection of contrast medium. **E** and **F**, Final result after excimer laser coronary angioplasty (ELCA), adjunctive balloon angioplasty, and stenting.

a 3-cm radiopaque, shapeable, coil tip for visualization under fluoroscopy. Further improvements in the wire, such as remote tip control, are anticipated.

A Spectranetics CVX-300 XeCl excimer laser was used. The fluence used during a laser guidewire procedure was 60 mJ/mm^2, with a pulse repetition rate of 25 Hz. Upon encountering resistance with the wire, the laser was activated in pulse trains for a maximum of 5 seconds. During laser activation, the laser guidewire was advanced at a rate of approximately 1 mm per second, typically during a simultaneous (contralateral) coronary artery injection of contrast medium to visualize the distal true lumen. Biplane angiography was used to guide the alignment of the wire with the target segment. Whenever the laser guidewire encountered additional intraluminal resistance during laser activation, for example, in calcified lesions, the pulse repetition rate was increased to 40 Hz, thus increasing the laser guidewire ablation rate.

Procedural Data

Typically, an initial attempt was made to cross the occlusion using conventional mechanical guidewires (*eg*, a Schneider [Bülach, Switzerland] J 0.014 in, ACS 0.010 in, 0.014 in Hi-Torque Floppy, or a 0.014 in Extra Support Wire), with a balloon catheter for additional backup support (*eg*, a Medtronic [Eindhoven, the Netherlands] 18 K, Schneider Speedy, Cordis Passage [Cordis Europa, Roden, the Netherlands]). If unsuccessful, a second attempt was made with the laser guidewire. After successful guidewire crossing, angioplasty was performed either by balloon angioplasty or a combination of excimer laser coronary angioplasty (ELCA), using the Spectranetics 1.4-mm or 1.7-mm Vitesse-C (Spectranetics, Colorado Springs, CO) rapid exchange coronary catheters with adjunctive balloon angioplasty. ELCA procedures were performed using a saline flush to facilitate removal of contrast medium and blood prior to and during laser activation, thereby diminishing vascular wall damage resulting from shock wave formation [18]. Usually, placement of one or more stents was required to obtain an optimal procedural result. Following a successful angioplasty patients were kept on a heparin infusion for 24 hours, maintaining the activated prothrombin time (APTT) between 60 and 90 seconds.

All patients who had successful procedures were asked to return for a 3-month clinical and a 6-month angiographic follow-up. In case of a failed procedure, patients were referred for elective coronary artery bypass surgery (CABG).

All data are given as mean ± the standard deviation unless otherwise indicated. Statistical significance was accepted for *P* values less than 0.05. For group analysis we used an unpaired two-tailed *t*-test.

Results

Procedural Data

Data were prospectively collected for 100 consecutive patients with a TIMI 0 flow chronic total coronary occlusion in at least one coronary artery, who underwent an interventional procedure using the laser guidewire. Of these patients, 15 appeared to have TIMI 1 flow at the time of the procedure. A possible explanation for this change in TIMI flow could be a difference in catheterization hardware, as smaller gauge catheters are usually used for diagnostic angiography while larger and more selectively positioned guiding catheters are used for angioplasty procedures. An alternative explanation might be the resolution of thrombus with time at the site of the occlusion. These patients were consequently excluded from the current analysis. In the remaining group

Table 8-1. Baseline Clinical Characteristics*

Number of Patients, *n*	85
Age, *y*	58 ± 9
Male gender, *n(%)*	70(82)
Previous myocardial infarction, *n(%)*	56(67)
Previous mechanical wire attempt, *n(%)*	62(73)

**Thrombolysis In Myocardial Infarction 0 patients.*

Table 8-2. Baseline Lesion Characteristic I*

Left anterior descending artery, *n*(%)	33(38)
Circumflex artery, *n*(%)	8(9)
Right coronary artery, *n*(%)	46(53)
Stump morphology	
Central funnel, *n*(%)	47(54)
Blunt stump, *n*(%)	26(30)
Eccentric funnel, *n*(%)	14(16)
Major side branch, *n*(%)	32(37)
Bridging collaterals, *n*(%)	20(23)

**Thrombolysis In Myocardial Infarction 0 patients.*

there were 87 occlusions in 85 patients. The baseline clinical characteristics are given in Table 8-1, the baseline angiographic data in Tables 8-2 and 8-3.

In all patients an initial attempt was made to cross the occlusion mechanically, either by using conventional guidewires ($n = 62$), or by making use of the mechanical properties of the laser guidewire ($n = 23$). The duration of the attempt to cross the occlusion using a mechanical guidewire was 34 ± 30 minutes. The duration of a subsequent attempt using the laser guidewire was 40 ± 34 minutes. The total fluoroscopic time was 97 ± 48 minutes with a total procedural duration of 2 hours and 54 minutes ± 58 minutes. The amount of contrast medium used during the procedure was 559 ± 190 cm^3.

TABLE 8-3. BASELINE LESION CHARACTERISTICS II

Age of occlusion	Median (range)
Angiographic age, *wk*	13 (2–728)
Clinical age, *wk*	28 (2–728)
Measurements*	Mean (± SD)
Length of occlusion, *mm*	21 ± 11†
Reference diameter, *mm*	2.85 ± 0.53

*Mean ± SD.
†Range, 7–56 mm.

Laser Guidewire Success

In 85 patients (87 occlusions) an attempt was made with the laser guidewire, resulting in 52 patients (54 occlusions) in whom the occlusion was successfully crossed (62% laser guidewire success). In the patients with a primary mechanical wire attempt the laser guidewire was less successful than in those cases in which the laser guidewire was the wire of first choice, although this difference did not reach statistical significance: 58% ($n = 36$) versus 70% ($n = 16$), $P = 0.3$ (Fig. 8-2).

Univariate analysis of the available clinical, lesion related, and procedural parameters was performed to assess whether any of these variables were associated with an increased procedural success rate. The results are given in Table 8-4. Those parameters typically predictive of procedural success in chronic total occlusion are the duration of occlusion, the stump morphology, the presence of bridging collaterals, and vessel size (reference diameter). As shown, only the length of occlusion was significantly related to the outcome of the procedure, 19 ± 9 mm (success) versus 24 ± 12 mm (failure) ($P = 0.03$, 95% CI of the difference: 0.5 to 9.5 mm).

Procedural Complications

Perforation of the laser guidewire, defined as misalignment of the laser guidewire with the vessel wall boundaries, occurred in 12 patients (14%). In one case,

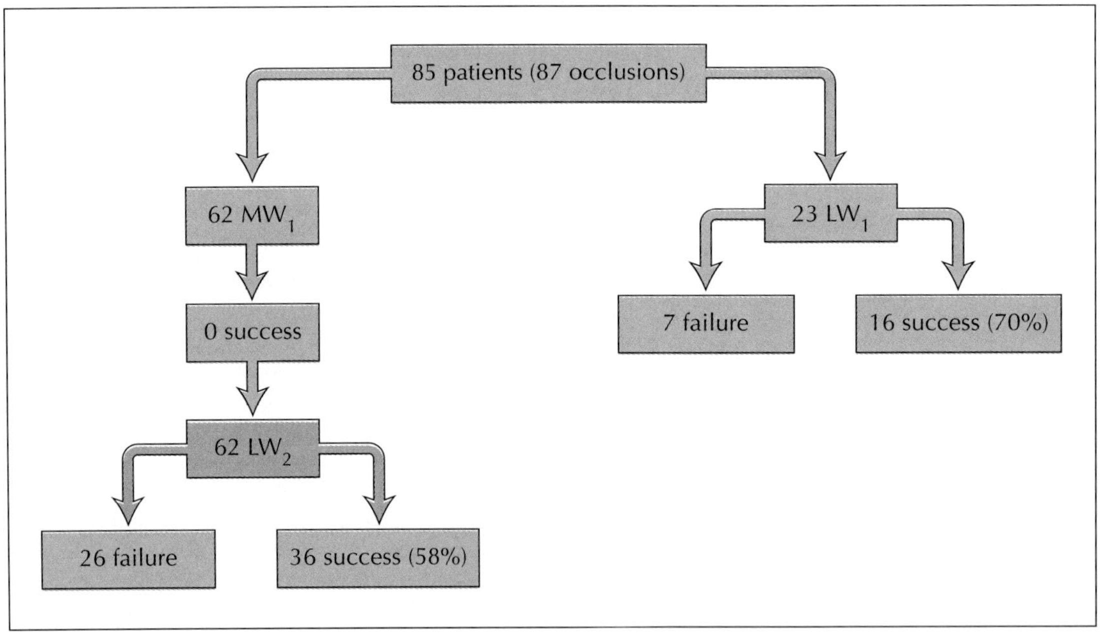

Figure 8-2. Breakdown of the results. All patients who entered the study had an initially failed mechanical attempt at recanalization. MW—an attempt at recanalization using mechanical guidewires; LW—a laser guidewire attempt.

the wire position was mistakenly thought to be intraluminal. Consequently, the inflation of a 1.5 mm diameter balloon catheter resulted in extravasation of contrast medium, leading to tamponade, which could be managed by pericardiocentesis. In the remaining cases the laser guidewire perforation was the reason for terminating the procedure. Systemic anticoagulation was reversed, and the patients were monitored by transthoracic echocardiography and continuous hemodynamic assessment. As there were no clinical sequelae in these patients, our current tendency is to consider a mere misalignment of the laser guidewire with the vessel wall boundaries as a relatively benign event, thus allowing for continuation of the procedure after withdrawal of the wire into the proximal part of the coronary artery.

Due to distal dissection, adjunctive angioplasty failed to restore TIMI 3 flow in three patients. As a result, procedural success was obtained in 49 patients (58%).

Clinical Events

In five patients (6%) a diagnosis of subacute reocclusion was confirmed angiographically within 24 hours after a successful procedure. Two of these patients experienced a non-Q–wave MI (CPK of 228 U/L and 799 U/L, respectively). Repeat angioplasty was performed in four cases and was successful in two. The remaining patient underwent elective CABG. As a result, the overall clinical success rate was 52% (44 out of 85 patients). There were no deaths, Q-wave MIs, or emergency CABGs.

Follow-up

Three patients were lost to follow-up (they resided outside the Netherlands). At clinical follow-up the mean angina class (Canadian Cardiovascular Society classification) was reduced from 2.9 ± 0.5 to 1.4 ± 0.7.

By May 1996, 6-month angiographic follow-up was completed in 31 of 32 eligible patients (97%). Of these, 26 patients had a patent vessel (84%), one patient a functional reocclusion (TIMI 1 flow), and four patients a TIMI 0 flow reocclusion. In those patients with a patent target vessel the mean reference diameter was 2.90 ± 0.51 mm with a minimal lumen diameter (MLD) of 2.02 ± 0.60 mm and a residual percentage diameter stenosis of 32 ± 13. It should be noted that *none* of the patients with reocclusion at follow-up angiography were stented during the initial angioplasty.

The Learning Curve

To get an impression of the learning curve with this new technology, the laser guidewire success rate and the procedural fluoroscopic time were analyzed per calendar year. The results are given in Table 8-5. As shown, the 1994 introduction of the steerable second generation laser guidewire, which allowed for the treatment of more tortuous lesions, had a clear impact on the results. Although the laser guidewire technique seems to have a rather long learning curve, the steady increase in the success rate (currently above 80%) compares favorably with recent reports on the success rates with other (mechanical) techniques for recanalization [19,20].

Table 8-4. Univariate Analysis of Lesion-, and Procedure-Related Parameters Relevant to Procedural Success

	Success	Failure	Significance Level
Lesion localization, *n(%)*			
LAD	22(42)	10(30)	NS
LCX	5(10)	2(6)	NS
RCA	25(48)	20(61)	NS
Age of occlusion, *wk*			
Angiographic	12	12.5	NS
Clinical	28	21	NS
Length of occlusion, *mm*	19 ± 9	24 ± 12	$P = 0.03$
Bridging collaterals, *n(%)*	13(25)	6(18)	NS
Central stump, *n(%)*	31(60)	15(46)	NS
Major side branch, *n(%)*	20(39)	12(36)	NS
Proximal reference diameter, *mm*	2.83 ± 0.52	2.75 ± 0.45	NS

LAD—left coronary artery; LCX—left circumflex artery; NS—no significance; RCA—right coronary artery.

Discussion

Recanalization of chronic totally occluded coronary arteries has remained the "stepchild" of interventional cardiology over the past decade. The initial low procedural success rates and poor long-term outcome of percutaneous techniques have kept chronic total occlusions predominantly within the domain of the cardiac surgeon. The introduction of a new laser guidewire especially designed for this indication initiated a reevaluation of this strategy in our institution. In order to be an acceptable alternative, laser guidewire–assisted angioplasty needs to be a safe and more successful procedure than angioplasty using conventional guidewires. However, it should be taken into account that angiographically unfavorable lesions were deliberately not excluded while the laser guidewire technology was and still is a technique "under construction."

When analyzing the initial laser guidewire experience, three distinctive periods can be distinguished. The procedural results of the first year were dominated by the experience with the first generation nonsteerable laser guidewire, which was nonsteerable. This technical limitation resulted in the selection of relatively less tortuous segments. The replacement of the nonsteerable by the steerable second generation laser guidewire resulted in a "second learning curve." Therefore, an overall laser guidewire success rate of 64%, or rather the current success rate of more than 80%, should be considered encouraging. It is of interest that a univariate analysis of those parameters that typically influence procedural success rates of angioplasty for chronic total occlusion in this study found that only lesion length was related with a poor outcome. This suggests that these parameters, which are often used for patient selection, have less value in the setting of angioplasty using a laser guidewire.

Laser guidewire perforation occurred in 14% of cases. The absence of clinical sequelae suggests that a laser guidewire perforation *per se* might be a benign phenomenon. However, it should be emphasized that angiographic confirmation of the intraluminal position of the wire tip prior to any device utilization is absolutely essential for the avoidance of tamponade. The absence of death, Q-wave MI, and emergency CABG in this patient cohort further indicates that recanalization of chronic occlusions using a laser guidewire is a relatively safe procedure.

In accordance with previous publications [11,21] we found a marked clinical improvement at the time of follow-up in patients who underwent a successful procedure and in whom the vessel remained patent. The angiographic reocclusion rate of 16% is consistent with previously reported results [22••]. It is suspected that the phenomenon of reocclusion occurs early, within the first 24 to 48 hours following the procedure. Furthermore, it seems to occur predominantly in those patients who are not stented or have a suboptimal final result. A strategy of early catheterization to diagnose and prevent early reocclusion may therefore be indicated. Whether a systematic use of intracoronary stents to optimize the final result will yield a significant reduction in the incidence of reocclusion [23–25] and a more favorable angiographic outcome at follow-up, needs to be confirmed in future randomized trials.

With the successful development of new technologies for percutaneous interventions, total coronary occlusion seems no longer to be the exclusive domain of the cardiac surgeon. In March 1995 the TOTAL (Total Occlusion Trial with Angioplasty using a Laser guidewire) study, a randomized, multicenter study evaluating the safety and efficacy of the laser guidewire as compared with conventional guidewires, was initiated. It is hoped that this study will succeed in delineating the true potential of the laser guidewire.

In conclusion, it is our impression that laser guidewire–assisted angioplasty, despite being technically demanding, is a relatively safe and successful technique.

Table 8-5. Learning Curve Analysis

Year	Patients, *n*	LW success rate, *n(%)*	AFT, *min**
1993	9	7(78)	102 ± 38
1994	29	15(52)	108 ± 48
1995	31	16(52)	99 ± 44
1996	16	14(88)	76 ± 53
Total	85	52(61)	97 ± 48

** ± SD.*
AFT—average fluoroscopic time; LW—laser wire.

References and Recommended Reading

Recently published papers of particular interest have been highlighted as:

- • Of special interest
- •• Of outstanding interest

1. Kahn JK: Angiographic suitability for catheter revascularization of total coronary occlusions in patients from a community hospital setting. *Am Heart J* 1993, 126:561–564.
2. Savage R, Hollman J, Gruentzig AR, *et al.*: Can percutaneous transluminal coronary angioplasty be performed in patients with total occlusion? *Circulation* 1982, 66:1319 (A).
3. Heyndrickx GR, Serruys PW, van den Brand M, *et al.*: Transluminal angioplasty after mechanical recanalization in patients with chronic occlusion of coronary artery [abstract]. *Circulation* 1982, II-5/1319.
4. Meyer B, Gruentzig AR: Learning curve for percutaneous transluminal coronary angioplasty: skill, technology or patient selection. *Am J Cardiol* 1984, 53:65C–66C.
5. Holmes DR, Vlietstra RE, Reeder GS, *et al.*: Angioplasty in total coronary artery occlusion. *J Am Coll Cardiol* 1984, 3:845–849.
6. Serruys PW, Umans V, Heyndrickx GR, *et al.*: Elective P.T.C.A. of totally occluded coronary arteries not associated with acute myocardial infarction; short-term and long-term results. *Eur Heart J* 1985, 6:2–12.
7. Kereiakes DJ, Selmon MR, McAuley BJ, *et al.*: Angioplasty total coronary artery occlusion: experience in 76 consecutive patients. *J Am Coll Cardiol* 1985, 6:526–533.
8. DiScascio G, Vetrovec GW, Cowley MJ, Wolfgang TC: Early and late outcome of percutaneous transluminal coronary angioplasty for subacute and chronic total coronary occlusion. *Am Heart J* 1986, 111:833–839.
9. Melchior JP, Meyer B, Urban P, *et al.*: Percutaneous transluminal coronary angioplasty for chronic total coronary occlusions. *Am J Cardiol* 1987, 59:53–58.
10. Bell MR, Berger PB, Bresnahan JF, *et al.*: Initial and long-term outcome of 354 patients after coronary balloon angioplasty of total coronary occlusions. *Circulation* 1992, 85:1003–1011.
11. Ivanhoe RJ, Weintraub WS, Douglas JS Jr, *et al.*: Percutaneous transluminal coronary angioplasty of chronic total occlusions: primary success, restenosis and long-term clinical follow-up. *Circulation* 1992, 85:106–115.
12. Stewart JT, Denne L, Bowker TI, *et al.*: Percutaneous transluminal coronary angioplasty in chronic coronary artery occlusion. *J Am Coll Cardiol* 1993, 21:1371–1376.
13. Stone GW, Rutherford BD, McConahay DR, *et al.*: Procedural outcome of angioplasty for total coronary artery occlusion: an analysis of 971 lesions in 905 patients. *J Am Coll Cardiol* 1990, 15:849–865.
14. The TIMI Study group. The Thrombolysis In Myocardial Infarction Group (TIMI) trial. Phase 1 findings. *N Engl J Med* 1985, 31:932–936.
15. • Hamburger JN, Serruys PW: Laser guidewire. In *Handbook of Cardiovascular Interventions*. Edited by Sigwart U, Bertrand M, Serruys PW. New York: Churchill Livingstone; 1996.

In this chapter, the laser guidewire technique is described for the first time.

16. Hamburger JN, Gijsbers GHM, Verhoofstad GGAM, van Marle J, *et al.*: Excimer laser coronary angioplasty: a physical perspective to clinical results. In *Current Review of Interventional Cardiology* edn 2. Edited by Topol EJ, Serruys PW. Philadelphia: Current Medicine; 1995:159–172.
17. Leeuwen van TG, Meertens JH, Velema E, *et al.*: Intraluminal vapor bubble induced by excimer laser pulse causes microsecond arterial dilation and invagination leading t o extensive wall damage in the rabbit. *Circulation* 1993, 87:1285–1263.
18. Deckelbaum LI, Strauss BH, Bittl JA, *et al.*: Effect of intracoronary saline infusion on dissection during excimer laser coronary angioplasty: a randomized trial. *JACC* 1995, 26:1264–1269.
19. Kinoshita I, Katoh O, Nariyama J, Otsuji S, *et al.*: Coronary angioplasty of chronic total occlusions with bridging collateral vessels: immediate and follow-up outcome from a large single-center experience. *J Am Coll Cardiol* 1995, 26:409–415.
20. Rees MR, Michalis LK: Activated-guidewire technique for treating chronic coronary artery occlusion. *Lancet* 1995, 346:943–944.
21. Finci L., Meyer B, Favre J, *et al.*: Long-term results of successful and failed angioplasty for chronic total coronary artery occlusion. *Am J Cardiol*> 1990, 66:660–662.
22. •• Violaris AG, Melkert R, Serruys PW: Longterm luminal renarrowing after successful elective coronary angioplasty of total occlusions: a quantitative angiographic analysis. *Circulation* 1995, 91:2140–2150.

Aside from what seems to be a subgroup of patients with early reocclusion, the late angiographic follow-up after successful recanalization of a chronic total occlusion compares favorably with the late outcome after dilatation of a stenosis.

23. Katoh O, Tsuchikane E, Awata N, Kobayashi T: Multivariate predictors of restenosis and reocclusion after coronary stenting of chronic total occlusions. *J Int Card* 1996, 8:48–69.
24. Moussa I, Di Mario C, Blengino S, *et al.*: Coronary stenting of chronic total occlusions without anticoagulation: immediate and long-term outcome. *J Int Card* 1996, 8:53–89.
25. Thomas MR, Wainwright RJ, Hancock J, *et al.*: Coronary stenting following successful angioplasty for total occlusions: preliminary results of a randomised trial. *J Int Card* 1996, 8:58–107.

Chapter 9

Laser Thrombolysis in Acute Myocardial Infarction

Kenton Gregory

Lasers can ablate all types of intravascular thrombi. Because thrombi strongly absorb light at many different wavelengths, most high-energy pulsed– and continuous-wave lasers can achieve an efficient vaporization or tissue removal (ablation) [1–13]. Although many lessons can be learned from the development of laser systems to remove atherosclerotic plaque, the optical and material properties of thrombus are markedly different, which create new issues and opportunities for laser thrombolysis [4]. The problem of inadvertent normal tissue destruction and resultant perforation using current laser angioplasty systems for removal of atherosclerotic lesions may be largely avoided by systems specifically designed for thrombus ablation.

Ultimately, lasers may be used as a sole therapy for acute or chronic thrombosis or as an adjunctive therapy with mechanical devices or fibrinolytic drugs. Lasers might be used to remove acute coronary thrombi in cases where current fibrinolytic or mechanical thrombolytic devices are either contraindicated or have failed. In the case of acute myocardial infarction (AMI), current available therapies have difficulty with large-volume thrombi or thrombi that have a high platelet content [14–19]. Lasers can very efficiently remove both large volumes of thrombi and platelet thrombi [2–5,20].

Background

Tissue Optics

An understanding of the interaction of light, vascular constituents, and thrombi is requisite before practical applications of lasers for thrombolysis can be developed or deployed [21–23]. In its most elementary aspect, four possible events can occur as photons are incident upon tissues: reflection, scattering, transmission, and absorption. A portion of all light that is incident on tissue is reflected. Reflected light has no effect on the tissue, but is obviously important if this light is captured by the retina or other imaging media. Transmitted light passes through the tissue without effect. Only photons that are absorbed by molecules in the tissue will have an effect on target tissue. Grotthuss observed in 1815 that "only those radiations which are absorbed by the reacting system result in change." Scattered photons "bounce" around in the tissue and are ultimately reflected, transmitted, or absorbed and have negligible direct effect on tissues except for changing light distribution within the tissue.

Absorption of photons by molecules in tissue can result in one or more primary light-tissue phenomena. When photons are absorbed within the molecular bonds, the vibrational state increases, which results in heat. If enough photons or photons of sufficient energy are absorbed and the vibrational energy is increased above the threshold, vaporization can be achieved that will result in tissue removal. When molecular bonds absorb a photon or photons, the bonds can be altered, which then results in chemical reactions or interactions. This stoichiometric process is generally a low power effect. Molecules absorbing photons in tissues can be boosted to a high energy state and, in order to return to the baseline energy state, this energy can be released via production of a photon that is always at a longer wavelength than the absorbed photon. The released photon, or fluorescent photon, is characteristic of the absorbing molecule. A spectral distribution of these fluorescence molecules can make up a unique signature of a tissue and can be used for diagnostic purposes [24–26]. As laser power or photon energy increases, the bonds absorbing the photons can be broken, resulting in photoablation that results in tissue removal. At very high energy, molecules absorbing photons can release sufficient energy so that electrons are released from the atom, which can produce a free electron flux or an optical plasma. This phenomenon has been reported with ablation of calcified atherosclerotic plaques. Calcified lesions have a high concentration, or population, of free electrons, which contribute to formation of optical plasmas. Optical plasmas have not been reported during laser thrombolysis at clinically relevant energy levels.

Optical properties of arterial and venous thrombi are generally governed by three major absorbing regions as shown in Figure 9-1. In the ultraviolet portion of the spectrum, tissue proteins and nucleic acids are the predominate absorbers. In the visible wavelengths, hemoglobin is overwhelmingly the most dominant absorber. In the near to mid-infrared region, water molecules dominate the absorption. The optical properties of arterial and venous thrombi of varying ages have similar absorption properties [2,4]. Lasers emitting light in ultraviolet, visible, and infrared regions of sufficient power and energy are all capable of ablating or removing thrombi.

Once thrombi absorb photons of sufficient energy to result in vaporization, prominent secondary effects can occur and may dominate the tissue removal process as well as collateral effects on surrounding

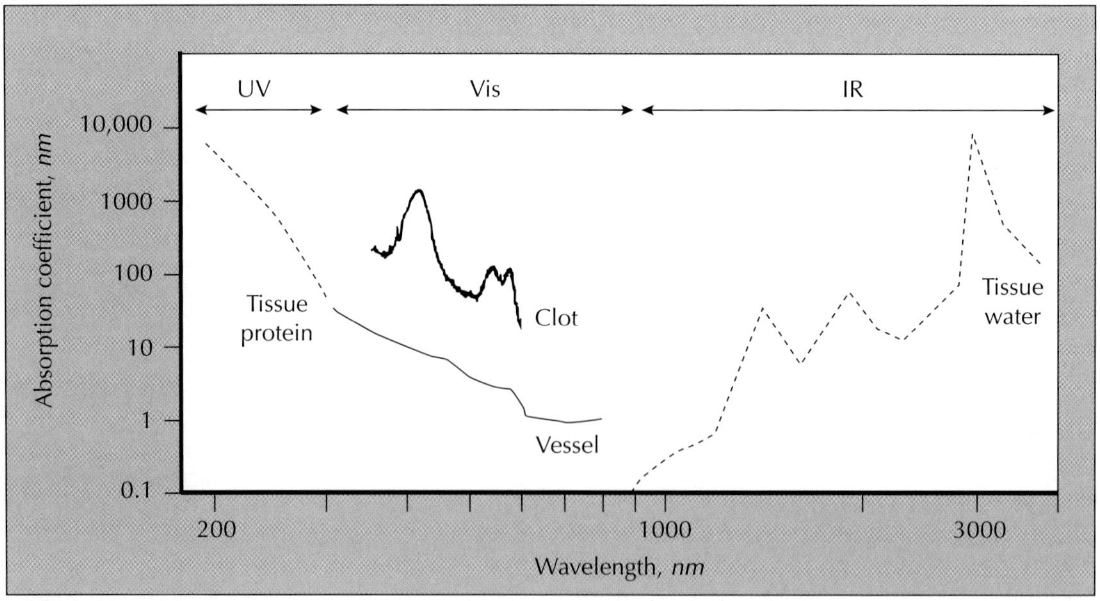

Figure 9-1. Absorption spectra of thrombus and artery. The absorption by thrombus is almost two orders of magnitude higher than artery absorption in the visible region of the electromagnetic spectrum. Therefore the minimum energy per unit area required to ablate thrombus is much less than that for artery. This gives lasers operating in the visible region the potential to selectively remove thrombus without injuring the vessel wall. IR—infrared; UV—ultraviolet; Vis—visible.

vascular structures. Once tissue is vaporized, two types of vapor bubbles occur [27,28]. The first type, a short-lived elastic expansion of water vapor, occurs because of absorption and heating of adjacent protein or hemoglobin molecules or, in the case of holmium lasers, direct absorption of energy by water molecules. This bubble expands and collapses in a period of 400 to 500 µs. A series of photographs of bubble formation following laser ablation of thrombus using ultra-fast flash photography is shown in Figure 9-2. Water vapor bubble expansion can result in bubbles that can reach 2 to 3 mm in diameter at clinically relevant energy levels. As these bubbles collapse, a pressure or acoustic wave is created. This pressure wave is directly related to the amount of energy in the laser pulse [27–31]. Depending on this energy and the absorption coefficient, these pressure waves can reach hundreds of atmospheres in the near vicinity of the bubble collapse. This effect has been shown to cause significant dissections and possibly perforations in pulsed laser angioplasty systems that are being used clinically for the ablation of atherosclerotic plaque. Fortunately, if laser wavelength, pulse width, and energy levels are properly selected for laser thrombolysis, the pressure transients can be reduced by orders of magnitude and reduce the chance of undesired damage to arterial walls.

A second type of vapor bubble is more long lived and is created through break-up of molecules into CO_2, water, and small complex gases [32]. These gas bubbles last milliseconds to seconds or minutes within the blood stream. These long-lived bubbles have a very small volume and have not been shown to cause significant gas embolism effects in tissue.

Early Studies

The use of lasers to ablate thrombi was first reported by Lee [1,13], who showed that thrombi could be vaporized using continuous-wave argon ion lasers emitting light at 454 and 514 nm. Removal of coronary artery thrombi in a canine model was attempted by Abela and Crea [33,34] using a similar laser system via conventional fused silica (quartz) fibers, which resulted in perforation in the majority of the studies. Gross thermal destruction of thrombi and segments of the arterial wall were described [34].

To avoid thermal damage to surrounding structures during laser thrombolysis, investigators moved to high-energy pulsed lasers that emitted light in pulse durations spanning from nanoseconds to hundreds of microseconds. Research by Srinivasan, Isner, and others [32,35,36] have shown that pulsed lasers can vaporize materials and tissues and limit thermal diffusion and damage to surrounding structures. Laser pulses less than 100 µs in duration can generate large thermal transients resulting in tissue vaporization without significant thermal diffusion to surrounding structures. Whereas pulsed laser systems reduced tissue necrosis and charring during laser ablation of target lesions, potential ablation of normal adjacent tissues commonly occurs due to inadvertent light exposure to the structures.

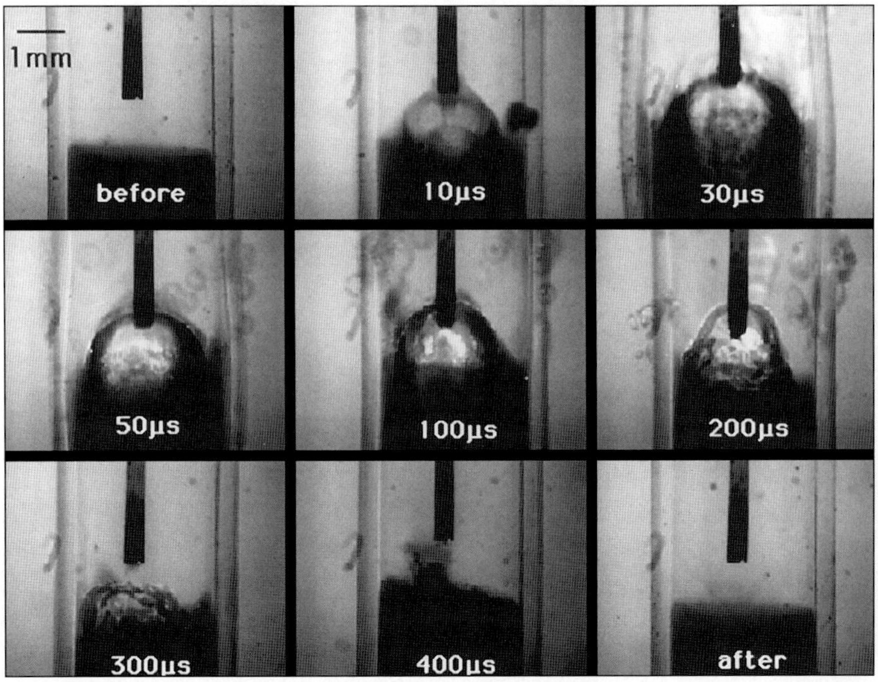

Figure 9-2. Bubble dynamics during pulsed laser ablation. The thrombus absorbs the laser energy and some of it is vaporized forming a vapor bubble. The bubble expands and collapses rapidly, resulting in further disruption of the clot. Here, a gel-based clot model is ablated under water in 3-mm diameter silicone tubes representing arteries. Microsecond laser pulses of 50 mJ energy are delivered through a 300-µm fiber, and flash photographs of bubble action are taken at various times after the ablative pulse. Each bubble shown is a separate event formed by identical pulses. The bubble expands and collapses within 400 µs. Significant material removal can be seen after bubble collapse. Some vessel dilation can be seen when the bubble is at its maximum size.

Selective Laser Thrombolysis

Selective photothermolysis, a concept pioneered by Parrish and Anderson for the treatment of skin lesions, offers the potential to vaporize intravascular thrombi with little or no optical or thermal effect on normal vascular wall constituents [37–41]. Parrish and Anderson safely removed pigmented skin lesions without damaging contiguous normal skin based on differing absorption properties of pigmented lesion and neighboring normal skin. LaMuraglia and Prince investigated the potential of selective photothermolysis to treat intravascular lesions [2–4,42]. To establish the feasibility for selective treatment of acute arterial thrombi, optical properties of fresh arterial thrombi were studied in an animal model of mixed platelet and fibrin arterial thrombus as described by Yasuda and colleagues [43]. Arterial thrombi (1 to 6 hours in age) and the arterial vessels were analyzed in a spectrophotometer. Reflectance and transmission were measured and absorption coefficients were calculated at wavelengths from 300 to 800 nm. The characteristic waveband of oxyhemoglobin is apparent in the visible spectra, and high absorption in the ultraviolet waveband as well as mid to near infrared is shown in Figure 9-1. In the waveband between 410 and 600 nm there is a marked difference in absorption between thrombi and arterial wall. Lasers emitting in this waveband can be configured to selectively ablate thrombus [5].

Optical Catheters

Optical catheters for intravascular delivery of laser energy for laser angioplasty for atherectomy have evolved over the past 10 years from single quartz (fused silica) fibers to bundles of thin (< 50 μm) fibers arranged around a central guidewire lumen. Although this design imparts more flexibility, these catheters require contact with target lesions and physically confine vaporization products (gases and high velocity particulates), which maximizes cavitation phenomena and increases the likelihood of undesired collateral damage to surrounding tissues from secondary physical ablation phenomena. Moreover, it is difficult to exclude blood from the target area, which then can absorb laser energy and increase unwanted laser-induced cavitation damage [44].

To overcome these limitations and concerns, a new method of laser energy delivery was developed in which laser pulses are transmitted down flowing streams of optical fluid rather than optical fibers [45,46]. The fluid simultaneously flushes away blood and transmits light distal to the catheter tip to the target lesion. The catheters are simple plastic tubes that can be easily and inexpensively manufactured. A schematic drawing of a fluid-core optical catheter is shown in Figure 9-3. Physical confinement of vaporization products by catheter contact is thus avoided, which allows a more benign interaction of light, catheter, target tissue, and adjacent vessel wall. Conveniently, all forms of iodinated contrast media have near-identical optical properties as quartz in visible wavelengths so that laser pulses can be transmitted down streams of contrast media. A photograph of a fluid-core optical catheter transmitting a laser pulse to a target in a water bath is shown in Figure 9-4. An angiogram is produced with each train of laser pulses to allow fluoroscopic visualization of the catheter, the laser target site, and the distal vasculature.

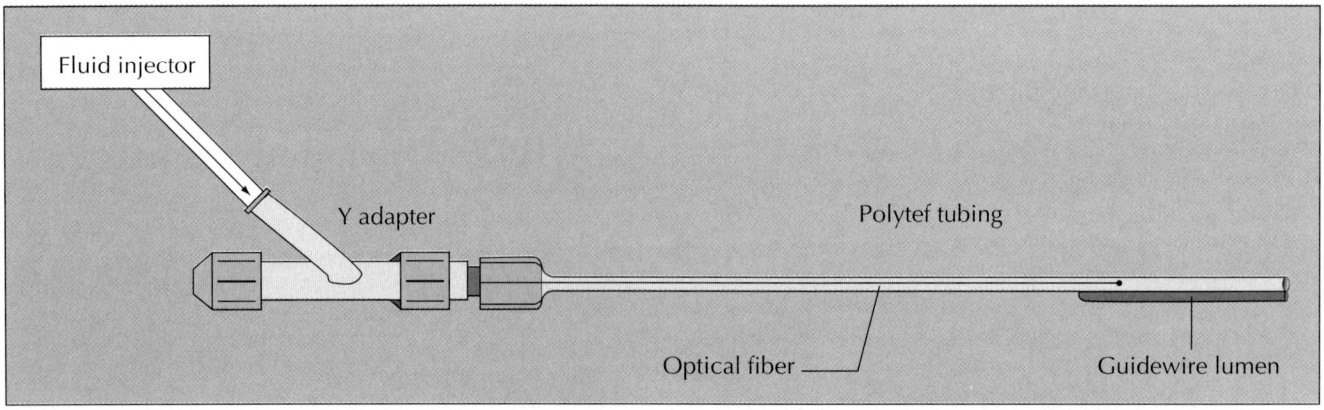

Figure 9-3. A fluid-core laser thrombolysis catheter. During the laser thrombolysis procedure, light is delivered by a fluid stream that is optically transparent. The light is launched into the stream by a quartz fiber inside the catheter tubing. The index of refraction of the tubing is less that of the fluid; therefore light is transmitted by total internal reflection. The catheter is open-ended, allowing the optical fluid to flow out and clear the path for transmission to the thrombus. Further, the fluid used (contrast media) is radiopaque, making real-time monitoring possible by fluoroscopy.

Pulsed-Dye Lasers

Lasers for selective laser thrombolysis should emit light within the waveband of 450 to 600 nm. To eliminate or minimize thermal diffusion and subsequent thermal injury to adjacent vascular structures, the laser should emit light in pulses no longer than 100 μs. High energy pulses shorter than 0.1 μs are more difficult to launch into optical fibers because of the high energy density. These criteria limit the field of available lasers. Fortunately, pulsed-dye lasers satisfy these criteria, and extensive development and clinical experience with these lasers for dermatologic applications have resulted in practical and relatively low-cost units. Laser light is generated in these lasers by excitation of a flowing column of fluorescent dye with a flashlamp. Dye lasers can produce a wide range of wavelengths by changing the dye in the laser. Pulsed-dye lasers emitting light at 480 or 577 nm in 1 to 2 μs pulses at energies up to 250 mJ have been developed specifically for laser thrombolysis.

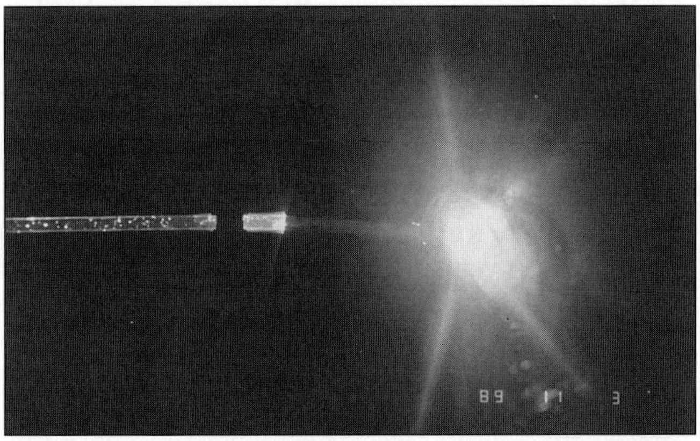

Figure 9-4. A fluid-core optical catheter transmitting a 50-mJ pulse at 480 nm in a water bath to a target 1 cm distal to the catheter tip. Iodinated contrast fluid was used as the optical fluid. Internal reflection of light within the fluid stream in the water bath occurs secondary to differing index of refraction and minimizes divergence of the beam.

Preclinical Investigations

Selective laser thrombolysis was investigated as a means of removing acute coronary artery thrombi in a canine model of AMI [5]. A mixed platelet and fibrin thrombus was formed in a macerated coronary artery segment associated with a 90% distal stenosis. Twenty-two coronary artery segments were treated with selective laser thrombolysis with a pulsed-dye laser (Palomar Medical Tech, Inc., Beverly, MA) and a fluid-core optical catheter in 22 dogs during an AMI. Thrombus removal and reperfusion occurred in all animals without perforation, vasospasm, or evidence of embolism. Thrombi were removed in all animals using 200 to 600 laser pulses, requiring a maximum of 2 minutes of laser activation. Vessels were harvested up to 2 hours after laser thrombolysis and scanning electron microscopy was performed. Platelet adhesion and aggregation on the laser-treated vascular surfaces were less than what was observed with control vessels [20]. Photomicrographs of an untreated control vessel and a vessel harvested 2 hours after selective laser thrombolysis are shown in Figure 9-5.

Clinical Studies of Selective Laser Thrombolysis

Initial clinical studies to evaluate the feasibility and safety of selective laser thrombolysis in the treatment of AMI were carried out at Providence St. Vincent Hospital (Portland, OR) and St. Joseph's Hospital (Atlanta, GA) as a phase I Food and Drug Administration (FDA)-approved clinical trial [47].

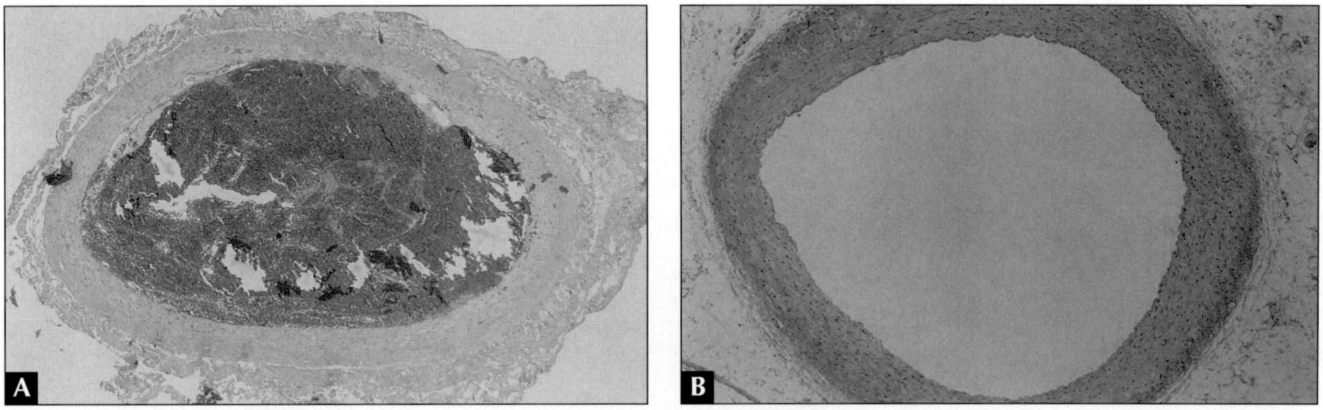

Figure 9-5. Photomicrographs of an untreated thrombotic canine coronary artery (**A**) and a coronary artery harvested 2 hours after selective laser thrombolysis (**B**).

Patients who had failed or had contraindications to fibrinolytic therapy were treated. Patients underwent angiography and only those with thrombus burdens thought to be substantial were chosen. Patients with small thrombus burden as shown by angiographic appearance were treated with balloon angioplasty. The pulsed-dye laser emitting 480-nm optical radiation in 1-µs pulses at 3 Hz was used. Patients received 150 to 800 laser pulses at 60 mJ per pulse. The laser was coupled to a fluid-core optical catheter system (Baxter LIS, Irvine, CA) delivered through conventional 8-F percutaneous transluminal coronary angioplasty guiding catheters with 0.014-inch guidewires using a monorail-type lumen in the optical catheter. After the thrombus was removed, balloon angioplasty or a Simpson Atherocath (DVI, Santa Clara, CA) was used to treat the underlying plaque to fully enlarge the lumen.

All 20 patients treated had a successful result (defined as TIMI class 2 or better coronary blood flow and < 50% lumenal stenosis at the end of the procedure). No perforation, vasospasm, or embolic events were observed. All patients survived to hospital discharge without evidence of thrombotic reocclusion. Photographs of angiograms from a patient with an acute inferior MI secondary to right coronary artery thrombotic occlusion are shown in Figure 9-6. From this small first series of patients, it was concluded that selective laser thrombolysis for treatment of large volume thrombus recalcitrant to conventional therapies may be safe and feasible in AMI. A multicenter study with expanded clinical indications and improved optical catheters has now been approved to further assess safety and feasibility.

Holmium Laser Thrombolysis

Most high-energy pulsed lasers can vaporize thrombus due to the rich content of chromophores that absorb light in most of the optical spectrum. Holmium lasers, developed especially for laser angioplasty, have also been used to ablate thrombotic lesions in patients with AMI [12,48]. Holmium lasers emit light at 2.1 µm (2100 nm), which is absorbed mostly by water molecules. Tissue is removed mostly through explosive vaporization of water. Because vascular tissues also have a high water content, selective ablation of thrombus through selective absorption is not possible (*see* Figure 9-1). The pulse duration of holmium lasers is 250 µs, longer than the thermal relaxation time for tissue such that thermal diffusion to surrounding tissues occurs. Thermal injury occurs but is limited to 50 to 200 µm in depth to adjacent vessel wall in investigations using holmium lasers for plaque ablation.

Topaz and colleagues [12,48] have reported holmium laser treatment of 14 patients with AMI. The laser delivered between 50 and 200 pulses at pulse energies between 250 and 600 mJ per pulse via an optical catheter composed of fused silica optical fibers arranged around a central guidewire channel. Topaz has reported a 100% success rate with holmium laser angioplasty for acute coronary thrombosis without perforation or other significant adverse events.

Excimer Laser Thrombolysis

Excimer laser angioplasty systems have also been evaluated for their potential to remove thrombotic lesions [6,7]. Excimer lasers emitting ultraviolet light in 100 to 200 ns pulses (0.1 to 0.2 µs) easily ablate thrombus by protein absorption of ultraviolet light. Because both thrombus and vessel wall constituents have a high protein content, selective absorption of light may not occur; thus thrombus must be removed through cautious direction of the catheter. The pulse width of the excimer laser pulse is well under the thermal relaxation time of the tissue so that thermal diffusion and thermal injury does not occur.

Although in vitro and in vivo studies show promise for excimer laser thrombolysis, initial clinical experience for the treatment of subacute coronary artery and coronary artery bypass graft thrombosis has been

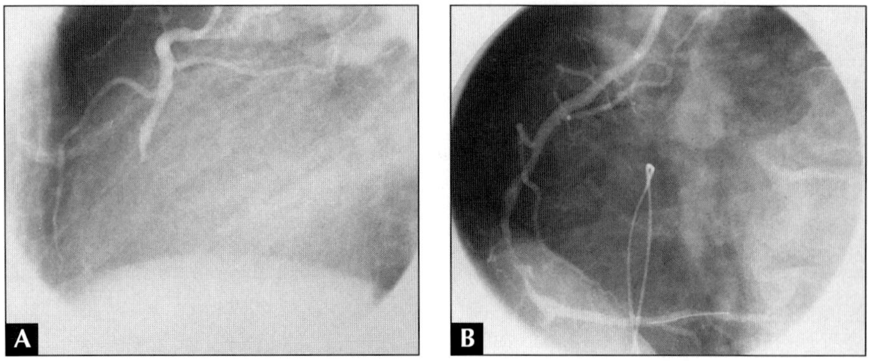

Figure 9-6. Angiograms of a 53-year-old man suffering an acute inferior myocardial infarction that rethrombosed after a streptokinase infusion before (**A**) and after (**B**) selective laser thrombolysis. The coronary artery thrombus has been removed, leaving a high-grade, ulcerated lesion in the proximal right coronary artery that was subsequently successfully treated with balloon angioplasty

mixed. Thrombus was shown to be removed, but in some cases embolization of thrombus occurred and acute vascular occlusion was reported [6,7].

Conclusions

Lasers have the potential for rapidly and safely removing intravascular thrombi. Early clinical trials indicate feasibility and safety. The place for lasers in the clinician's armamentarium against thrombus may be in the treatment of coronary artery and coronary bypass thrombosis—both acute and subacute—in cases where large thrombus burden or platelet content reduce the effectiveness of fibrinolytic or mechanical thrombus-removing therapies. The treatment of extracardiac vascular thrombotic syndromes such as stroke, pulmonary artery, and peripheral thrombosis is also under investigation.

Acknowledgment

I would like to thank Deborah Tuke Bahlman, RN for her patience and expert assistance in the preparation of this chapter.

References

1. Lee G, Ikeda RM, Stobbe D: Effects of laser irradiation on human thrombus: demonstration of a linear dissolution-dose relation between clot length and energy density. *Am J Cardiol* 1983, 52:876–877.
2. LaMuraglia GM, Anderson RR, Parrish JA, *et al.*: Selective laser ablation of venous thrombus: implications for a new approach in the treatment of pulmonary embolus. *Lasers Surg Med* 1988, 8:486–493.
3. LaMuraglia GM, Ortu P, Fillmore D, *et al.*: Selective laser photoablation enhances thrombolytic graft recanalization. *Surg Forum* 1990, 41:363–364.
4. LaMuraglia GM, Prince MR, Nishioka N: Optical properties of human arterial thrombus, vascular grafts and sutures: implications for selective laser thrombus ablation. *IEEE J Quantam Electronics* 1990, 26:2200–2206.
5. Gregory KW, Guerrero JL, Girsky M, *et al.*: Coronary artery laser thrombolysis in acute canine myocardial infarction [abstract]. *Circulation* 1989, 80:(suppl II):344.
6. Rosenfield K, Pieczek A, Losordo DW, *et al.*: Excimer laser thrombolysis for rapid clot dissolution in lesions at high risk for embolization: a potentially useful new application for excimer laser [abstract]. *J Am Coll Cardiol* 1992, 19 (suppl A):104.
7. Estella P, Bittl JA, Landzberg JM, Ryan TJ: Intracoronary thrombus increases the risk of excimer laser coronary angioplasty. *Circulation* 1992, 86:654.
8. Chasteney EA, Ravichandran PS, Furnary AP, *et al.*: Selective laser thrombolysis for arterial bypass thrombosis. *Lasers Surg Med* 1994, 6(suppl):44.
9. Chasteney EA, Ravichandran PS, Furnary AP, *et al.*: Laser thrombolysis for bypass graft thrombosis [abstract]. *J Am Coll Cardiol* 1994, 1(suppl):374.
10. Anderson RR, Parrish JA: Selective photothermolysis: precise microsurgery by selective absorption of pulsed radiation. *Science* 1983, 220:524–527.
11. Pettit GH, Saidi IS, Tittel FK, *et al.*: Thrombolysis by excimer laser photoablation. *Lasers Life Sci* 1993, 5:185–197.
12. Topaz O, Vetrovec G: Laser for optical thrombolysis and facilitation of balloon angioplasty in acute myocardial infarction following failed pharmacologic thrombolysis. *Cathet Cardiovasc Diagn* 1995, 36:38–42.
13. Lee G, Ikeda R, Kozina J, Mason DT: Laser dissolution of coronary atherosclerotic obstruction. *Am Heart J* 1981, 102:1074–1075.
14. Hartzler GO, Rutherford BD, McConahay DR: Percutaneous transluminal coronary angioplasty with and without thrombolytic therapy for acute myocardial infarction. *Am Heart J* 1983, 106:965–973.
15. O'Keefe JH, Rutherford GD, McConahay DR, *et al.*: Early and late results of coronary angioplasty without antecedent thrombolytic therapy for acute myocardial infarction. *Am J Cardiol* 1989, 64:1221–1230.
16. Rothbaum DA, Linnemeier TJ, Landin RJ, *et al.*: Emergency PTCA in acute myocardial infarction: a three year experience. *J Am Coll Cardiol* 1987, 10:264–272.
17. Ellis SG, O'Neill WW, Bates ER, *et al.*: Implications for patient triage from survival and left ventricular functional recovery analysis in 500 patients treated with coronary angioplasty for acute myocardial infarction. *J Am Coll Cardiol* 1989, 13:1251–1259.
18. Grines CL, Browne KF, Vandormael M, *et al.*: Primary angioplasty in myocardial infarction (PAMI) trial [abstract]. *Circulation* 1992, 86(suppl):641.
19. Hopkins J, Savage M, Zalunski A: Recurrent ischemia in the zone of prior myocardial infarction: results of coronary angioplasty of the infarct related vessel [abstract]. *Am Heart J* 1988, 115:14–19.
20. Gregory KW, Flotte T, Michaud N, *et al.*: Laser-induced inhibition of platelet adhesion. *Circulation* 1989, 80 (suppl 2):523.
21. Cheong WF, Prahl SA, Welch AJ: A review of the optical properties of biological tissues. *IEEE J Quantum Electronics* 1990, 26:2166–2185.

22. Keijzer M, Jacques SL, Prahl SA, Welch AJ: Light distributions in artery tissue: Monte Carlo simulations for finite-diameter laser beams. *Lasers Surg Med* 1989, 9:148–154.

23. Jacques SL: Role of tissue optics and pulse duration on tissue effects during highpower laser irradiation. *Appl Opt* 1993, 32:2447–2454.

24. Deckelbaum LI, Lam JK, Cabin HS, *et al.*: Discrimination of normal and atherosclerotic aorta by laser-induced fluorescence. *Laser Surg Med* 1987, 7:330–335.

25. Leon MB, Lu DY, Prevosti LG: Human arterial surface fluorescence: atherosclerotic plaque identification and effects of laser atheroma ablation. *J Am Coll Cardiol* 1988, 12:94–102.

26. Leon MB, Prevosti LG, Smith PD, *et al*: Probe and fire laser angioplasty: fluorescence atheroma detection and selective laser atheroma ablation. *Circulation* 1987, 76(suppl IV): IV-409.

27. Vogel A, Lauterborn W: Acoustic transient generation by laser-produced cavitation bubbles near solid boundaries. *J Acoust Soc Am* 1988, 84:719–731.

28. Vogel A, Lauterborn W, Timm R: Optical and acoustic investigations of the dynamics of laser-produced cavitation bubbles near a solid boundary. *J Fluid Mechanics* 1989, 206:299–238.

29. Sathyam US, Shearin A, Prahl SA: Visualization of microsecond laser ablation of porcine clot and gelatin under a clear liquid. In *Proceedings of Lasers in Surgery: Advanced Characterization Therapeutics and Systems VI,* vol. 2671. Edited by Anderson RR, Katzir A. San Jose: Society of Photo-optical Instrumentation Engineers; 1996:28–35.

30. Shangguan H, Casperson LW, Shearin A, Prahl SA: Investigation of cavitation bubble dynamics using particle image velocimetry: implications for photoacoustic drug delivery. In *Proceedings of Lasers in Surgery: Advanced Characterization Therapeutics and Systems VI,* vol. 2671. Edited by Anderson RR, Katzir A. San Jose: Society of Photo-optical Instrumentation Engineers; 1996:104–115.

31. Sathyam US, Shearin A, Prahl SA: The effect of spot size, pulse energy and repetition rate on microsecond ablation of gelatin under water. In *Proceedings of Laser-Tissue Interaction VI,* vol. 2391. Edited by Jacques SL. San Jose: Society of Photo-optical Instrumentation Engineers; 1995:336–344.

32. Isner JM, Donaldson RF, Deckelbaum LI, *et al.*: The excimer laser: gross, light microscopic and ultrastructural analysis of potential advantages for use in laser therapy of cardiovascular diseases. *J Am Coll Cardiol* 1985, 6:1102–1109.

33. Abela GS, Normann SJ, Cohen DM, *et al.*: Laser recanalization of occluded atherosclerotic arteries in vivo and in vitro. *Circulation* 1985, 71:403–411.

34. Crea F, Fenech A, Smith W, *et al.*: Laser recanalization of acutely thrombosed coronary arteries in live dogs. *J Am Coll Cardiol* 1985, 6:1052–1056.

35. Srinivasan R, Leigh W: Ablative photo-decomposition action of far-ultra-violet9193nm) laser radiation on poly (ethylene terophythalate) films. *J Am Chem Soc* 1982, 104:6784–6785.

36. Linkser R, Srinivasan R, Wayne JJ, Alonso DR: Far ultra-violet laser absorption of atherosclerotic lesion. *Lasers Surg Med* 1984, 3:201–208.

37. Parrish JA, Deutsch TF: Laser photomedicine. *IEEE J Quantum Electronics* 1984, 12:1386–1396.

38. Anderson RR, Jaenke KF, Parrish JA: Mechanisms of selective vascular changes caused by dye lasers. *Lasers Surg Med* 1983, 3:211–215.

39. Parrish JA: New concepts in therapeutic photomedicine: photochemistry, optical targeting and the therapeutic window. *J Invest Dermatol* 1983, 77:45–50.

40. Anderson RR, Parrish JA: Microvascular can be selectively damaged during dye lasers: a basic theory and experimental evidence in human skin. *Lasers Surg Med* 1981, 1:263–276.

41. Anderson RR, Parrish JA: Selective photothermolysis: precise microsurgery by selective absorption of pulsed radiation. *Science* 1983, 220:524–527.

42. Prince M: Selective laser ablation of diseased tissue: investigations on a safe method of opening occluded arteries [PhD dissertation]. Cambridge, MA: MIT; 1988.

43. Yasuda T, Gold HK, Fallon JT, *et al.*: A canine model of coronary artery thrombosis with superimposed high grade stenosis for the investigation of re-thrombosis after thrombolysis. *J Am Coll Cardiol* 1989, 13:1409–1414.

44. Gregory KW, Prince, MR, LaMuraglia GM, *et al.*: Effect of blood upon the selective ablation of atherosclerotic plaque with a pulsed dye laser. *Lasers Surg Med* 1990, 10:533–543.

45. Gregory KW, Anderson RR: Iodinated contrast fluid can replace quartz in laser catheters. *Circulation* 1989, 80(suppl 2):107.

46. Gregory KW, Anderson RR: Liquid core light guide for laser angioplasty. *IEEE J Quantum Electronics* 1990, 26:2289–2296.

47. Gregory KW, Block PC, Knopf WD, *et al.*: Laser thrombolysis in acute myocardial infarction [abstract]. *J Am Coll Cardiol* 1993, 21:289.

48. Topaz O, Rozenbaum EA, Battista S, *et al.*: Laser facilitated angioplasty and thrombolysis in acute myocardial infarction complicated by prolonged or recurrent chest pain. *Cathet Cardiovasc Diagn* 1993, 28:7–16.

Ultraviolet Light for Restenosis

Chapter 10

Robert A. VanTassel
Michael E. McClurken

Ultraviolet (UV) light has long been known to cause significant photochemical reactions in biologic molecules. UV light is classified into three regions based on wavelength: UVC, 200 to 290 nm; UVB, 290 to 320 nm; and UVA, 320 to 400 nm. The upper limit of the UVA band is the lower limit of the visible range. Above 320 nm, little light is absorbed by protein or nucleic acids, unless photosensitizing agents are present. The most commonly used laser angioplasty systems operate at 308 nm in the UVB band [1]. UVB is sometimes referred to as sunburn radiation because wavelengths in this band are absorbed by both proteins and nucleic acids. The UVC band is often referred to as germicidal because germicidal lamps emit mainly at 254 nm. Proteins and nucleic acids, such as DNA, absorb most strongly in the UVC band, as shown in Figure 10-1. Wavelengths from the sun below 290 nm are strongly absorbed by stratospheric ozone and virtually none reaches the surface of the earth [2].

The absorption coefficient of UVC in skin as well as in normal and atherosclerotic human arterial tissue has been reported by several investigators and implies that roughly 50% of the incident UV radiation is absorbed in the first 15 to 50 µm [1,3,4]. At low doses (< 10 mJ/cm^2), it is likely that cell replication can be inhibited by affecting only the DNA and the ability of the cells to reproduce. Studies of DNA films have shown that the absorption of UV radiation leads predominantly to the formation of thymine dimers, or intrastrand DNA-DNA cross-links that block both transcription and translation, leading to cell death [5,6]. At higher doses (> 100 mJ/cm^2), it is more likely that a combination of effects on DNA plus direct effects on proteins is responsible for cell death. Investigators have demonstrated that UV radiation can destroy the integrity of cell membranes, cross-link the type I and IV collagen present in arterial walls, and seriously damage the proteins present in the extracellular matrix [7–10].

In vitro cell culture studies on mouse embryo cells have demonstrated that the cytotoxicity of UVC radiation depends on the wavelength and is proportional to the DNA absorption spectra [11]. For single-cell-thickness cultures of human fibroblasts, a dose of 1.5 mJ/cm^2

results in a fractional survival of 10% [12]. The effect of a broad range of wavelengths on cultures of rat aorta smooth muscle cells was studied and showed that 266 nm had an effect on cell survival, whereas wavelengths of 355 nm, 532 nm, and 1064 nm had no effect [13]. Subablative UVC from a pulsed laser at 262 nm was also shown to inhibit neointimal hyperplasia in balloon-injured rat carotid arteries [14]. A subset of the porcine data presented later shows that UV light can create an acellular medium and result in favorable remodeling in injured vessels [15,16].

Other restenosis reduction efforts involving UV light are the light-activated release of nitric oxide from vascular smooth muscle cells [17] and UVA-activated psoralen photodynamic therapy [18,19]. Both of these therapies have shown promise in reducing restenosis in experimental models.

The use of ionizing radiation to inhibit neointimal hyperplasia after balloon angioplasty has been studied extensively in several animal models. Several investigators have shown that γ radiation from an intracoronary iridium (^{192}Ir) source inhibits neointimal proliferation in pigs after balloon injury [20–23]. Interestingly, some of these investigators observed medial hypocellularity and fibrosis from γ radiation at a dose of 20 Gy, whereas others did not observe fibrosis at a lower dose of 14 Gy. Others have previously demonstrated a positive proliferative effect from externally applied γ radiation [24,25].

Because less than 1% of the γ radiation incident on the lumen is absorbed in the arterial wall, with the remainder penetrating deeply, investigators have also studied β radiation as a safer, more practical alternative to γ radiation. The use of a pure β emitter such as strontium/yttrium (^{90}Sr/Y) that penetrated from 2 to 3 mm resulted in a significant reduction in luminal area stenosis compared with controls at 14 days' and 6 months' follow-up in a balloon-injured porcine model. Although almost 20-fold more β than γ was absorbed at the same depth, the investigators found little difference between their β and previous γ results [26]. Similar results have been found using a hypercholesterolemic rabbit stenosis model [27]. The use of both γ and β radiation in conjunction with stents has been studied in experimental animals, showing generally good results [28–31]. γ radiation was used after stent implantation in the superficial femoral arteries of 13 patients, with follow-up at 3 to 27 months showing no restenosis in the stented area [32]. A number of investigators are performing feasibility studies in humans to assess the clinical viability of γ radiation. γ radiation was used before stenting of femoropopliteal lesions in four patients followed for 23 to 30 months [33]. γ radiation was successfully used on 11 patients after angioplasty to prevent restenosis of narrowed dialysis arteriovenous grafts [34]. Finally, a randomized study is underway to study the impact of γ radiation therapy in reducing restenosis after coronary stenting [35].

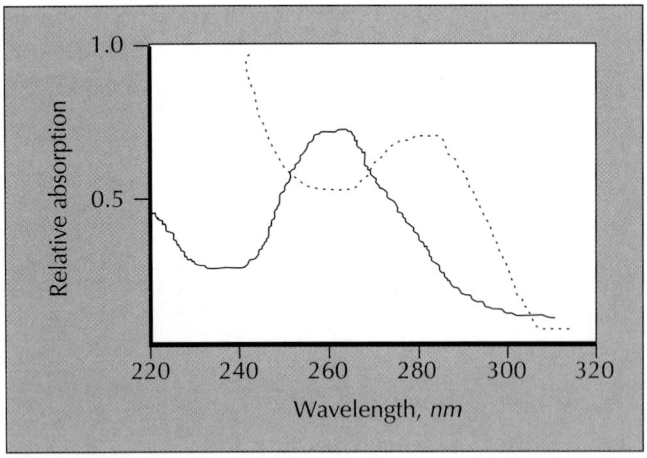

Figure 10-1. Absorption spectra of protein (*dashed line*) and DNA (*solid line*).

METHODS

To assess the effect of UVC on porcine coronary arteries and the safety of such a treatment, a series of animal studies was devised. A delivery system was developed and is shown schematically in Figure 10-2. UV light at a wavelength of 275 nm was generated by a continuous-wave argon ion laser. The light was coupled into a fiberoptic catheter called the light guide, which was placed through a Y-adapter into the guidewire lumen of a modified angioplasty catheter. Light emanated from a 4-mm-long diffusion zone at the tip of the light guide and exited through the modified angioplasty catheter's inner shaft and saline-filled balloon. Slight overdilatation of the vessel by the balloon provided sufficient contact with the vessel lumen to allow light to reach the media. An intravenous pump provided a continuous slow saline flush between the light guide and the lumen of the delivery catheter to prevent backflow of blood, which could obstruct UV light.

The light guide was often moved while delivering light to provide a more uniform dose along the longitudinal surface of the balloon. The light guide was stationary, pulled once from distal to proximal during an inflation, or reciprocated back and forth. This is shown schematically in the close-up of the balloon in Figure 10-2.

The key study parameters of six chronic porcine studies are summarized in Table 10-1. These studies were performed sequentially over a 6-month period as part of the product development efforts of Angiomedics II Inc. (Plymouth, MN). Because of the evolutionary nature of the development process, several key parameters of the studies were changed in significant ways as results were obtained and analyzed.

Continuous-wave UV light at 275 nm was delivered for all the studies. Delivery catheters were SciMED percutaneous transluminal coronary angioplasty (PTCA) catheters, either model MVP or Cobra (Scimed Life Systems, Inc., Maple Grove, MN), modified to provide a more UV-transparent polyethylene inner shaft and to provide marker bands in the desired position. When prior balloon injury was used, treated sites received prior balloon injury of the same amount as the controls. "Sham" treatments were performed for some of the studies to determine the effect of performing multiple treatment occlusions (up to eight) without UV light being delivered. The speed of the light guide motion varied from 1 mm/sec to 5 mm/sec.

For nonionizing radiation such as UV light, dose is typically expressed as the fluence, or total energy delivered per unit area. For this report, dose is reported in units of mJ/cm^2. Because the first law of photobiology is that photochemical events occur only when a photon strikes a molecule, a photobiologic response should be proportional to the total number of incident photons and hence the total energy. Total energy is the product of power and exposure time. Dose was therefore varied either by adjusting the power output of the laser or by varying the number of exposures. The maximum power output of the laser was approximately 600 mW, although most experiments were performed at lower power.

Dose distributions along the vessel in vivo were estimated from bench measurements made using representative delivery catheters and light guides attached to a special micrometer-driven fixture plus a calibrated integrating sphere and spectrometer. The diagram shown in balloon close-up in Figure 10-2 was representative for studies 2, 3, and 6, with reciprocating light guides and balloons with marker bands in the cones. For these studies, the dose distribution along the length of the treated site was generally uniform near the middle of the balloon but tapered off near each end. The peak dose is the number noted as the dose for this report.

For study 1, a largely unmodified Scimed MVP PTCA catheter was used with a center marker band present that blocked light and resulted in a notched dose distribution. For studies 4 and 5, the light guide was not moved but held fixed in the distal portion of the balloon. The dose distribution was nonuniform, but the plateau in the region of the peak dose was long enough, about 3 to 4 mm, to be detected by the tissue sections, which were cut every 2 mm.

All porcine studies were performed at the Mayo Foundation in Rochester, Minnesota, and were approved by the Mayo Foundation Animal Care and Use Committee. Domestic cross-bred swine (18 to 30

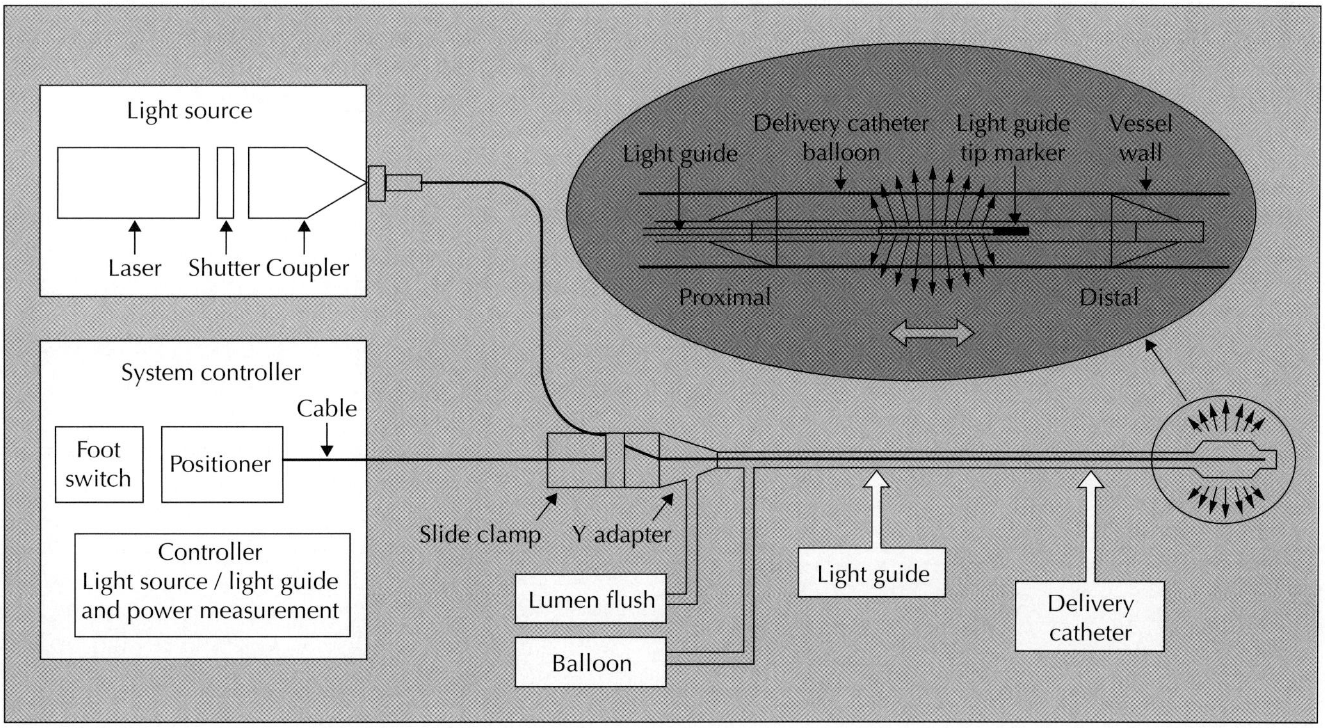

Figure 10-2. Schematic diagram of the ultraviolet delivery system.

kg) were given aspirin (650 mg) and verapamil (120 mg) orally at least 12 hours before the procedure. They were sedated with a mixture of 10 cc ketamine (100 mg/mL) and 1.5 cc xylazine (100 mg/mL) by intramuscular injection. Additional ketamine/xylazine mixture was administered intravenously during the procedure as needed. Limb lead electrocardiogram was monitored throughout the procedure.

After placement of an 8-F introducer sheath in the left carotid artery by surgical cutdown, each animal received 10,000 units of heparin intra-arterially. An 8-F guide catheter was introduced and positioned in the coronary ostia, with angiography performed to visualize the three candidate coronary vessels: the left anterior descending, the right coronary artery, and the left circumflex. A single treatment or control site was sought within each of these vessels and chosen primarily based on luminal diameter estimated from fluoroscopy plus comparison to the guide catheter diameter, with a range of 2.5 to 3.3 mm being acceptable. Acceptable sites were found in all three vessels for most animals.

Balloon injury was performed as previously described and shown in Table 10-1, using a 2-cm-long Scimed MVP PTCA catheter. The goal of the injury was to rupture the internal elastic lamina (IEL). If balloon injury was to be followed by UV light treatment a 0.014-in exchange guidewire was used to place the injury catheter. In the case of study 1, the same balloon catheter was used to perform both the balloon injury and the UV treatment.

Placement of the delivery catheter was followed by incremental low-pressure inflations, 1 atm at a time, with contrast material injections after each inflation to estimate the vessel diameter at occlusion and ensure good contact between the balloon and tissue during subsequent treatment. Using the estimated vessel diameter, the laser output power was adjusted to achieve the desired dose, measuring the output from the tip of the light guide when inserted into the spectrometer using a special sterile sleeve. After the power was adjusted, the exchange guidewire was removed and replaced with the light guide, with several hardware adjustments made, including the connection of the light guide to the stepper motor-driven mechanism that moved the light guide. The proper motion and position of the light guide in the region of the balloon was confirmed with fluoroscopy with the UV light turned off.

The delivery catheter balloon was brought to the proper predetermined inflation pressure, and the UV light was turned on synchronous with motion of the light guide. After the timed course of light delivery was completed, either 20 or 30 seconds, the light was shut off, the light guide motion stopped, and the balloon quickly deflated. To allow adequate distal perfusion, at least 30 seconds was allowed to elapse before an additional treatment inflation could be performed.

TABLE 10-1. SUMMARY OF STUDY PARAMETERS FOR THE PORCINE STUDIES

Study number	1	2	3	4	5	6
Animals, *n*	6	8	4	5	4	4
Treated sites, *n*	6	9	12	11	10	10
Control sites, *n*	6	4	0	2	2	1
Type of control	Injury only	Injury only	—	Sham treat*	Sham treat*	Sham treat*
Prior balloon injury? (Y/N)	Y	Y	Y	N	N	N
Injury over-dilatation, %	30	45	30	—	—	—
Injury dilatations, *n*	1	3	3	—	—	—
Minimum dose, *mJ/cm²*	3600	840	180	480	1300	3500
Maximum dose, *mJ/cm²*	41,000	89,000	3400	16,000	16,000	17,000
Treatment inflations, *n*	1,4,8	2–38	1,3	1	3	3,4,8
Duration of treatment inflation, *s*	20	60	30	30	30	30
Light guide motion	1-way	1-way	Reciprocal	Fixed	Fixed	Reciprocal
Delivery catheter balloon length, *cm*	2	3	2	2	2	1
Marker bands, *n*	1	2	2	1	1	2
Position of marker bands	Center	Cones	Cones	Center	Center	Cones

**The treatment balloon was inflated as if ultraviolet (UV) was being delivered, but the UV was not turned on.*

After each treatment, both the delivery catheter and the light guide were removed, visually inspected, and tested for light power output. When all vessel sites had been addressed, all hardware was removed from the animal, and the carotid cutdown was repaired. A submuscular injection of 10,000 U of heparin was performed, and the animal was returned to routine care.

All pigs were sacrificed 21 days after the procedure. The animals were first heparinized, a lethal dose of a euthanizing solution was given, the chest was opened, and the heart was excised. The entire coronary system was pressure fixed at 70 mm Hg in 10% buffered formalin for a minimum of 12 hours. All treatment and control sites were excised along with some adjacent myocardium and a portion of both proximal and distal normal vessel. Segments were embedded and sectioned at 2-mm intervals, affixed to glass slides, and stained with hematoxylin and eosin (H & E), Verhoeff-van Gieson elastin, and Masson trichrome.

Morphometric analysis was performed on all tissue sections. Because extensive medial necrosis and hypocellularity was routinely observed, an attempt was made to quantify the acellular media cross-sectional area. This was done by using an optical microscope equipped with a calibrated eyepiece to estimate the vessel diameter, average intimal thickness, and average medial thickness from sections stained with Verhoeff-van Gieson elastin. The average thickness of the acellular media layer was measured from sections stained with H & E. Percent area stenosis and the arc of internal elastic lamina rupture were estimated by eye from sections stained with Verhoeff-van Gieson elastin.

Results: Injured and Treated

Hardware Performance: Delivery of Ultraviolet Light After Balloon Injury

For study 1, the delivery catheter balloon had a center marker band, and the "notch" of reduced dose in the center usually resulted in less acellular media and percent area stenosis in the center. For study 2, the delivery catheter balloon had no center marker band, but the balloon was lengthened from 2 to 3 cm. None of the sites in study 2 showed a media effect that exceeded 2 cm in length, indicating that the 3-cm-long balloon was an ineffective means of obtaining good occlusive contact between the balloon and the lumen. For study 3, the effect on stenosis extended about 2 cm in several cases, the length of the delivery balloon, but the media effect was usually confined to a much shorter length.

A thin white film of well-adhered denatured protein was usually found to be coating the balloon after treatment. This film absorbed as much as 50% of the UV light in some cases and often formed after only a single treatment. The film is believed to form as a result of UV light irradiating blood plasma proteins. The presence of the film makes dosimetry difficult, although later a dose-response relationship is demonstrated. Posttreatment measurements of the balloon output power were not made for studies 1 and 2, so the actual dose may have been lower. Posttreatment measurements of balloon output power were made for studies 3 through 6, and the doses for these studies reflect the impact of varying amounts of film.

Percent Area Stenosis After Balloon Injury

Using a two-tailed student's *t*-test for unpaired data, the treated sites from study 1 had significantly greater area stenosis ($P < 0.0005$), although neither the number of sections with IEL rupture nor the maximum arc of ruptured IEL were significantly different ($P < 0.10$). It appears, however, that the treated sections had greater vessel injury, possibly owing to the multiple numbers of inflations for several of the treated sites.

Using the same statistical methods for study 2, the treated sites also had significantly greater percent area stenosis ($P < 0.005$), although neither the number of sections with IEL rupture nor the maximum arc of ruptured IEL were significantly different ($P < 0.25$).

For study 3, the results were similar. The treated sites had considerable percent area stenosis even though the dose was much lower than for either study 1 or 2. No additional injured controls were performed for study 3, but using the controls of study 2 the treated sites of study 3 resulted in significantly greater percent area stenosis ($P < 0.0005$). Again, there was no significant difference in either the number of sites with ruptured IEL or the maximum arc of IEL rupture.

Figure 10-3 shows a bar chart of the results of the three studies with balloon injury. Although there were considerable differences in terms of dose, balloon length and type, extent of injury, and light guide motion, all three studies demonstrated a statistically significant increase in percent area stenosis after treatment compared to controls. The similarity of the results for study 3 to the other two studies is interesting considering that the average dose for study 3 was at least an order of magnitude less, and the amount of acellular media area was also considerably less.

Remodeling After Treatment of Injured Vessels

Gregoire and colleagues [16] used computer-assisted morphometry to analyze changes in the area within the boundary of the external elastic lamina (EEL) versus neointimal area using the tissue sections from studies 3, 4 and 5. They demonstrated a significant trend toward increasing EEL area with increasing neointimal area if the IEL had been ruptured (Fig. 10-4).

Histopathologic Analysis of Injured and Treated Vessels

Internal elastic lamina rupture with stenosis and acellular media

The typical response of an injured vessel to UV treatment is shown in Figure 10-5*A*. This is a section from a vessel in study 1 that received a peak dose of 3600 mJ/cm^2. The section has been stained with Verhoeff-van Gieson elastin to show the IEL rupture. The same section stained with H & E is shown in Figure 10-5*B*, demonstrating pink areas of acellular media as well as intimal hyperplasia that includes some thrombus and hemorrhage. The same section is shown in Figure 10-5C, stained with Masson trichrome to highlight in blue the fibrous tissue that has replaced portions of the media. No figure showing the response to balloon injury alone is shown because this has already been well described in the literature [20,21,23,26]. None of the 10 control vessel sites that were balloon injured exhibited percent area stenoses greater than 35%, even when significant IEL rupture resulted.

Internal elastic lamina rupture with stenosis and without acellular media

Significant intimal hyperplasia still occurred even when the dose was lower and no acellular media was observed. For example, this can be seen in the Verhoeff-van Gieson stained section shown in Figure 10-6*A*. For this site, the dose was 1300 mJ/cm^2 and the section shown has a percent area stenosis of about 80% with an IEL rupture arc of about 90°. The same section stained with H & E is shown in Figure 10-6*B*. The intimal hyperplasia is characterized by smooth muscle cells, and no significant hypocellularity or medial fibrosis is evident.

Results: Uninjured and Treated

Hardware Performance: Treatment of Uninjured Vessels

Studies 4, 5, and 6 did not involve prior balloon overdilatation injury, and the intent was not to rupture the IEL. This was done to isolate the effects of the UV light apart from balloon injury and to achieve better contact between the delivery catheter balloon and the vessel lumen. Because it is well-known how little intimal hyperplasia results when the IEL is not ruptured, only five control sites were performed, using up to eight inflations with no UV light delivered.

For study 4, a single treatment inflation with slight vessel overdilatation was used with the light guide stationary in the distal half of the balloon.

For study 5, three treatment inflations were used with slight vessel overdilatation and with the light guide also stationary in the distal half of the balloon. Study 5 was intended to be similar in dose to study 4, but with three treatment inflations at one third the power of study 4. The purpose was to compare the results of studies 4 and 5 to check if reciprocity was holding (*ie*, to see if the results were dependent on total dose or on power level). A greater media effect with less percent stenosis was typically seen for study 5 versus study 4. Subsequent bench experiments indicated that study 4 may have resulted in comparatively less tissue effect because of the presence of diluted blood in the saline purge of the gap between the light guide and the lumen of the delivery catheter.

For study 6, from three to eight treatment inflations were used with greater vessel overdilatation of 6% to 11% and the light guide reciprocating back and forth. For study 6, the balloons were only 1 cm in length to

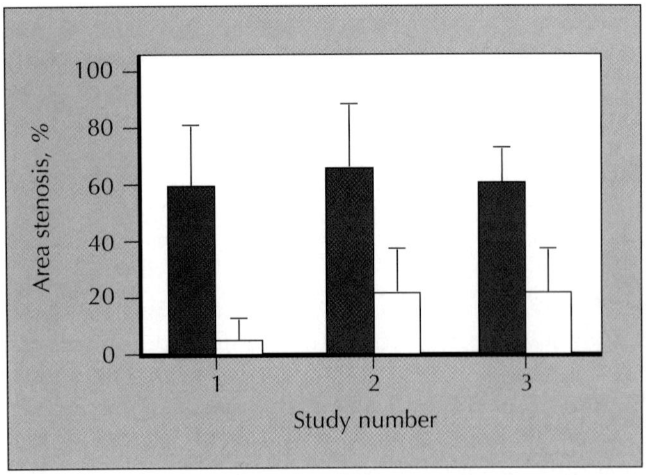

Figure 10-3. Summary of results for percent area stenosis for injured and treated (*solid*) and injured controls (*open*). Error bars are + 1 SD.

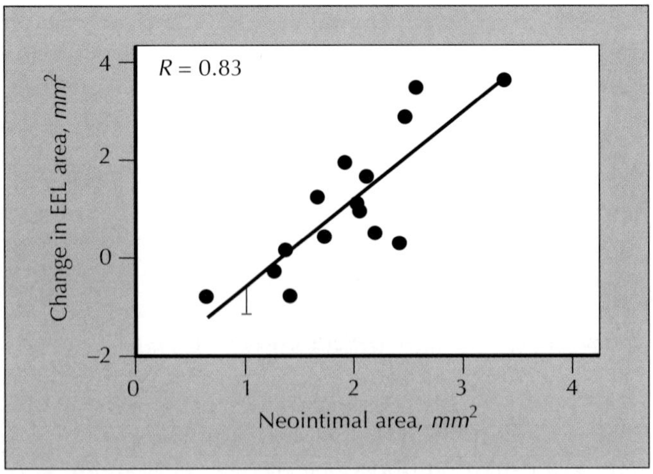

Figure 10-4. Remodeling of injured and treated vessels. Data from studies 3, 4, and 5.

try to minimize the amount of unintentional IEL damage because of treatment inflations. A film was usually found on the outer surface of the delivery catheter balloon, just as with studies 1, 2, and 3.

Percent Area Stenosis After Treatment of Uninjured Vessels

Because of the small number of controls for uninjured vessels, the five controls were lumped together for the purpose of statistical comparison. Treated sites from study 4 had significantly greater percent area stenosis than controls ($P < 0.005$). Clearly, treatment with UVC can result in significant stenosis even in the absence of IEL rupture.

All sites in study 5 were treated using three inflations. Compared to the lumped controls, the percent area stenosis for study 5 was significantly greater but just barely ($P < 0.05$). Comparing the results of studies 4 and 5 using a student's *t*-test shows that the percent area stenosis was significantly less for study 5 ($P < 0.005$). The amount of IEL damage as measured by both the number of sites with ruptures and the maximum arc of rupture was also significantly less, although just barely so ($P < 0.05$). It is not readily apparent whether the reduction in percent stenosis was due to the possible presence of diluted blood blocking light in study 4, the difference in IEL damage, or the difference in power at the same dose. The section with the maximum stenosis for the site was not usually associated with an isolated IEL rupture.

Compared with the lumped controls, the percent area stenosis with study 6 was significantly greater ($P < 0.01$). Compared to study 4, the percent area stenosis is less but not significant statistically ($P > 0.05$). The amount of IEL damage is similar to that of study 5, indicating that the shorter 1-cm-long balloon may not have contributed to less damage.

Figure 10-7 shows a bar chart of the results of the three studies on uninjured vessels. Although there were considerable differences between studies 4, 5, and 6 in terms of dose, balloon length and type, and light guide motion, all three studies demonstrated a statistically significant increase in stenosis after treatment compared with controls.

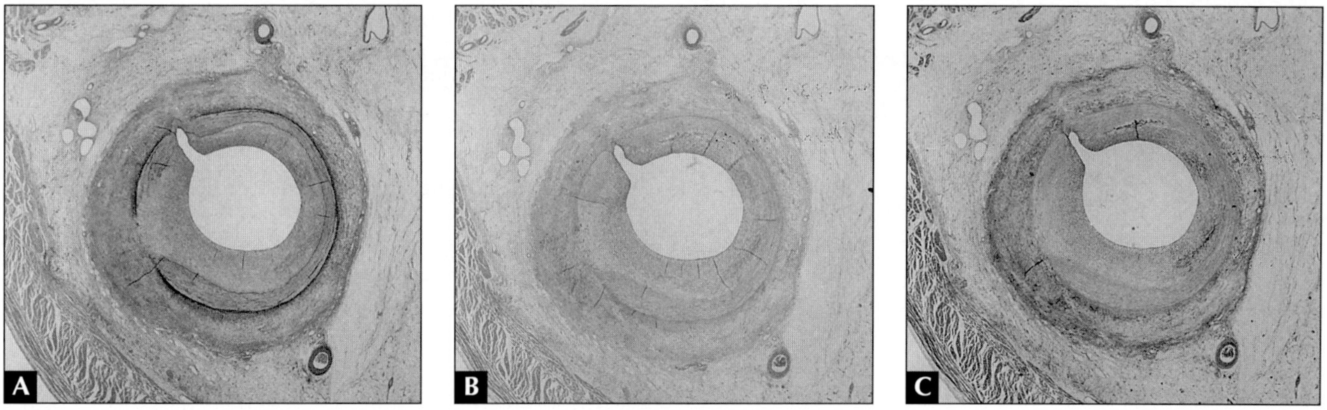

Figure 10-5. Tissue section from an animal in study 1 showing the response to a dose of 3600 mJ/cm^2. **A**, Verhoeff-van Gieson. **B**, Hematoxylin and eosin. **C**, Trichrome.

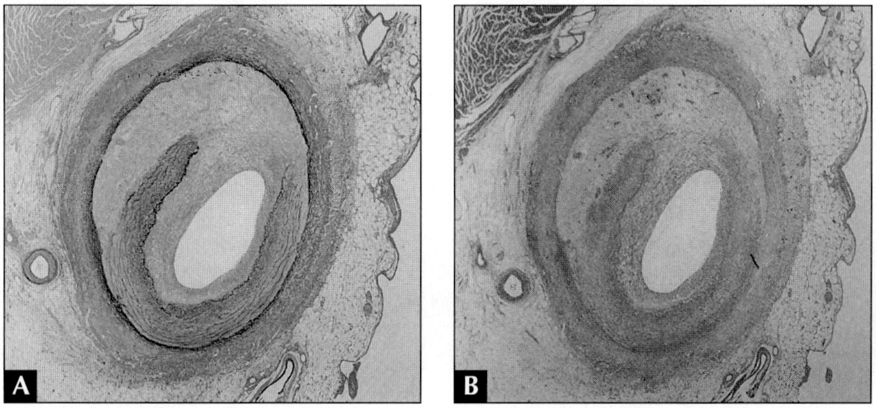

Figure 10-6. Tissue section from an animal in study 5 showing the response of an injured vessel to a low dose of 1300 mJ/cm^2. **A**, Verhoeff van Gieson. **B**, Hematoxylin and eosin. Note the absence of acellular media on the hematoxylin and eosin–stained section.

Histopathologic Analysis of Uninjured and Treated Vessels

No internal elastic lamina rupture without stenosis and with acellular media

Figure 10-8 shows the "ideal" result that was sought for all the studies. This vessel from study 5 received a dose of 15,000 mJ/cm^2 from a stationary light guide with UV exposures during three inflations. No intimal hyperplasia were present. The Verhoeff-van Gieson stain shows that although there is no IEL damage, the lamina has been flattened, showing none of the usual waviness seen in nontreated vessels. The media is also about 50% thinner than either proximal or distal sections that were not exposed to UV light. The H & E stained section shows that the media is completely acellular. The Masson trichrome section shows that the entire media has been completely replaced with dense fibrous tissue.

For all six studies, this type of result was never obtained for any section in which the IEL had been ruptured. Only 10 vessels of the total 58 vessels treated in all six studies displayed one or more sections with a percent area stenosis of 10% or less corresponding to a completely circumferential acellular media effect. Five of these were from study 5, four were from study 6, and one was from study 1. Peak dose was 3500 to 16,000 mJ/cm^2.

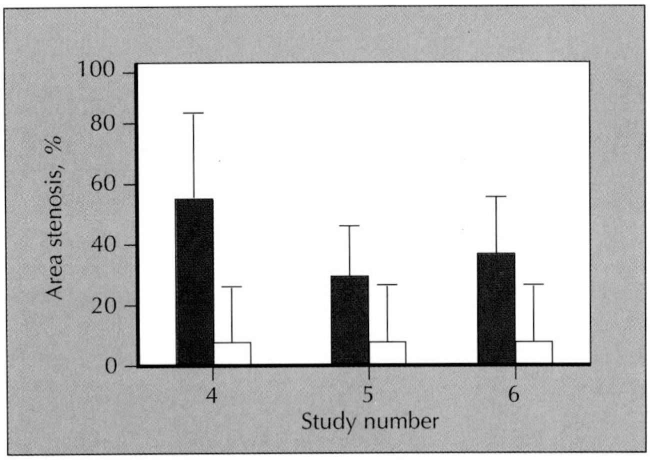

Figure 10-7. Summary of results for percent area stenosis for uninjured and treated (*shaded*) and uninjured controls (*open*). Error bars are + 1 SD.

No internal elastic lamina rupture with stenosis and acellular media

More often, the presence of acellular media did not correspond to low stenosis for uninjured sites. Figure 10-9 shows a section stained with H & E from a site in study 6 that had a relatively high amount of acellular media from a dose of 11,100 mJ/cm^2 but yet still had a significant area stenosis of about 50%. Note that the acellular media extends circumferentially almost completely around the lumen, and the media is thickened on one side.

No internal elastic lamina rupture with stenosis and without acellular media

Stenosis occurred even when the dose was too low to result in significant acellular media. Several sites from study 4 showed this result, from doses in the range of 480 to 1700 mJ/cm^2, with percent area stenosis ranging from 15% to 90%.

Dosimetry

The effect of UV light on tissue can been examined by analyzing the maximum acellular media area versus peak dose for each vessel site. Because the axial dose distribution was often quite variable, it is reasonable to presume that the tissue section with the maximum amount of acellular media corresponds to the peak dose for the vessel site. The first two studies were excluded from this analysis because their doses were not corrected for the presence of film on the balloon. All the data from studies 3, 4, 5, and 6 are shown plot-

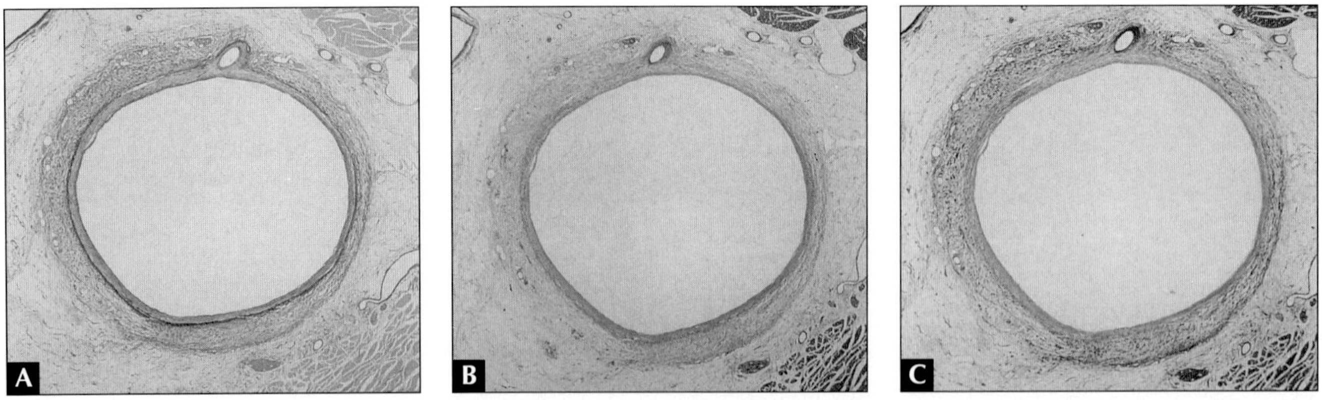

Figure 10-8. Tissue section from an animal in study 5 showing the response to a dose of 15,000 mJ/cm^2. **A**, Verhoeff-van Gieson. **B**, Hematoxylin and eosin. **C**, Trichrome. The percent area stenosis was zero for this section.

ted in Figure 10-10, maximum acellular media area (AMA) versus peak dose. Doses that resulted in zero acellular media have been excluded from this plot. The results shown in Figure 10-10 clearly indicate that increasing dose usually resulted in increasing acellular media area.

Other Events

There were no intraoperative incidences of significant spasm, arterial rupture, or thrombosis. One pig developed ventricular fibrillation during a prolonged procedure. One animal died 12 hours postoperatively secondary to guide catheter trauma that caused a periadventitial hemorrhage seen at necropsy. Tissue sections from this animal stained with H & E showed a significant amount of acellular media 12 hours after treatment. The one site that completely occluded (study 2) had been treated with 38 treatment inflations, the last of which ended unexpectedly with a longitudinal balloon rupture at nominal pressure, possibly causing additional trauma to the vessel. No coronary artery section demonstrated evidence of coronary ectasia, aneurysm formation, or rupture.

Discussion

The minimum dose required for sunburn is approximately 20 mJ/cm^2. The lowest dose delivered in this study was 180 mJ/cm^2, and this dose did not produce medial necrosis. Minimal medial necrosis appears at approximately 400 mJ/cm^2, and complete medial necrosis occurs at 3000 mJ/cm^2. Clearly, all doses above 3000 were excessive and not necessary to produce cellular changes. Doses above 3000 mJ/cm^2 caused excessive cellular damage and resultant intimal hyperplasia. The mechanism of the changes at this dose level are almost certainly a combination of DNA effects plus the direct effects on proteins as described previously. Unfortunately, many of the experiments cited were complicated by the possibility of heat production, unrecognized UV absorption by blood and balloon film, and possible contrast contamination. Accurate uniform delivery of UV light is extremely difficult, and the asymmetry noted in the histologic sections most likely reflects these concerns.

Circumferential Asymmetry

Most often, the medial necrosis was of varying depth and circumferentially asymmetric, with necrotic zones often directly adjacent to normal medial tissue. There were no gradual transitions of medial cell density from normal to necrotic but either clearly defined bands of necrosis or normal media. This was most likely due to the delivery system. The inner shaft of the delivery catheter that provides the lumen for the light guide was most likely off center and up against the balloon over most of the balloon length. This was confirmed by bench tests and is not surprising because the inner shaft is radially unsupported in the region of the balloon, and only a slight balloon curvature is needed to push it completely off to one side. The doses presented in this report are radial averages. In the worse case, the "hot" spot radial dose could have been about four times greater than the radial average and the "cold" spot about 40% less than the radial average. The extent of the "hot" spot would at most extend around one quadrant of the circumference.

Film and Thrombus

It was also difficult to deliver UVC consistently to vessels. The thin white film found on most treatment balloons was most likely denatured plasma protein formed as a result of UVC irradiating the thin layer of blood or plasma trapped between the balloon and the vessel wall. Bench experiments have shown that UVC

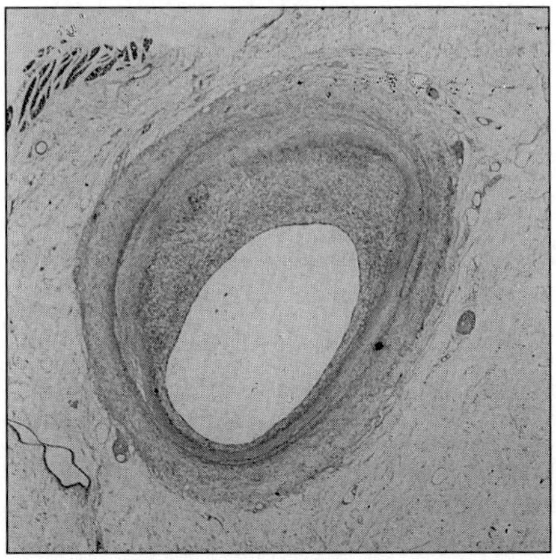

Figure 10-9. Tissue section from an animal in study 6 showing the response to a dose of 11,100 mJ/cm^2. Note significant acellular media and significant intimal hyperplasia, plus lack of intraepithelial lymphocyte rupture. Hematoxylin and eosin stain.

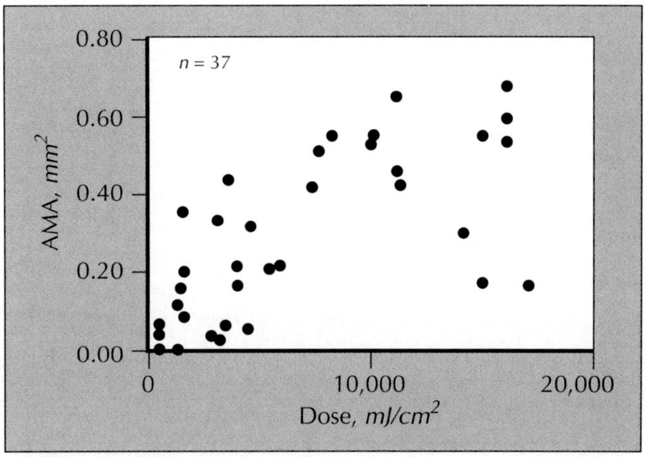

Figure 10-10. Dosimetry plot of acellular media area (AMA) versus peak dose.

is strongly absorbed by undiluted blood, with 50% absorption occurring over less than 20 μm. Although the film was observed on balloons used to treat both injured and uninjured vessels, most of the medial necrosis was observed for uninjured sites. This difference may have been due to the presence of a thin localized layer of adherent thrombus that can form soon after injury at the site of rupture of the IEL. Even if thin, a layer of thrombus could significantly reduce the dose that reaches the media.

Thermal Injury

The vast majority of the energy of UV light that is incident on tissue goes into heating. The three major types of thermal balloon angioplasty devices (laser, microwave, or radiofrequency) have all produced similar histologic results. The primary signs of thermal damage are 1) medial necrosis, 2) thinning of the vessel wall, and 3) straightening of elastic tissue, particularly the IEL [36]. All of these signs were observed from UVC treatment.

The PLOSA (Physiologically Controlled Low-Stress Angioplasty) thermal angioplasty system, based on a radiofrequency-heated balloon and thermal conduction into the media, operated at the lowest temperature of the three types of thermal angioplasty devices and has produced histologic results that are similar to UVC results. Porcine coronaries treated with the PLOSA system at 50°, 60°, or 70°C for either 30 or 60 seconds resulted in full transmural medial necrosis for all heated segments. Deep to the adventitia, there was a direct relationship between the depth of periadventitial myocardial necrosis and both the temperature and the duration of the treatment inflation. A mean depth of periarterial myocardial necrosis of about 35 μm resulted from a single 30-second exposure to 50°C. A mean depth of periarterial myocardial necrosis of about 130 μm resulted from a single 30-second exposure to 60°C. The temperature threshold for full straightening of elastic tissue in porcine coronaries was about 70°C [37].

Bench experiments have shown that the UVC system is capable of generating peak luminal "hot" spot temperatures of up to 60°C at the most extreme conditions used in the six studies. The duration of these temperatures, however, was short because the light guide was moving at a speed of at least 1 mm/sec for four of the six studies. Furthermore, if UVC had resulted in 60°C over one quadrant of the circumference for a significant amount of time, we should have observed medial necrosis penetrating to a depth of almost 500 μm caused by just a single 60-second exposure. Even the highest power levels with multiple exposures never resulted in medial necrosis deeper than 120 μm.

Experiments on porcine and human skin have shown that even though cellular injury can occur at temperatures as low as 44°C, up to 6 hours of heating at this temperature is required to produce irreversible injury [38,39]. As temperatures rise above 45°C, cellular death starts to occur with increasingly shorter heating intervals [38–40].

The light guide was stationary only for studies 4 and 5. At the highest doses of study 4 (14,000 to 16,000 mJ/cm^2), the peak "hot" spot temperature may have been only as high as 44°C for three 30-second exposures. In addition, the medial necrosis at three of the four highest dose sites in study 5 was completely circumferential, which is unlikely to have been the result of a thermal "hot" spot. UVC also produced a significant level of medial necrosis at power levels that were certainly too low to have caused thermal damage. The lower doses in study 5 also produced significant medial necrosis although the maximum temperature rise could have only been a few degrees under worse-case conditions. The presence of significant medial necrosis at power levels much too low to be caused by thermal damage leads to the conclusion that UV light alone was the cause.

Recent Efforts

Work has focused on the development of an improved delivery catheter to address the issues of centering and formation of film on the balloon. A multisegmented inner balloon covered by a microporous outer balloon addresses these issues. A multisegmented inner balloon provides improved centering of the light guide in the lumen to improve radial dose uniformity and minimize any potential for thermal effects. Another investigator has used a similar balloon with four segments to improve the luminal centering of a β source [27,41]. A continuous saline flush of 500 mL/h through the outer porous balloon helps keep blood from the balloon/lumen interface and minimize the buildup of the film of denatured protein. A higher-power continuous-wave laser provides UVC at 254 nm, enabling shorter treatment times while still avoiding thermal damage.

Conclusions

UV light adversely effects the porcine coronary artery when delivered at doses higher than 3000 mJ/cm^2. Tissue effects at this level are represented by acellular media, intimal hyperplasia, and a thickened adventitia. At a lower dose, in which only the DNA effects may be seen, no adverse media changes are noted, and this is reflected in less intimal hyperplasia. With the advent of new, more reliable delivery systems, which ensure accurate delivery uniformly to the entire arterial wall, further studies with lower dosing are clearly warranted.

References

1. Leon MB, Smith PD, Bonner RF: Laser angioplasty delivery systems: design considerations. In *Lasers in Cardiovascular Disease*. Edited by White RA, Grundfest WS. Chicago: Year Book Medical Publishers, 1987:44–63.
2. Kochevar IE: Basic principles in photomedicine and photochemistry. In *Clinical Photomedicine*. Edited by Lim HW, Soter NA. New York: Marcel Dekker, 1993:1–18.
3. Prince MR, Deutsch TF, Mathews-Roth MM, *et al.*: Preferential light absorption in atheromas in vitro: implications for laser angioplasty. *J Clin Invest* 1986, 78:295–302.
4. Anderson RR: Optics of the skin. In *Clinical Photomedicine*. Edited by Lin HW, Soter NA. New York: Marcel Dekker, 1993:27–31.
5. Carrier WL, Snyder RD, Regan JD: Ultraviolet-induced damage and its repair in human DNA. In *The Science of Photomedicine*. Edited by Regan JD, Parrish JD. New York: Plenum Press, 1982:91–112.
6. Smith KC: UV radiation effects: DNA repair and mutagenesis. In *The Science of Photobiology*, edn 2. Edited by Smith KC. New York: Plenum Press, 1989:111–138.
7. Kochevar IE: UV-induced protein alterations and lipid oxidation in erythrocyte membranes. *Photochem Photobiol* 1990, 52:795–800.
8. Kato Y, Nishikawa T, Kawakishi S: Formation of protein-bound 3,4-dihydroxyphenylalanine in collagen types I and IV exposed to ultraviolet light. *Photochem Photobiol* 1995, 61:367–372.
9. Mayne R: Collagenous proteins of blood vessels. *Arteriosclerosis* 1986, 6:585–593.
10. Grossweiner LI, Smith KC: Photochemistry. In *The Science of Photobiology*, edn 2. Edited by Smith KC. New York: Plenum Press, 1989:47–78.
11. Papadopoulo D, Muel B, Latarjet R: Relative efficiencies of three ultraviolet radiation wavelengths for cell killing and transformation in mouse cells in vitro. *Int J Radiat Biol* 1983, 44:241–249.
12. Green H, Boll J, Parrish JA, *et al.*: Cytotoxicity and mutagenicity of low intensity, 248 and 193 nm excimer laser radiation in mammalian cells. *Cancer Res* 1987, 47:410–413.
13. Clarke RH, Isner JM, VanTassel RA, *et al.*: Wavelength-dependent cytotoxicity of laser light on vascular smooth muscle: implications for restenosis prevention [abstract]. *Circulation* 1991, 84(suppl II):360.
14. Pastore CJ, DeJesus ST, VanTassel RA, *et al.*: Low dose, subablative ultraviolet (UV-C) laser irradiation from a Q-switched, frequency-quadrupled ND:YLF diode laser inhibits neointimal hyperplasia in balloon-injured rat carotid arteries [abstract]. *J Am Coll Cardiol* 1994, 23:472A.
15. Gregoire J, Edwards WD, Jeong MH, *et al.*: Transcatheter short wave ultraviolet laser energy creates acellular media in porcine coronary arteries: an in vivo study [abstract]. *J Invas Cardiol* 1996, 8:84.
16. Gregoire J, Edwards WD, Jeong MH, *et al.*: Porcine coronary arteries exposed to short wave ultraviolet laser energy exhibit favorable remodeling [abstract]. *J of Invas Cardiol* 1996, 8:84.
17. Kubaszewski E, Peters A, McClain S, *et al.*: Light-activated release of nitric oxide from vascular smooth muscle of normotensive and hypertensive rats. *Biochem Biophys Res Commun* 1994, 200:213–218.
18. Sumpio BE, Phan SM, Gasparro FP, *et al.*: Control of smooth muscle cell proliferation by psoralen photochemotherapy. *J Vasc Surg* 1993, 17:1010–1016.
19. March KL, Patton BL, Wilensky RL, *et al.*: 8-Methoxypsoralen and longwave ultraviolet irradiation are a novel antiproliferative combination for vascular smooth muscle. *Circulation* 1993, 87:184–191.
20. Wiedermann JG, Marboe C, Amols H, *et al.*: Intracoronary irradiation markedly reduces restenosis after balloon angioplasty in a porcine model. *J Am Coll Cardiol* 1994, 23:1491–1498.
21. Wiedermann JG, Marboe C, Amols H, *et al.*: Intracoronary irradiation markedly reduces neointimal proliferation after balloon angioplasty in swine: persistent benefit at 6-month follow-up. *J Am Coll Cardiol* 1995, 25:1451–1456.
22. Wiedermann JG, Leavy JA, Amols H, *et al.*: Effects of high-dose intracoronary irradiation on vasomotor function and smooth muscle histopathology. *Am J Physiol (Heart Circ Physiol 36)* 1994, 267:H125–H132.
23. Waksman R, Robinson KA, Crocker IR, *et al.*: Endovascular low-dose irradiation inhibits neointima formation after coronary artery balloon injury in swine. *Circulation* 1995, 91:1533–1539.
24. Schwartz RS, Koval TM, Edwards WD, *et al.*: Effect of external beam irradiation on neointimal hyperplasia after experimental coronary artery injury. *J Am Coll Cardiol* 1992, 19:1106–1113.
25. Gelman J, Healy G, Qingsheng C, *et al.*: The effect of very low dose irradiation on restenosis following balloon angioplasty. A study in the atherosclerotic rabbit [abstract]. *Circulation* 1991, (suppl II):331.
26. Waksman R, Robinson KA, Crocker IR, *et al.*: Intracoronary low-dose β-irradiation inhibits neointima formation after coronary artery balloon injury in the swine restenosis model. *Circulation* 1995, 92:3025–3031.
27. Verin V, Popowski Y, Urban P, *et al.*: Intra-arterial β irradiation prevents neointimal hyperplasia in a hypercholesterolemic rabbit restenosis model. *Circulation* 1995, 92:2284–2290.
28. Waksman R, Robinson KA, Crocker IR, *et al.*: Intracoronary radiation before stent implantation inhibits neointima formation in stented porcine coronary arteries. *Circulation* 1995, 92:1383–1386.
29. Mazur W, Ali NM, Dabaghi SF, *et al.*: High dose rate intracoronary radiation suppresses neointimal proliferation in the stented and ballooned model of porcine restenosis [abstract]. *Circulation* 1994, 90(suppl I):I652.

30. Fischell TA, Kharma BK, Fischell DR, *et al.*: Low-dose beta-particle emission from 'stent' wire results in complete, localized inhibition of smooth muscle cell proliferation. *Circulation* 1994, 90:2956–2963.

31. Carter AJ, Laird JR, Hoopes TG, *et al.*: Histology after placement of beta-particle emitting stents: insights into inhibition of neointimal formation [abstract]. *J Am Coll Cardiol* 1996, 198A.

32. Bottcher HD, Schopohl B, Liermann D, *et al.*: Endovascular irradiation—a new method to avoid recurrent stenosis after stent implantation in peripheral arteries: technique and preliminary results. *Int J Radiat Biol Phys* 1994, 29:183–186.

33. Liermann D, Bottcher HD, Kollath J, *et al.*: Prophylactic endovascular radiotherapy to prevent intimal hyperplasia after stent implantation in femoropopliteal arteries. *Cardiovasc Intervent Radiol* 1994, 17:12–16.

34. Waksman R, Crocker IR, Kikeri D, *et al.*: Endovascular low dose radiation for prevention of restenosis following angioplasty for treatment of narrowed dialysis arterio venous grafts [abstract]. *J Am Coll Cardiol* 1996, 27:14A.

35. Teirstein PS, Massulo V, Jani S, *et al.*: A randomized clinical trial of radiation therapy to reduce restenosis following coronary stenting—early results [abstract]. *J Am Coll Cardiol* 1996, 27:15A.

36. Fram DB, McKay RG: "Hot" balloon angioplasty: radiofrequency, neodymium:YAG, and microwave. In *Textbook of Interventional Cardiology*. Edited by Topol EJ. Philadelphia: WB Saunders, 1994:819–839.

37. Fram DB, Aretz TA, Mikan JF, *et al.*: In vivo radiofrequency thermal balloon angioplasty of porcine coronary arteries: histological effects and safety. *Am Heart J* 1993, 126:969–978.

38. Moritz AR, Henriques FC Jr: Studies of thermal injury: II. The relative importance of time and surface temperature in the causation of cutaneous burns. *Am J Pathol* 1947, 23:695–720.

39. Moritz AR: Studies of thermal injury: III. The pathology and pathogenesis of cutaneous burns: An experimental study. *Am J Pathol* 1947, 23:915–941.

40. Cheong W, Spears JR: Laser balloon angioplasty. *Crit Rev Biomed Eng* 1991, 19:113–146.

41. Verin V, Popowski Y, Urban P, *et al.*: Yttrium-90, a new β emitter for prevention of post angioplasty restenosis: tissue dosimetry and importance of intraarterial centering [abstract]. *J Am Coll Cardiol* 1996, 8:321A.

Chapter 11

Excimer Laser Angioplasty: Results from Recent Randomized Clinical Trials

J.J. Piek
Y.E.A. Appelman

Coronary revascularization by percutaneous techniques has demonstrated an enormous growth since its introduction in 1977. In 1995, the total number of coronary angioplasty procedures was 994,000 and exceeded the number of coronary bypass surgery procedures (740,000). At present, balloon angioplasty is still the most commonly applied percutaneous transluminal technique for coronary revascularization. However, balloon angioplasty remains cumbersome in complex coronary lesions such as long, diffusely diseased vessels, aorto-ostial lesions, totally occluded vessels, and vein graft lesions. The recognized limitations of balloon angioplasty led to the introduction of alternative procedures, including laser angioplasty. The clinical application of the first generation of continuous-wave laser systems in the mid-1980s was rather limited because it required straight, noncalcified arterial segments. Furthermore, the risk of vessel perforation was substantial due to the thermal damage. The pulsed laser system was subsequently introduced to reduce the heating of the surrounding tissue in contrast to the continuous-wave laser light delivery. Initial experiments using excimer laser showed that ablation of aortic tissue resulted in a smooth ablation crater with very limited damage to the adjacent tissue [1] (Fig. 11-1). This characteristic of excimer laser was considered to be ideal for laser angioplasty. The introduction of multifiber over-the-wire laser catheters made possible the use of this excimer laser in the clinical setting for removal of atherosclerotic plaque in coronary arteries (Fig. 11-2).

In 1988, Litvack and colleagues [2] reported the first percutaneous coronary angioplasty performed with a pulsed xenon chloride excimer laser system, which operates at a wavelength of 308 nm. The initial results of excimer laser coronary angioplasty (ELCA) in several institutions in the United States were centrally collected in the so-called ELCA registry. The initial report of this registry included a total number of 1151 lesions, and the results were presented for the first time at the meeting of the American Heart Association in November 1990. The procedural results in type A and B1 lesions according to the modified American College of Cardiology–American Heart Association criteria were similar to balloon angioplasty. However, the primary success rate and procedural complications in type B2 and C lesions were favorable to balloon angioplasty. It was concluded that the promising initial results warranted a randomized trial in order to establish the role of excimer laser angioplasty as an alternative approach in the treatment of obstructive coronary artery disease.

THE AMSTERDAM-ROTTERDAM TRIAL

The multicenter AMRO (Amsterdam-Rotterdam) trial was started in September 1991 and completed in November 1993 [3••]. Patients with stable angina pectoris and coronary lesions of the native arteries longer than 10 mm on visual assessment, including total or functional occlusions, were included in the trial. Patients with unstable angina or a myocardial infarction (MI) within the previous 2 weeks were excluded. Furthermore, patients with relative contraindications for laser angioplasty such as extreme tortuosity of the vessel, highly eccentric lesions, or angulated lesions of more than 45° were excluded.

The excimer laser systems (wavelength of 308 nm) used were the Dymer 200+ (Advanced Interventional Systems Inc., Irvine, CA), with a pulse duration of 210 ns and a repetition rate of 20 Hz, delivered by multifiber over-the-wire laser catheters with a diameter of 1.3, 1.6, or 2.0 mm and a fluence of 45 to 65 mJ/mm^2, and the CVX-300 system (Spectranetics, Colorado Springs, CO), with a pulse duration of 135 ns at a repetition rate of 25 Hz, delivered by 1.4-, 1.7-, or 2.0-mm laser catheters, with a similar fluence. The 1.3-mm laser catheter was used after its introduction in 1992. The 1.3- and 1.4-mm laser catheter was used for vessels with a diameter of 1.8 to 2.3 mm, the 1.6- and 1.7-mm laser catheter for vessels with a diameter of 2.3 to 3.0 mm, and the 2.0-mm laser catheter for vessels with a diameter of 3.0 mm or more.

Heparin was administered intravenously to maintain the activated clotting time for more than 400 seconds and was continued for at least 12 hours after the procedure. After crossing the lesion with the guidewire, the laser catheter was advanced at a speed of about 1 mm/s. Quantitative coronary angiography was performed before and after the procedure and at 6-month follow-up. The angiograms were analyzed in a central core laboratory with the computer-assisted cardiovascular angiography analysis system.

A total of 308 consecutive patients (325 lesions) were randomly assigned to laser angioplasty (151 patients; 158 lesions) or balloon angioplasty (157 patients; 167 lesions). Additional balloon angioplasty was required in 98% of the procedures allocated to laser angioplasty in order to obtain an optimal angiographic result (Fig. 11-3). The angiographic success rate by visual assessment was 80% (126 lesions) in patients treated with excimer laser angioplasty compared with 79% (132 lesions) in patients treated with balloon angioplasty. The clinical events occurring during the procedure and 6-month follow-up are shown

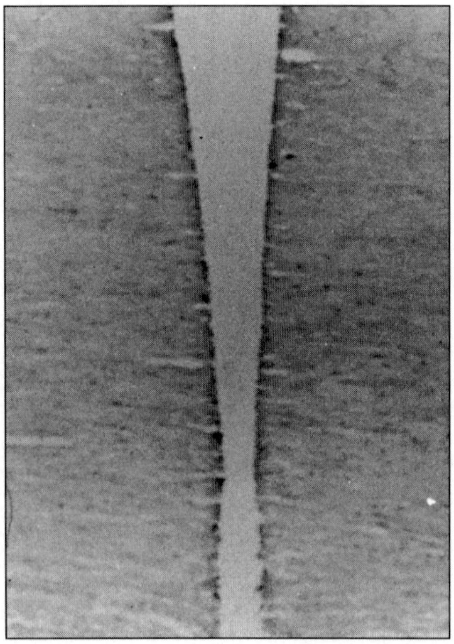

Figure 11-1. Histologic effect of an incision with a 308-nm excimer laser on atherosclerotic aorta irradiated in air. The margins are regular, without carbonization or blast injury.

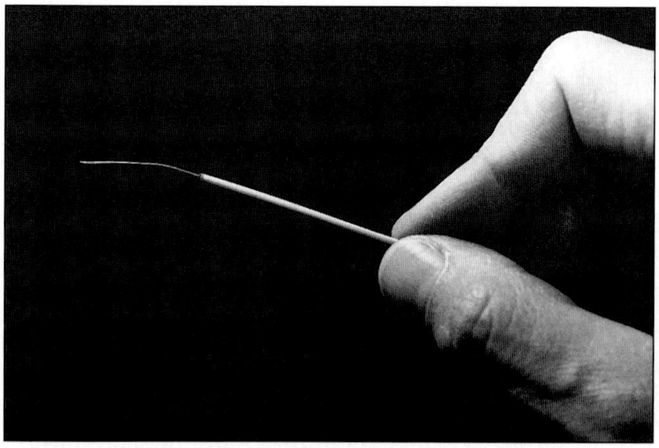

Figure 11-2. A flexible multifiber over-the-wire excimer laser catheter.

in Table 11-1. There were no deaths. The incidence of MI, coronary bypass surgery, and repeated angioplasty was similar in both groups. Most non–Q-wave MIs were small in both groups (maximal creatine kinase–myocardial band concentration < 20 U/L). Intimal dissections after completion of the procedure occurred in 74 lesions (46.8%) in the patients treated with excimer laser angioplasty. Most of these dissections (91%) were type A, B, or C, and are characterized by their benign nature. The dissection rate was similar in patients treated with balloon angioplasty (54.5% [91 lesions] of the patients), with 90% of dissections being type A, B, or C. The angiographic results are summarized in Table 11-2. The net gain in minimal lumen diameter was similar in both groups. The net gain in the excimer laser angioplasty group was the result of a

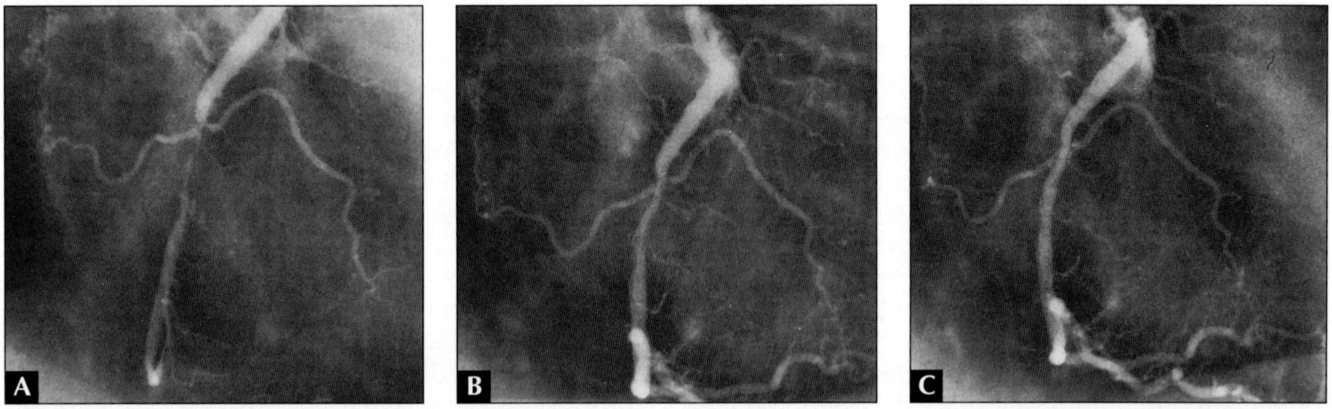

Figure 11-3. Cineangiogram frames from an excimer laser angioplasty procedure. **A**, The initial angiogram revealed a long narrowed segment in the right coronary artery. **B**, The angiogram displaying the coronary lesion after treatment with a 1.6-mm excimer laser catheter. **C**, The final angiographic result after adjunctive balloon angioplasty showing a small dissection and a minimal residual stenosis of the coronary lesion.

TABLE 11-1. CLINICAL EVENTS DURING ELCA AND BA AND DURING 6 MONTH FOLLOW-UP

	ELCA, *n(%)**	BA, *n(%)*†	Relative risk, (95% CI)	*P* value
Death	0	0	—	—
MI	7(4.6)	9(5.7)	0.81 (0.31–2.12)	0.67
Q-wave	4(2.6)	3(1.9)	1.39 (0.32–6.10)	0.72
Periprocedural	2(1.3)	2(1.3)	1.04 (0.15–7.2)	0.97
Follow-up	2(1.3)	1(0.6)	2.08 (0.19–22.70)	0.54
Non–Q-wave	3(2.0)	6(3.8)	0.52 (0.13–2.04)	0.50
Periprocedural	3(2.0)	3(1.9)	1.04 (0.21–5.07)	0.96
Follow-up	0	3(1.9)	0.15 (0.01–2.85)	0.09
CABG	16(10.6)	17(10.8)	0.98 (0.51–1.87)	0.95
Periprocedural	7(4.5)	3(1.9)	2.43 (0.64–9.21)	0.18
Follow-up	9(6.0)	14(8.9)	0.67 (0.30–1.50)	0.32
Repeat angioplasty	32(21.2)	29(18.5)	1.15 (0.73–1.80)	0.55
Periprocedural	2(1.3)	3(1.9)	0.69 (0.12–4.09)	0.68
Follow-up	30(19.9)	26(16.6)	1.20 (0.75–1.93)	0.45
Primary clinical endpoints‡	50(33.1)	47(29.9)	1.11 (0.80–1.54)	0.55

**Total number of patients, 151.*
†Total number of patients, 157.
‡The occurrence of either death or myocardial infarction (MI) or coronary artery bypass grafting (CABG) or repeat angioplasty.
BA—balloon angioplasty, ELCA—excimer laser coronary angioplasty.

small but nonsignificant increase in the acute gain minus a significant greater late loss compared with the balloon angioplasty group. This phenomenon is illustrated in the cumulative frequency distribution curve of the minimal lumen diameter (Fig. 11-4).

The results of this randomized study indicate no additional clinical or angiographic benefit of excimer laser angioplasty compared with balloon angioplasty in the treatment of longer (> 10 mm) coronary lesions. The more recent data from the ELCA registries indicate an increased use of additional balloon angioplasty, which is consistent with the results of the AMRO study [4•].

The additional balloon angioplasty results in a larger acute gain but is followed by a significantly greater late loss in minimal lumen diameter in the excimer laser angioplasty group compared with the balloon angioplasty group (*see* Fig. 11-4). The greater late loss in minimal lumen diameter resulted in a higher restenosis rate after excimer laser angioplasty: 51.6% in the excimer laser group versus 41.3% in the balloon angioplasty group. The adage "bigger is better" relates to the angiographic alterations observed following balloon angioplasty and new percutaneous techniques for coronary revascularization such as directional atherectomy or coronary stenting. In this respect, the propensity of excimer laser angioplasty for the development of restenosis seems to be a unique feature of this device. This phenomenon may be related to an accelerated degree of neointimal response due to mechanical effects of rapid vapor bubble formation during laser application or a negative influence on the geometric remodeling process after intracoronary interventions [5].

It is difficult to compare the results of this study with the results of the nonrandomized ELCA registries [4•,6]. Most of these registries focus on the initial results after excimer laser surgery and have reported completeness of angiographic follow-up in 73% to 88% of the patients after successful excimer laser angioplasty. In the AMRO trial, the clinical follow-up was completed in 98% of the patients in both groups, and the angiographic follow-up was completed in 93% of the patients in the excimer laser group and 91% of the patients in the balloon angioplasty group. Furthermore, patients included in the registries had a variety of coronary lesions and the reported procedural success rates relate to those procedures in which the coronary lesion was successfully crossed with the guidewire. This explains why success rates in this randomized study based on the intention-to-treat analysis

TABLE 11-2. QUANTITATIVE ANALYSIS OF ELCA AND BA

	ELCA*	BA†	Difference (95% CI)	*P* value
Reference diameter, *mm* §	2.51 ± 0.47‡	2.47 ± 0.59	—	—
Length, *mm*	17.69 ± 5.58	18.82 ± 7.15	—	—
Diameter stenosis, %				
Before angioplasty	68.5 ± 18.3	68.9 ± 18.6	—	—
After angioplasty	37.6 ± 10.3	37.9 ± 8.9	-0.4 (-2.8–2.0)	0.76
At follow-up	56.1 ± 23.3	52.6 ± 23.4	3.4 (-2.4–9.3)	0.25
Restenosis, %	51.6	41.3	10.3 (-2.0–22.6)	0.13
MLD, *mm*				
Before angioplasty	0.77 ± 0.44	0.77 ± 0.47	—	—
After angioplasty	1.69 ± 0.41	1.59 ± 0.34	0.10 (0.01–0.19)	0.05
At follow-up	1.17 ± 0.71	1.25 ± 0.68	-0.08 (-0.25–0.93)	0.34
Net gain, *mm*¶	0.40 ± 0.69	0.48 ± 0.66	-0.08 (-0.25–0.09)	0.34
Acute gain, *mm***	0.92 ± 0.53	0.82 ± 0.50	0.10 (-0.03–0.23)	0.15
Late loss, *mm*††	0.52 ± 0.70	0.34 ± 0.62	0.18 (0.15–0.35)	0.04

**Total number of lesions, 124.*
†Total number of lesions, 126.
‡Values are mean ± SD.
§Reference values are the interpolated diameters of normal vessels.
¶Minimal lumen diameter (MLD) at follow-up minus MLD before the initial procedure.
***MLD after the initial procedure minus MLD before the initial procedure.*
††MLD after the initial procedure minus MLD at follow-up.
BA—balloon angioplasty; ELCA—excimer laser coronary angioplasty.

are lower than reported in the excimer laser angioplasty registries, whereas the results of the per protocol analysis are comparable with the registry data. Moreover, quantitative coronary analysis was performed by an independent core laboratory, whereas most angiographic results in the registries were based on visual assessment or semiquantitative assessment.

The results of the AMRO trial indicate that excimer laser angioplasty yields no additional benefit in long coronary lesions. The indications for excimer laser angioplasty were recently reviewed; the conclusions were that long (> 20 mm) lesions, aorta-ostial lesions, and total coronary occlusions were considered favorable for this treatment modality. However, the results of a subanalysis of the AMRO trial do not support these assumptions [7]. Approximately 25% of the patients had coronary lesions larger than 20 mm in length or one third of the patients had a functional or total coronary occlusion. The clinical and angiographic outcome in this patient subset did not indicate a favorable result after excimer laser angioplasty. In fact, the restenosis rate was higher after excimer laser angioplasty compared with balloon angioplasty in longer (> 18 mm in length) coronary lesions (52% vs 32%; P = 0.02). Nevertheless, the study protocol did not include the use of saline infusion, which may improve the result of excimer laser angioplasty [8].

The Excimer Rotational Balloon Angioplasty Comparison

The ERBAC (German Excimer Rotational Balloon Angioplasty Comparison) study was a single-center randomized trial comparing balloon angioplasty, excimer laser angioplasty, and rotational atherectomy in type B or C *de novo* coronary lesions of native arteries suitable for these three techniques. The trial started in 1991 and was completed in 1994. The final results of this trial have not yet been published. The results of an interim analysis demonstrated a procedural success rate, evaluated on an intention-to-treat basis, of 84% for balloon angioplasty, 89% for excimer laser angioplasty, and 93% for rotational atherectomy [9]. The in-hospital complication rate (death, emergency coronary bypass surgery, MI) was 7.0% for balloon angioplasty, 5.7% for excimer laser angioplasty, and 1.5% for rotational atherectomy. There were no significant differences between balloon angioplasty and excimer laser angioplasty with respect to the incidence of death or Q-wave MI during a 6-month follow-up period. However, revascularization procedures of the target vessel were more frequently required following excimer laser angioplasty (47% vs 31% after balloon angioplasty; P = 0.02). The restenosis rate was similar in both groups (52% after balloon angioplasty and 53% after excimer laser angioplasty). The angiographic analysis demonstrated, in accordance with the results of the AMRO study, a nonsignificant increase in acute gain of the minimal luminal diameter followed by a significantly greater late loss in the excimer laser angioplasty group. The ERBAC study, which was performed in the same time period as the AMRO trial, did not include a flushing protocol during excimer laser angioplasty. These preliminary results of the ERBAC study coincide with the results of the AMRO trial, showing no additional benefit of excimer laser angioplasty with respect to the clinical and angiographic outcome.

In Vitro and In Vivo Experiments

Recent insights from clinical studies have provided additional information with respect to laser–tissue interaction during excimer laser angioplasty. Intravascular angioscopy of the morphologic changes induced by pulsed excimer laser light in peripheral and coronary arteries has revealed dissections, intima flaps, fractures of plaques, and tissue remnants corresponding to angiographic findings of haziness and dissections [10]. Moreover, intravascular ultrasound imaging has demonstrated that the recanalization process following ELCA is the result of mechanical dilation of the atheroma rather than of tissue removal [11]. With the clinical randomized trials ongoing, in vitro studies with excimer laser systems made it clear that this tech-

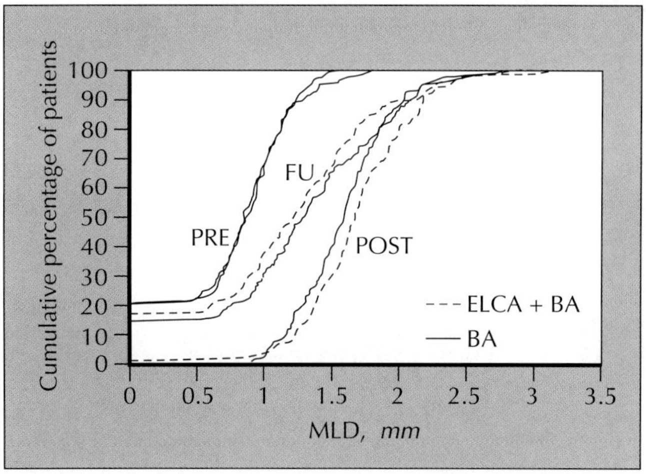

Figure 11-4. Cumulative frequency distribution curves. Minimal luminal diameters (MLDs) are shown before the initial intervention (PRE), after the initial intervention (POST), and at follow-up angiography (FU) for 151 patients treated with excimer laser coronary angioplasty (ELCA) followed by additional balloon angioplasty (BA) and 157 patients treated with BA. All patients were included in the Amsterdam-Rotterdam trial.

nique was not as "smooth and clear cut" as previously anticipated. The relatively high incidence of dissections after the application of pulsed laser light in a clinical setting were caused by mechanical trauma related to the relatively large and stiff laser catheters of the first generation.

Experimental models have indicated that the dissections caused by the currently used pulsed laser catheters were not related to the catheters but to the pulsed laser energy delivery itself. It was demonstrated that the excimer laser reaches a substantial increase in temperature within a very short time span due to

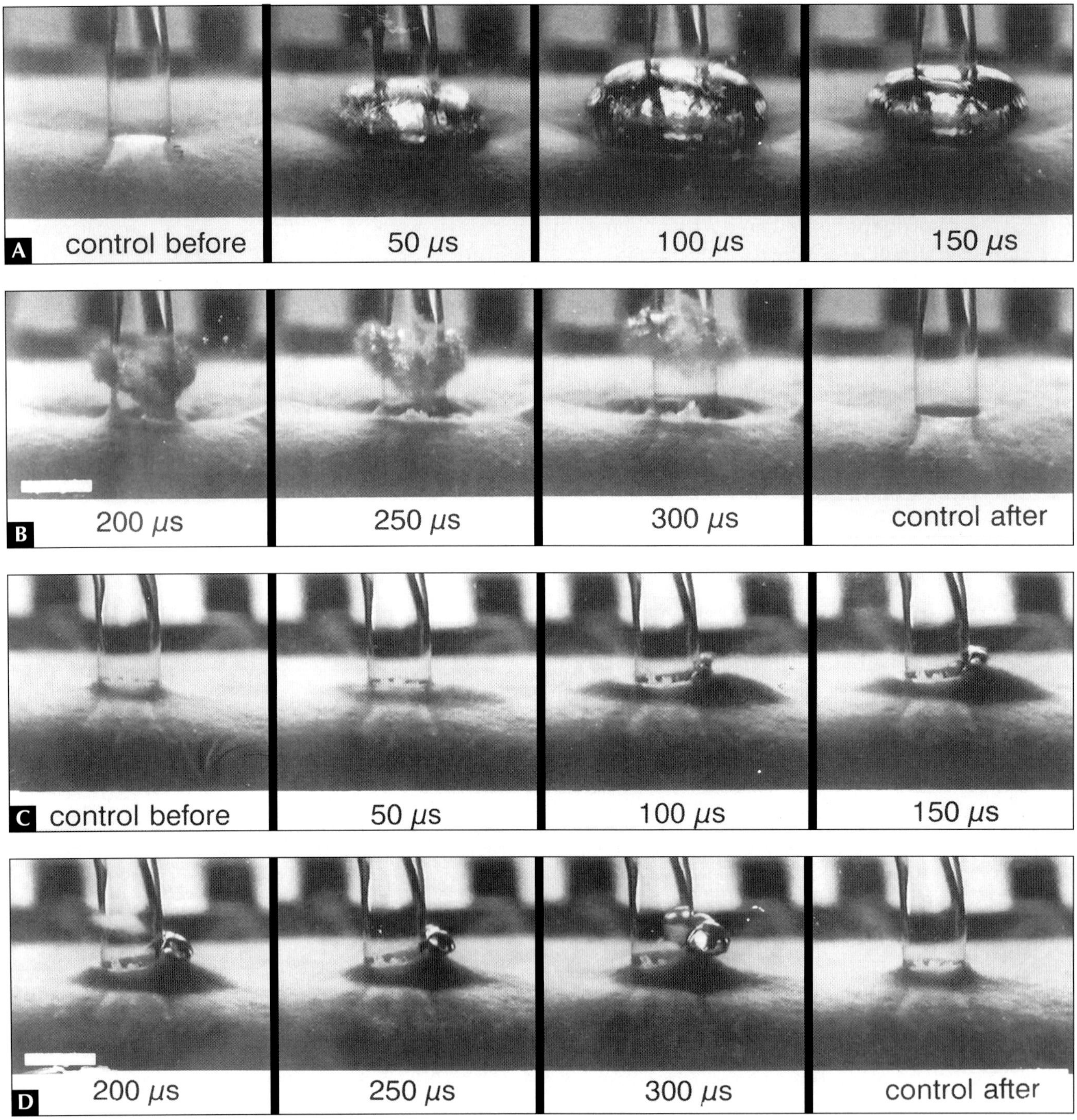

Figure 11-5. Time-lapse photographs of the interaction between a 34 mJ (53 mJ/mm^2) excimer laser pulse in light contact mode (**A** and **B**) and with the 900-μm diameter fiber tip buried in the porcine aorta as a result of force contact (0.1 N) (**C** and **D**) (*Bar* indicates 1 mm.) (*From* Van Leeuwen and colleagues [5]; with permission.)

the short pulse duration—too short for surrounding tissue burning, but long enough for vaporization of water. This mechanism results in fast-expanding and imploding vapor bubbles forming within 250 μs after each pulse, accompanied by shock waves that cause damage of the vascular wall [5] (Fig. 11-5). Histology of the tissue samples of the in vitro studies on porcine aorta showed dissections of the intima and media, presumably caused by dilation of fast-expanding bubbles. Experiments in rabbit femoral and iliac arteries demonstrated that fast expanding and imploding vapor bubbles caused microsecond dilation and invagination of the adjacent vascular wall [12••] (Fig. 11-6). Histology showed extensive damage to the vascular wall and smooth muscle cell necrosis. The threshold energy density for fast-expanding bubble formation in porcine aorta appeared to be 20 mJ/mm^2. This finding indicates that fast-expanding bubble formation will most likely occur at energy densities used in the clinical setting (40 to 60 mJ/mm^2).

In addition, ablation of organic polymers by ultraviolet radiation is usually attributed to photochemical dissociation of the molecular bonds by ultraviolet photons. Due to the absorption of the photon energy, large molecules are divided into smaller components or in insoluble gas [13]. It was demonstrated that ultraviolet light was highly absorbed by blood and that, in particular, lipids of cell membranes were responsible for insoluble gas formation. Based on these findings, investigators considered that fast-expanding vapor bubble and insoluble gas formation together are responsible for damage of the vascular wall and, consequently, for the formation of dissections during excimer laser angioplasty. It was demonstrated that the mechanical distension of the vessel was a potent stimulus for smooth muscle cell proliferation as well as for an increased vasomotor tone contributing to restenosis or vasospasm. Furthermore, previous experiments using balloon angioplasty in a swine model demonstrated that the extent of vessel wall injury during the intervention was correlated with the degree of subsequent neointimal thickening [14]. Consequently, the higher restenosis rate after excimer laser angioplasty in the clinical randomized studies may be the result of such an exaggerated neointimal response.

Future Perspectives

These new insights in the mechanism of tissue interactions during excimer laser treatment have led to refinements in the technique to reduce the vascular wall damage. *In vitro* studies demonstrated a marked reduction of vapor bubble formation and pressure waves generated by laser ablation due to the hemodilution or replacement of blood with saline. Based on these results, a "flush and bathe" technique was advocated in order to replace blood and contrast medium with saline in the ablation field. Recently the initial results of a randomized study reported a remarkable reduction in the dissection rate following excimer laser

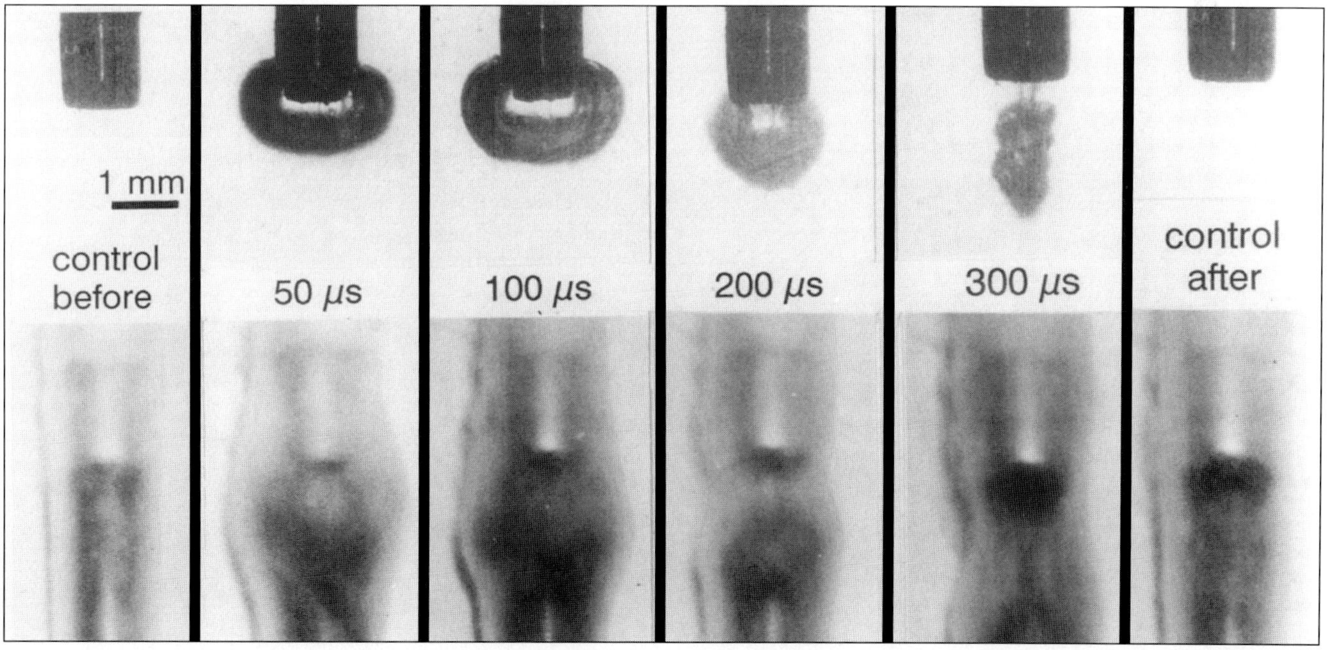

Figure 11-6. Time-resolved flash photographs of bubble expansion and implosion in hemoglobin solution (16% wt/vol) (*top*) and in *in vivo* microsecond dilation and invagination of the rabbit femoral artery (*bottom panel*). Output energy of 3.5-F multifiber catheter was 9 to 9.5 mJ per pulse (55 to 60 mJ/mm^2). The catheter tip and guidewire are visible through the arterial wall. (*From* Van Leeuwen and colleagues [12••]; with permission.)

angioplasty. However, the application of this saline technique was hampered by adequate removal of blood from the ablation site [8].

The use of lower energy densities during excimer laser angioplasty reduces the production of insoluble gas and, consequently, may reduce the quantity of vascular wall damage (Fig. 11-7) [15]. However, the production of fast-expanding and imploding vapor bubbles, the main cause of vascular wall damage, will still be present at energy densities of more than 20 mJ/mm^2 used in a clinical setting for effective tissue ablation.

Another approach for reduction of vascular wall damage is the concept of "multiplexing", or "smooth" ELCA. The principle is based on a sequential activation of catheter sections of the multifiber laser catheter to decrease the pulse energy at the same fluence. As a result, the overall size of the fast expanding and imploding vapor bubbles is reduced, which may reduce vascular wall damage. This technique is currently under investigation [16].

The currently used multifiber catheters in ELCA consist of a certain quantity of dead space between the fibers that is still present during activation at the level of the catheter–tissue interface. However, in vitro it was demonstrated that an increase of the beam diameter resulted in an increase of ablation efficacy. Thus, a modified laser catheter tip was constructed consisting of a laser catheter with a flat polished distal tip and a silica window in order to diffuse the light arising from the fibers. This resulted in an increased effective ablation area with a homogeneous light distribution at the window–tissue interface. In vitro experiments on porcine aorta immersed in saline demonstrated that the average ablation efficacy increased using the modified catheter with limited damage to the surrounding tissue as analyzed by electron microscopic control. The investigators concluded that homogeneous light distribution not only improves ablation efficacy, but also reduces damage to the vascular wall at a fluence well below the threshold for fast-expanding bubble formation. Nevertheless, at present, this modified laser catheter is only available for in vitro experiments [17].

Current laser angioplasty is limited to treatment of coronary lesions that can be crossed with a guidewire. The recent introduction of fiberoptic guidewires for primary laser recanalization of chronic total occlusions may expand the applications of the current laser angioplasty technology for other indications than evaluated in the clinical randomized trials. At present, a multicenter randomized clinical trial is being conducted to establish the role of this new device.

CONCLUSIONS

In conclusion, the results of the reported randomized clinical trials demonstrated no beneficial effect of excimer laser angioplasty compared with balloon angioplasty in the treatment of complex coronary lesions. Recent insights from *in vitro* and experimental studies require further careful clinical testing in order to define the role of excimer laser angioplasty for percutaneous coronary revascularization.

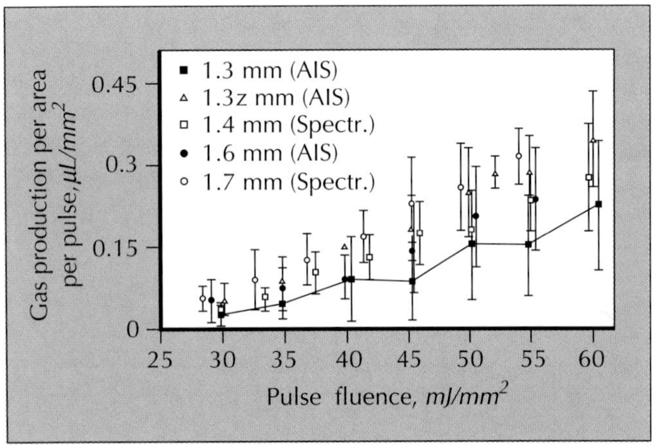

Figure 11-7. Relationship between gas production per fiber of cross-sectional area and energy fluence of the different sized laser catheters. Measurements are of porcine aortic tissue immersed in saline. The data are expressed as mean values ± SD. AIS—Advanced Interventional Systems, Irvine, CA; Spectr.— Spectranetics, Colorado Springs, CO.(*From* Appelman and colleagues [15]; with permission.)

REFERENCES AND RECOMMENDED READING

Recently published papers of particular interest have been highlighted as:
- • Of special interest
- •• Of outstanding interest

1. Grundfest WS, Litvack F, Forrester JS, *et al.*: Laser ablation of human atherosclerotic plaque without adjacent tissue injury. *J Am Coll Cardiol* 1985, 5:929–933.

2. Litvack F, Grundfest WS, Goldenberg T, *et al.*: Percutaneous excimer laser angioplasty of aortocoronary saphenous vein grafts. *J Am Coll Cardiol* 1989, 14:803–808.

3.•• Appelman YEA, Piek JJ, Strikwerda S, *et al.*: Randomised trial of excimer laser angioplasty versus balloon angioplasty for treatment of obstructive coronary artery disease. *Lancet* 1996, 347:79–84.

The final results of the clinical and angiographic outcome of the first randomized trial comparing excimer laser angioplasty with balloon angioplasty in long coronary lesions.

4.• Litvack F, Eigler N, Margolis J, for the ELCA investigators: Percutaneous excimer laser coronary angioplasty results in the first consecutive 3,000 patients. *J Am Coll Cardiol* 1994, 23:323–329.

The results of prospective nonrandomized registries demonstrating the safety and efficacy of excimer laser angioplasty in complex coronary lesions.

5. Van Leeuwen TG, Meertens JH, Valema E, *et al.*: Intraluminal vapor bubble induced by excimer laser pulse causes microsecond arterial dilation and invagination leading to extensive wall damage in the rabbit. *Circulation* 1993, 87:1258–1263.

6. Baumbach A, Oswald H, Kvasnicka J, and the coinvestigators of the European Coronary Excimer Laser Angioplasty Registry: Clinical results of coronary excimer laser angioplasty: report from the European Coronary Excimer Laser Angioplasty Registry. *Eur Heart J* 1994, 15:89–96.

7. Appelman YEA, Koolen JJ, Piek JJ, *et al.*: Excimer laser angioplasty versus balloon angioplasty in functional and total coronary occlusions. *Am J Cardiol* 1996, in press.

8. Deckelbaum LI, Natarajan MK, Bittl JA, for the Percutaneous Excimer Laser Coronary Angioplasty Investigators: Effect of intracoronary saline infusion on dissection during excimer laser coronary angioplasty: a randomized trial. *J Am Coll Cardiol* 1995, 26:1264–1269.

9. Vandormael M, Reifart N, Preusler W, *et al.*: Immediate and 6 month follow-up outcomes following excimer laser angioplasty, rotational atherectomy and balloon angioplasty for complex lesions: ERBAC randomized study [abstract]. *Eur Heart J* 1994;829A.

10. Larrazet FS, Dupouy PJ, Rande Dubois JL, Hirosaka A, Kvasnicka J, Geschwind HJ: Angioscopy after laser and balloon coronary angioplasty. *J Am Coll Cardiol* 1994, 23:1321–1326.

11. Honye J, Mahon DJ, Nakamura S, *et al.*: Intravascular ultrasound imaging after excimer laser angioplasty. *Cathet Cardiovasc Diagn* 1994;32:213-222.

12.•• Van Leeuwen TG, Meertens JH, Velema E, *et al.*: Intraluminal vapor bubble induced by excimer laser pulse causes microsecond arterial dilation and invagination leading to extensive wall damage in the rabbit. *Circulation* 1993, 87:1258–1263.

An *in vivo* experimental study showing the intraluminal vapor bubble formation after excimer laser pulse, inducing microsecond dilation and invagination of the adjacent arterial segment and causing dissections and extensive vascular wall damage.

13. Gijsbers GHM, Van den Broecke DG, Sprangers RLH, Van Gemert MJC: Effect of force on ablation depth for a XeCl excimer laser beam delivered by an optical fiber in contact with arterial tissue under saline. *Lasers Surg Med* 1992, 12:576–584.

14. Schwartz RS, Huber KC, Murphy JG, *et al.*: Restenosis and the proportional neointimal response to coronary artery injury. *J Am Coll Cardiol* 1992, 19:276–275.

15. Appelman YEA, Piek JJ, Verhoofstad GGAM, *et al.*: Tissue ablation and gas formation of two excimer laser systems: an in vitro evaluation on porcine aorta. *Lasers Surg Med* 1996, 18:197–205.

16. Xie DY, Hassenstein S, Oberhoff M, *et al.*: In vitro evaluation of ablation parameters of normal and fibrous aorta using smooth excimer laser coronary angioplasty. *Lasers Surg Med* 1993, 13:618–624.

17. Hamburger JN, Gijsbers GHM, Verhoofstad GGAM, *et al.*: Excimer laser coronary angioplasty: a physical perspective to clinical results. In *Current Review of Interventional Cardiology*, edn. 2 Edited by Topol EJ, Serruys PW. Philadelphia: Current Medicine; 1995:159–172.

Chapter 12

Homogeneous Light Distribution and High-Density Laser Techniques in Excimer Laser Coronary Angioplasty

Geert H.M. Gijsbers
Jaap N. Hamburger
Patrick W. Serruys

Excimer laser coronary angioplasty (ELCA) is used as a debulking method for stenosed coronary arteries. Prior to its clinical introduction in 1988, it was shown that a free xenon chloride (XeCl) excimer laser beam focused in air was able to remove tissue very accurately without substantial injury to adjacent tissue [1–3]. This finding led to the development of clinically usable XeCl laser systems that employ catheters with a silica fiberoptic bundle to guide the laser beam to the arteriosclerotic plaque.

Although thousands of patients have been treated with these laser systems and catheters [4–7,8•], the results show that the method does not yield a clear clinical advantage over the "gold standard" of coronary balloon angioplasty. ELCA was shown to debulk only a limited amount of plaque [9], is associated with major dissection formation and the occurrence of a ragged vessel wall [4,7,9–11], and does not result in a better clinical outcome [7,8•]. The reason for the limited debulking and the damage done to the coronary vessel wall is believed to be the formation of fast expanding water vapor bubbles and insoluble gas in a liquid environment in the confined space of a stenosed coronary artery [12•,13]. It is assumed that the expansion of the water vapor and gas disrupts tissue cells and structures, and that this very mechanism is responsible for tissue ablation. In the open-air experiments mentioned previously, the vapors and debris were unhampered and could escape out of the region of beam incidence, resulting in smooth crater walls. However, in a coronary artery, the fast expanding and collapsing bubbles (or "fast bubbles") are created in soft tissue [12•,13,14] and in blood and contrast media [14,15]. When a laser catheter contacts the atherosclerotic plaque, the fast bubble will forcefully find its way between the catheter tip and the adjacent tissue. This results in a fast dilatation and invagination of both the tissue and the coronary vessel wall, leading to microdissections in the tissue directly surrounding the catheter tip. Because hemoglobin and iodine-containing contrast media are strong absorbers of 308-nm ultraviolet light of the XeCl excimer laser, this process is strongly enhanced in the presence of blood or contrast medium.

As a result of photochemical dissociation, many microliters of insoluble gas are created in the coronary artery during ELCA [12•,16,17]. This gas is believed to enhance dissections created by fast bubbles and to further mechanically dilate a stenosed artery. This dilation could cause the catheter to cross past a lesion, but at the same time would reduce the amount of material that will be ablated because it will be displaced outside the laser beam that is emitted from a catheter.

The introduction of saline flush to ELCA has contributed to a reduction of dissection rate and severity. A bolus of saline that is injected into the region of the distal laser catheter tip removes the blood and contrast medium prior to the application of laser pulses, thus reducing the forceful expansion of vapor in blood and contrast medium. This technique results in fewer dissections during ELCA [18•]. Further reduction of adverse side effects of ELCA could possibly be obtained by weakening the force of fast bubbles and gas yield. This could be achieved by reducing the pulse energy density [12•,13,17].

However, experiments on porcine aorta showed that tissue penetration is not possible with current multifiber catheters at low pulse energy densities (*eg*, 30 mJ/mm^2). This observation was attributed to the dead space between individual fibers in a multifiber catheter, where there is no overlap of light at the catheter tip–tissue interface. Furthermore, there is a large non-light–emitting area at the catheter tip at the position of the guidewire lumen and the area outside the circular fiber bundle. As a result, the progression of a multifiber catheter is halted at low energy densities because of nonablated tissue remnants. Only at higher energy densities (≥ 50 mJ/mm^2) is the impact of the fast bubble great enough to remove tissue at the position of the dead space to allow the catheter to penetrate the tissue. However, the higher energy densities typically cause damage to the tissue directly surrounding the area of ablation [12•].

Preliminary experiments have shown that when XeCl excimer laser light from a multifiber catheter was homogenized at the catheter tip by means of a silica window (Fig. 12-1), it was possible to remove tissue at a very low pulse energy density (≈ 8 mJ/mm^2) with virtually no collateral damage to the adjacent tissue [12•]. Although these experiments were performed using only a limited number of pulses, we hypothesized that by using a beam delivery device with a homogeneous light distribution (HLD), vascular tissue can be ablated efficiently at low energy densities with a reduction of insoluble gas formation and fast bubble size. Further tests in our laboratory, using bare fibers that have an intrinsic HLD at the tip, have indeed proven that effective tissue penetration is possible at pulse energy densities as low as 10 mJ/mm^2.

Because part of the dead space of a catheter is positioned inside and outside the bundle of fibers, it is not clear whether the space between the individual fibers or the combined effect of all dead space is responsible for the inability to penetrate tissue at low energy densities. This problem has been investigated using test devices that are closely packed with fibers, leaving no dead space except the space between the fibers and the necessary thin outer coating. These devices are called *high-density* (HD) devices.

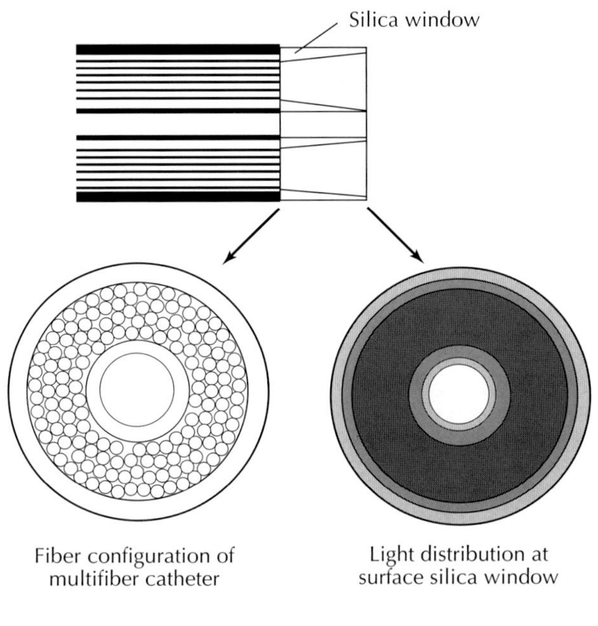

Figure 12-1. Method used to homogenize the light distribution emitted from a multifiber catheter. A silica window was mounted provisionally on top of a multifiber catheter. Light that was emitted from individual fibers overlapped at the surface of the window due to a slight divergence, thus creating a near homogeneous light distribution (HLD).

This chapter compares the performance of a standard multifiber laser catheter, an HLD device, and an HD device in terms of penetration capability and speed, insoluble gas yield and occurrence, and size of fast bubbles. The results of this comparison will indicate whether an HLD or an HD catheter offers a benefit compared with the currently used multifiber catheters.

Materials and Methods

The different test devices are shown in Figure 12-2. A 1.4-mm multifiber catheter (Spectranetics Vitesse-C; Spectranetics, Colorado Springs, CO) was used over a piece of 0.014-in guidewire pierced through the test tissue. The HLD device was a 1-mm bare fiber; the HD device was a circular bundle of closely packed fibers held together by epoxy and surrounded by a polyimide coating, also with a total outer diameter of 1 mm. A Spectranetics CVX-300 XeCl excimer laser (Spectranetics, Colorado Springs, CO), emitting a wavelength of 308 nm with a pulse repetition rate of 25 Hz, was used in all experiments.

The measurements of the advancement of the devices through tissue and the recording of fast bubbles were performed in the set-up shown in Figure 12-3*A*. Figure 12-3*B* shows the device used to measure the yields of insoluble gas generated by the laser pulses. All experiments were performed on fresh porcine aortic tissue immersed in saline.

Results

Advancement Capability and Efficiency

Figure 12-4 shows the advancement of the devices through fresh porcine aorta as a function of pulse energy density at the device tips. The advancement was determined from the linear movement of a device into the tissue during the application of a laser pulse train. This linear movement lasted until the porcine aorta was perforated or until no further device advancement was observed. To apply the same pressure on the devices, 10-g weights were added to the HLD and HD devices; an 18-g weight was added to the 1.4-mm catheter. In all cases, laser pulses at 25 HZ were given until the porcine aortic tissue was perforated or until no further device advancement was observed.

The 1.4-mm multifiber catheter was not able to perforate the porcine aortic wall at a pulse energy density of 30 mJ/mm^2. Although the catheter started to penetrate the tissue, it halted in the upper parts of the tissue. At 45 mJ/mm^2, the catheter was able to cross the medial layer but was often halted by the adventitial layer. At 60 mJ/mm^2, the catheter perforated the porcine aortic tissue sample very efficiently.

In contrast to the catheter, both the HLD and the HD devices were able to completely perforate the aortic tissue once advancement was observed. The minimum energy densities needed for device advancement were approximately 10 mJ/mm^2 for the HLD device and approximately 20 mJ/mm^2 for the HD device,

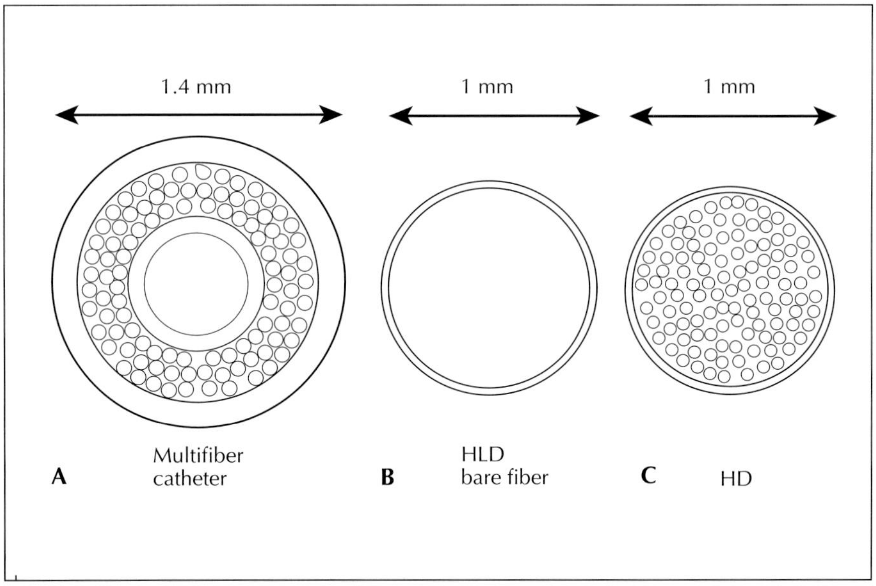

Figure 12-2. Test excimer laser coronary angioplasty (ELCA) beam delivery devices. **A**, This 1.4-mm multifiber catheter (Spectranetics Prima laser catheter; Spectranetics, Colorado Springs, CO) represents a standard ELCA catheter. It contains 96 fibers (diameter, 61 μm) grouped in a circle around the guidewire lumen, with a total light-emitting area of 0.28 mm^2. **B**, The homogenous light distribution (HLD) device is a single fiber with a light-emitting diameter of 0.9 mm (total light-emitting area, 0.64 mm^2) and an outer diameter of 0.99 mm (the outer diameter is due to the layers of lower index of refraction around the fiber). **C**, A similar-sized high-density (HD) device, containing 110 fibers of 61-μm diameter (total light-emitting area, 0.32 mm^2), with a total outer diameter of 1.0 mm and a light-emitting diameter of 0.9 mm.

which for both devices corresponded to a pulse energy of about 6.4 mJ per pulse.

Insoluble Gas Yield

The gas yields per unit of light-emitting area and per pulse as a function of pulse energy density are shown in Figure 12-5. The yields are presented in this way to enable swift comparison of the yields of the different devices. The gas yield per pulse was determined over the number of pulses in which a linear increase of gas volume during the application of a pulse train was present. Usually the gas production was abruptly halted or sharply decreased when the device perforated the tissue or was halted inside the tissue at too low an energy density.

It would be reasonable to expect that the gas yield per unit of area per pulse of all devices is the same at the same energy density, because every unit of area that is receiving light experiences the same amount of ultraviolet (UV) photons. However, this was not the case for the HLD and the HD devices. The gas yield per unit area of the HLD device was smaller than the yield of the HD device, both in the overlapping energy density range and at the minimum energy densities at which device penetration occurs (≈ 10 mJ/mm^2 for the HLD device and ≈ 20 mJ/mm^2 for the HD device). The

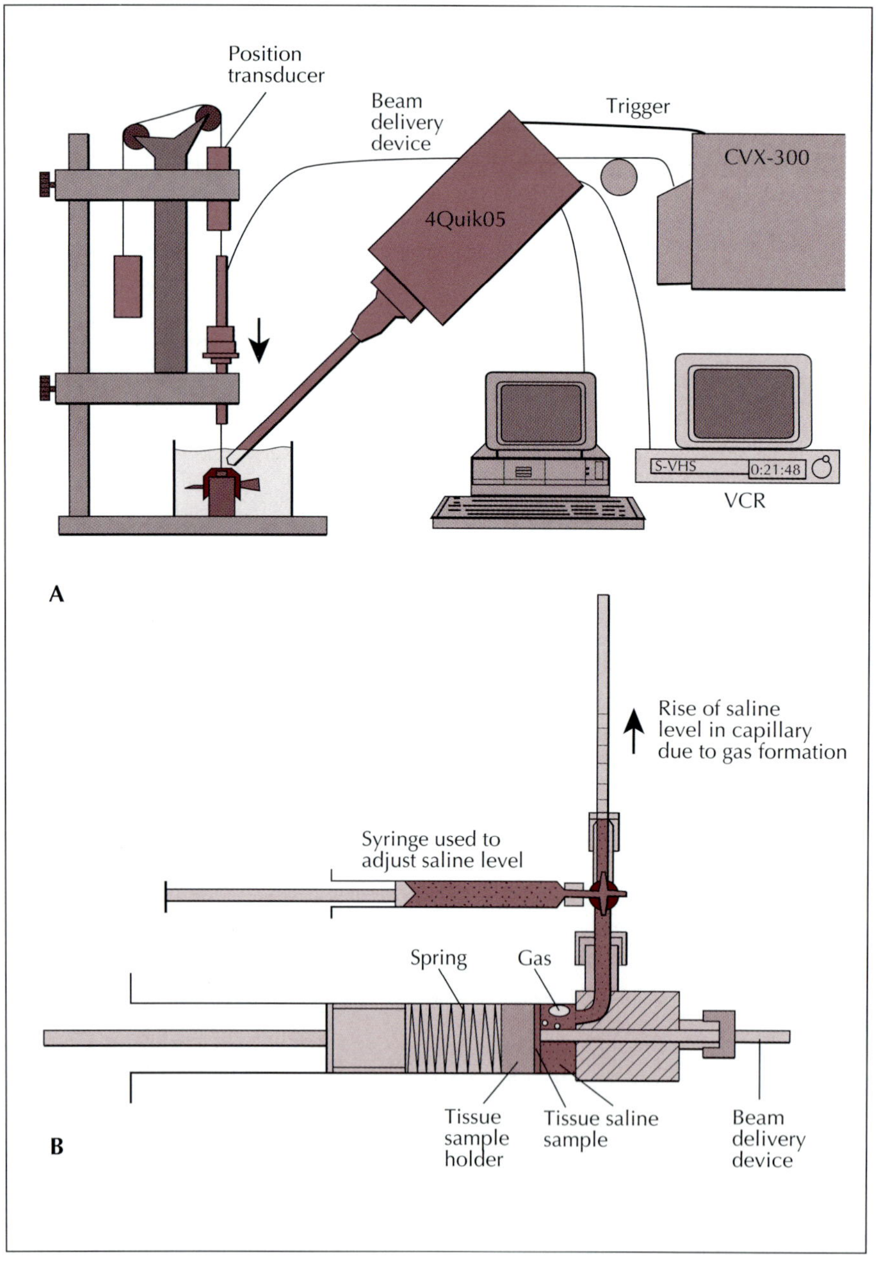

Figure 12-3. A, Set-up to record the advancement of a light-delivery device through a tissue sample and to visualize fast-expanding bubbles. In the device on the left, a beam-delivery device was mounted in a shaft. The device delivered pulses from the CVX-300 (Spectranetics, Colorado Springs, CO) excimer laser.Weights could be added to the shaft to control the pressure of the delivery device onto the tissue. The downward movement of the shaft during application of laser pulses was recorded by means of a position transducer. An image of the fast bubbles generated at the tip of a delivery device was obtained by an intensified CCD camera (4Quik05; Stanford Computer Optics, Palo Alto, CA) and a borescope. The mounted borescope enabled close-up imaging in the saline environment. The exposure time of the image intensifier was set to 5 μs to "time-freeze" the movement of the fast bubble. The delay time between the laser trigger to the camera and the moment of exposure was always set to a time (typically 40 μs) where the expansion of the fast bubble was maximal, as found in test experiments. **B**, Gas measurement set-up. Gas was created by laser pulses delivered by a device in contact with a tissue sample in a closed saline environment. The gas caused a rise of the saline level in the capillary proportional to the gas volume increase. A spring was used to adjust the pressure of the delivery device onto the tissue. VCR—video cassette recorder.

gas yield of the HD device was similar to the gas yield of the 1.4-mm catheter at an energy density greater than 40 mJ/mm^2. The very low gas yield of the 1.4-mm catheter at 30 mJ/mm^2 may be caused by the dynamics of tissue removal under individual fibers at the catheter tip. After the first few pulses, tissue under the individual fibers has been ablated, but the tissue bridges between fibers impede advancement of the tip. Interaction between light emitted from the fiber and fresh tissue is diminished, with consequent decrease in gas formation.

The low gas yield of the HLD device at approximately 30 mJ/mm^2 could be due to the fact that tissue in front of the tip was torn very effectively, leading to efficient penetration but not enough to cause ablation with accompanying gas yield.

To estimate the total gas yield for future HLD or HD catheters, we assumed that the gas yields per unit of area for such devices would be the same as the yields for the 1-mm HLD and HD devices, as shown in Figure 12-5. It was assumed that the catheters would have an outer diameter of 1.4 mm and a guidewire lumen with an inner diameter of 0.5 mm. The HLD catheter was assumed to exhibit a homogeneous light–emitting area between these diameters, with a total light-emitting area of 1.34 mm^2. The HD catheter was assumed to be filled with 61-μm fibers between the diameters. The total light-emitting area of 0.67 mm^2 of this device was taken to be half the area of the corresponding HLD device, as was the case with the 1-mm devices shown in Figure 12-2. The gas yields per pulse as a function of energy density (calculated

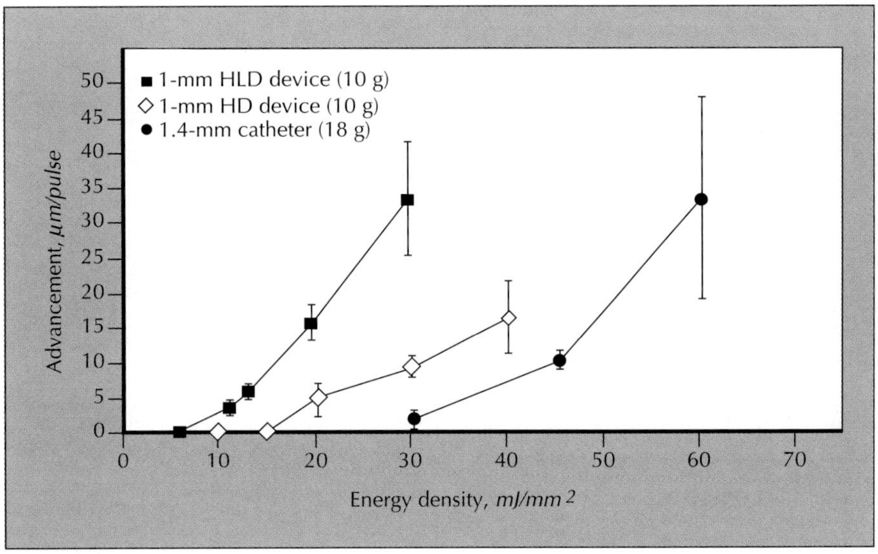

Figure 12-4. Advancement as a function of pulse energy density for the 1.4-mm catheter and the homogeneous light distribution (HLD) and high-density (HD) devices. (*T-bars* indicate ± SD [*n* = 10].)

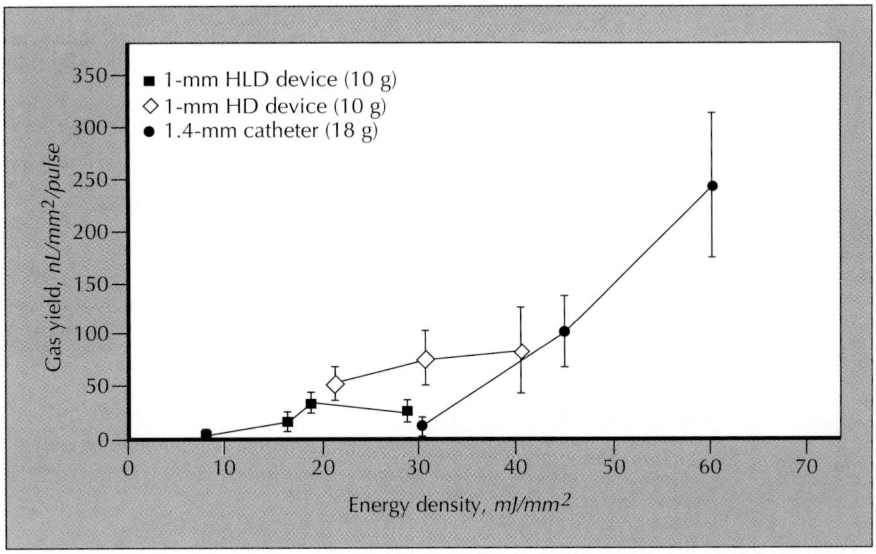

Figure 12-5. Gas yield per unit of emitting area per pulse as a function of pulse energy density for the 1.4-mm catheter and the homogenous light distribution (HLD) and high-density (HD) devices. (*T-bars* indicate ± SD [*n* = 10].)

from the data in Figure 12-5), are also shown in Figure 12-6. This graph illustrates that only the HLD catheter used at energy densities less than 15 mJ/mm^2 would lead to a substantially reduced gas yield per pulse as compared with the gas yield of a standard catheter at energy densities used clinically.

Fast Bubbles

Figure 12-7 presents the maximum bubble radii of the different devices as a function of energy density. It is obvious that all devices exhibit fast bubbles that expand considerably outside the circumference of the devices, even at pulse energy densities that are considered to be below the single pulse threshold for water vaporization ($\approx$ 20 mJ/mm^2) [13]. These bubbles are attributed to accumulation of heat generated by individual fibers with energy densities lower than the threshold. After a pulse, not all heat is diffused before the next pulse arrives. Several pulses can generate temperatures of up to 100°C. This heat will result in the instant formation of water vapor and, therefore, a fast bubble. Note that generation of insoluble gas was observed immediately after the first laser pulse, even at the lowest pulse energy densities that were used in this study.

Although fast bubbles could be observed at any pulse energy density where device advancement was seen, there was a qualitative difference between the effects of the bubbles at low energy densities and high energy densities. With the 1.4-mm catheter, the fast bubble lifted tissue lying flush against the circumference of the advancing catheter at 45 or 60 mJ/mm^2. This effect was absent with the HLD and HD devices at 10 and 20 mJ/mm^2, respectively. Although fast

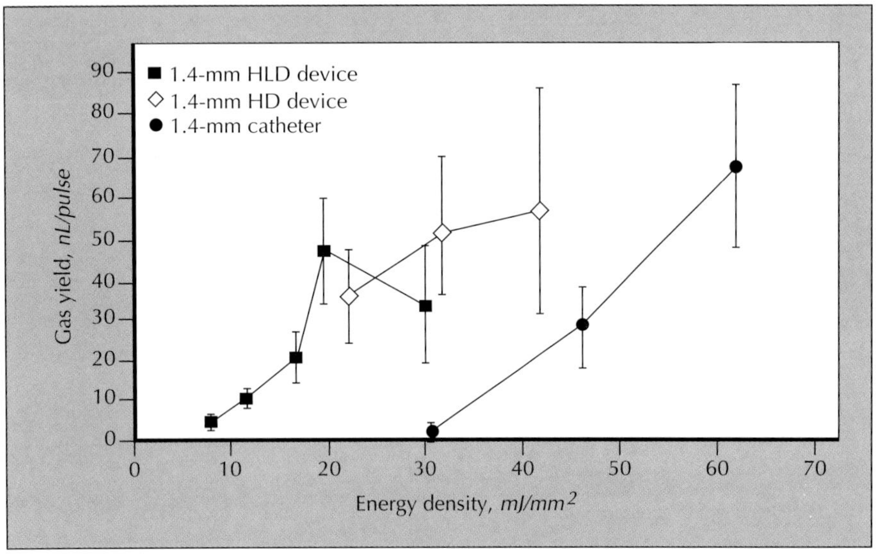

Figure 12-6. Gas yields per pulse as a function of pulse energy density for hypothetical homogenous light distribution (HLD) and high-density (HD) catheters together with the gas yield for a standard 1.4-mm catheter. The results are calculated from the results given in Figure 12-5 using light-emitting areas of 1.34 mm^2 for the HLD device, 0.67 mm^2 for the HD device, and 0.28 mm^2 for the 1.4-mm catheter.

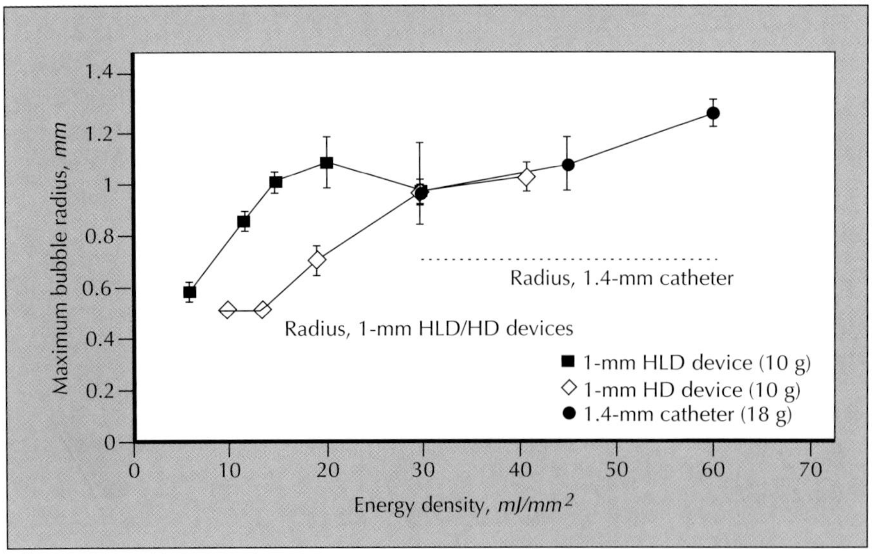

Figure 12-7. Maximum radii of fast bubbles as a function of pulse energy density for the 1.4-mm catheter and the homogeneous light distribution (HLD) and high-density (HD) devices. (*T-bars* indicate ± SD [*n* = 10].)

bubbles were seen here, they did not seem to be strong enough to lift the tissue: the bubbles simply moved over the surface without any visible mechanical effect on the tissue. At higher energy densities, the fast bubbles generated by the HLD and HD devices became more violent, and mechanical damage of the crater edges was observed.

As indicated previously, many pulses may be needed before a fast bubble is observed. Figure 12-8 shows the number of pulses needed to observe a fast bubble after the start of a pulse train at 25 Hz on fresh porcine aorta. The number of pulses needed to start penetration of a device under the same conditions are also given in these graphs.

As can be expected, the number of pulses required to start both fast bubble formation and tissue penetration decreased with increasing pulse energy density. Remarkably, however, in all cases it took more pulses to start penetration than to start fast bubble formation. This might indicate that the formation of expanding water vapor is a vital ingredient in the process of tissue penetration.

The fact that the tissue penetration was always lagging behind the occurrence of fast bubbles indicates that fast bubbles will always be present during ELCA, and will always cause some strain in the surrounding tissue. However, as mentioned previously, the fast bubbles did not inflict observable damage at the lowest energy densities at which tissue advancement was possible with the HLD and HD devices.

Discussion

It has been shown that device penetration is always accompanied by fast bubbles, because the advancement of any beam delivery device invariably follows the occurrence of fast bubbles, whereas insoluble gas formation is always seen to begin with the very first pulse in a pulse train.

Although part of the tissue components are weakened by photochemical decomposition, this process obviously is not sufficient to overcome the mechanical integrity of the tissue. This can only be done by the fast bubble, which disrupts and removes the tissue by its expansion. With current multifiber laser catheters, energy densities of 50 to 60 mJ/mm^2 had to be used to fully perforate fresh porcine aortic wall immersed in saline. Only at these energy densities were the mechanical effects strong enough to remove all tissue in front of the catheter to allow penetration—but with the consequence of violently tearing the tissue surrounding the catheter.

For a 1-mm single-fiber HLD device, a minimal pulse energy density of 10 mJ/mm^2 is sufficient to accomplish tissue penetration. For a fully packed 1-mm HD device, a minimal pulse energy density of 20 mJ/mm^2 is needed. The light-emitting area of the HLD device is twice the light-emitting area of the HD device; thus both energy densities represent the same total pulse energy.

These results show that the dead space between the fibers of the HD device requires a higher energy density under each fiber, compared with the HLD device, to allow the device to penetrate. This concept may be applied to current laser catheters, which have even more dead space between fibers than the HD device, as well as additional dead space at the outer rim and the guidewire rim. Our data have shown that an even greater energy density is needed under each fiber to overcome the tissue impediment implied by these dead spaces.

Although the pulse energy density needed for tissue penetration of the 1-mm HD device is twice the pulse energy density needed for the penetration of the 1-mm HLD device, the effects of fast bubbles are the same in both devices. At the lowest possible energy densities, the size of the bubbles and the times needed to start fast bubble formation and penetration are very similar for both devices.

Gas yields for both devices are not similar. As indicated in Figure 12-6, the gas yield of the HD device at 20 mJ/mm^2 is more than three times as large as the gas yield of the HD device at 10 mJ/mm^2.

Gas formation may enhance the deleterious effects of the fast bubble. In our experiments it was often observed that during penetration of the devices, the surface of the tissue is lifted like the inflation of a balloon. This effect was strongest with the 1.4-mm catheter. This process, which is attributed to the gas that accumulates around the device tips, can create severe effects. Often gas can be seen to escape from the tissue several millimeters away from the position of the device. The gas is able to disrupt the tissue layers away from the place where tissue removal is desired. As already stated, the adverse effects of insoluble gas are predicted to be smallest when using an HLD device at 10 mJ/mm^2, but even in this situation gas is observed to affect the tissue surrounding the fiber tip.

There are other effects of gas. In the video recordings made to measure the sizes of the fast bubbles, it was noted that when a pulse train was applied after the removal of a device, the resulting crater was usually smaller than the diameter of the device at the surface. Close examination of our video recordings of the penetration of the different devices revealed that after penetration of the devices into the tissue, the deeper part of the crater was much smaller in diameter than the device diameter. This effect was most pronounced with the 1.4-mm catheter, where the upper part of the crater also was considerably smaller than the catheter

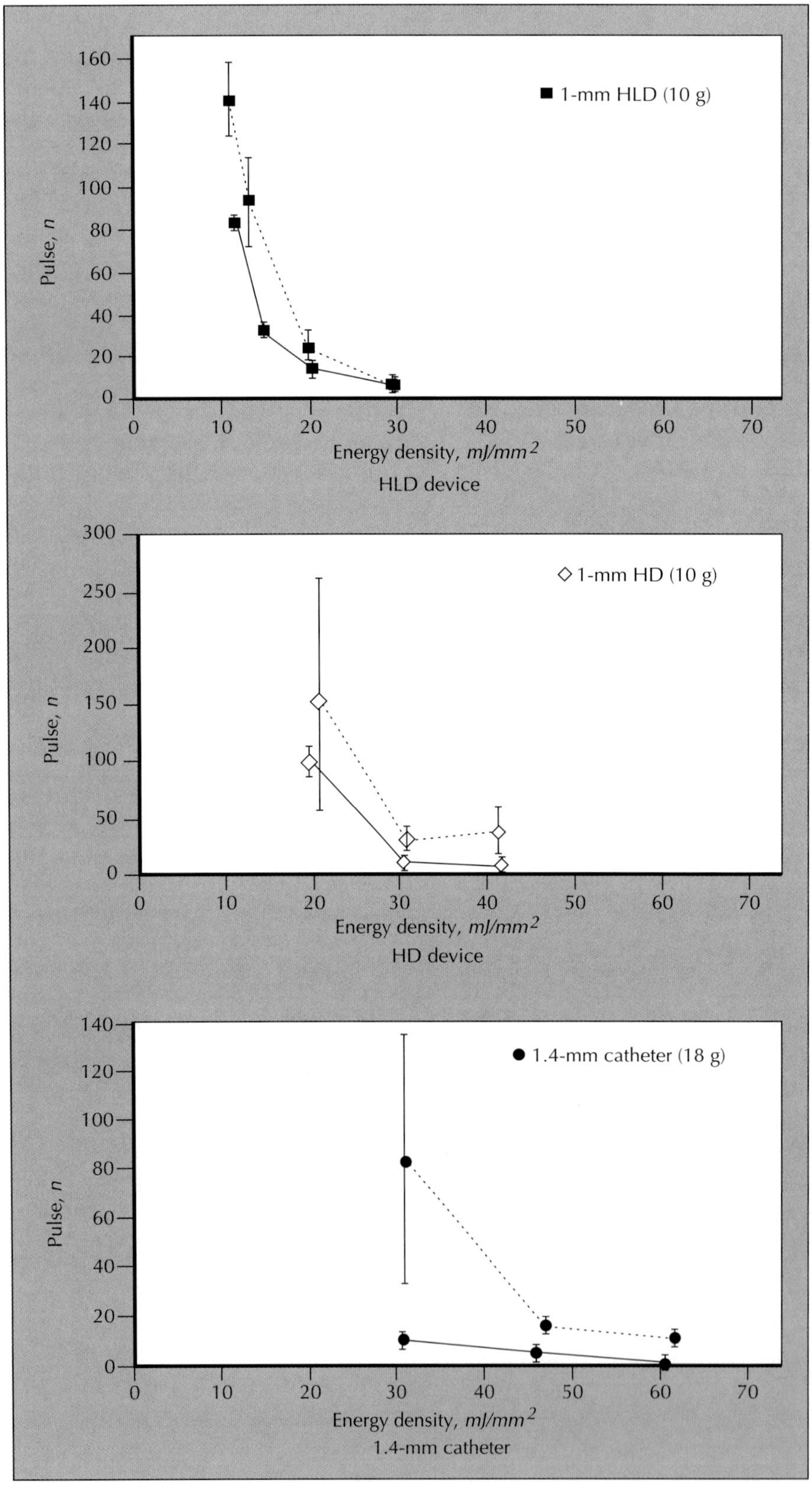

Figure 12-8. The number of pulses needed to start fast bubble formation (*solid lines*) and the number of pulses needed to start device penetration (*dashed lines*) as functions of pulse energy density. (*T-bars* indicate ± SD [*n* = 10].)

diameter. Further, these deeper parts had a ragged appearance.

We hypothesize that this effect is caused by the entrapment of the gas at the tip of the catheter. Once the fast bubble opens (or tears) the tissue, the gas that is pushed forward by the continuous pressure on the device enhances any tear in the tissue made by a fast bubble. Also, the device tip itself pushes away tissue. This facilitates penetration but leads to incomplete ablation. This hypothesis led to the idea that as much gas as possible should be removed from the area between the device tip and the tissue.

Some preliminary experiments have been performed with the 1.4-mm catheter and the 1-mm HLD device. In these experiments, the gas was allowed to escape by continuously moving the device up and down while continuously applying laser pulses (at 25 Hz). Figure 12-9 shows the results with the 1.4-mm catheter at 50 mJ/mm^2 used over a piece of guidewire. The crater on the left is the result of a continuous pulse train with continuous pressure applied to the catheter. The crater on the right is the result of applying laser pulses while alternately touching and lifting the catheter. The diameter of the crater made without lifting is considerably smaller than the catheter diameter, and tissue is still present in the crater. This difference is due to the processes described previously. The crater on the right shows much more tissue removal, apart from the tissue plug around the guidewire, and is much larger in diameter. In the video recordings with the triggered intensified CCD camera, it was seen that a crater was formed slowly, and that the gas at the bottom of the crater was "blown away" by the laser pulses during the lifting of the catheter. The crater thus created was nearly the size of the diameter of the catheter. When the catheter touched the tissue as it was lowered, it was observed that fast bubbles immediately lifted the edge of the crater. This process is probably responsible for the ragged appearance of the crater on the right.

The craters in Figure 12-10 were created in a similar fashion using the 1-mm HLD device at 10 mJ/mm^2. Again, the crater on the left, made without lifting the device, is much smaller than the device itself, and a rim can be seen around the crater that may be due to the inflation of the trapped gas. The crater on the right was made while touching and lifting the device. The crater edge is very sharp, with hardly any observable collateral damage.

Fast bubbles were also seen when the device touched the tissue, but in contrast to the bubbles created by the catheter, they did not affect the tissue; thus the edge of the crater was sharp. Although these results are preliminary, they indicate that the back-and-forth technique leads to a more thorough debulking of the tissue and to further reduction of collateral damage with the HLD device.

Conclusions

Decreasing dead space in an XeCl excimer laser beam delivery device leads to a decrease in the pulse energy density needed to penetrate tissue, as compared with the energy density of 50 to 60 mJ/mm^2 needed with current multifiber catheters. Optimal packing of fibers (the HD approach) over the full area of the device decreased the necessary pulse energy density to 20

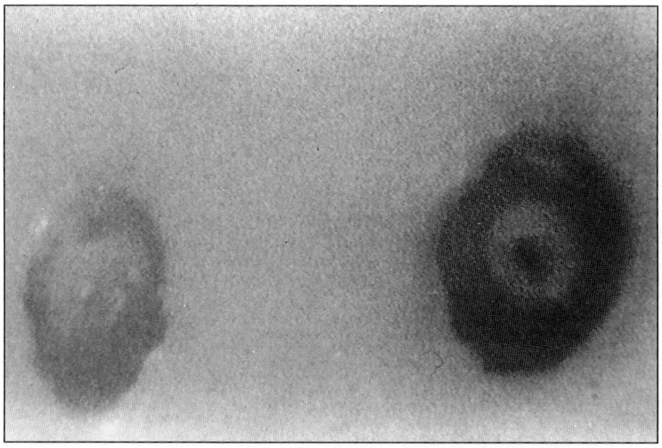

Figure 12-9. Craters made in porcine aortic tissue immersed in saline by means of a 1.4-mm laser catheter over a piece of 0.014-in guidewire pierced through the tissue. Laser pulse energy density was 50 mJ/mm^2, and laser pulses were applied at 25 Hz. **Left**, Continuous pulse train with constant pressure applied to the catheter. **Right**, continuous pulse train while the catheter was touching and lifting from the tissue.

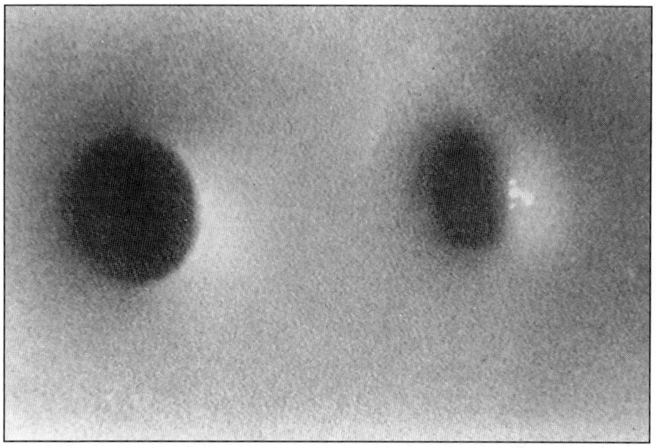

Figure 12-10. Craters made in porcine aortic tissue immersed in saline by means of a 1-mm homogenous light distribution (HLD) bare fiber. Laser pulse energy density was 10 mJ/mm^2, and laser pulses were applied at 25 Hz. **Left**, Continuous pulse train with constant pressure applied to the catheter. **Right**, Continuous pulse train while the catheter was touching and lifting from the tissue.

mJ/mm^2. A device having an HLD needs the smallest pulse energy density (10 mJ/mm^2). At these low energy densities, the effects of fast bubbles seem to be smaller than the effect of the bubbles generated by a standard laser catheter. In addition, the amount of insoluble gas was considerably smaller than the amount of gas created by the standard catheter.

We have seen that efficient removal of tissue is feasible at excimer laser pulse energy densities as low as 10 mJ/mm^2; however, even at this low energy density, tissue debulking is limited when the device is allowed to penetrate the tissue in one smooth motion. True debulking seems to be possible with any ELCA device only when a back-and-forth motion is used to allow gas to escape. This concept, which will affect catheter design and catheter employment techniques, needs to be addressed by further investigation.

ACKNOWLEDGMENTS

The authors express their gratitude to Sandjay Dhoenmoen for performing many of the experiments for this work. This work has in part been supported by a grant from the Dutch Sorbo Heart Foundation.

REFERENCES AND RECOMMENDED READING

Recently published papers of particular interest have been highlighted as:

- • Of special interest
- •• Of outstanding interest

1. Grundfest WS, Litvack IF, Goldenberg T, *et al.*: Pulsed ultraviolet lasers and the potential for safe laser angioplasty. *Am J Surg* 1985, 150:220–226.
2. Grundfest WS, Litvack IF, Forrester J, *et al.*: Laser ablation of human atherosclerotic plaque without adjacent tissue injury. *J Am Coll Cardiol* 1985, 5:929–933.
3. Litvack F, Grundfest WS, Goldenberg T, *et al.*: Pulsed laser angioplasty: wavelength power and energy dependencies relevant to clinical application. *Lasers Surg Med* 1988, 8:60–65.
4. Bittl JA, Sanborn TA, Tcheng JE, *et al.*: Clinical success, complications and restenosis rates with excimer laser angioplasty. *Am J Cardiol* 1992, 70:1533–1539.
5. Bittl JA, Sanborn TA: Excimer laser-facilitated coronary angioplasty: relative risk analysis of acute and follow-up results in 200 patients. *Circulation* 1992, 86:71–80.
6. Oswald H, Schernikau U, Baumbach A, *et al.*: Quantitative results of the European coronary excimer laser angioplasty registry [abstract]. *Eur Heart J* 1993, 14:2296.
7. Litvack F, Eigler N, Margolis J, *et al.*: Percutaneous excimer laser coronary angioplasty: results in the first consecutive 3000 patients. The ELCA Investigators. *J Am Coll Cardiol* 1994, 23:323–329.
8. • Appelman YEA, Piek JJ, Strikwerda S, *et al.*: Randomised trial of excimer laser coronary angioplasty versus balloon angioplasty for treatment of obstructive coronary artery disease. *Lancet* 1996, 347:79–84.

This study (the AMRO trial) is the first randomized trial in which ELCA followed by balloon angioplasty is compared with balloon angioplasty alone in 308 patients. The results show that there is no benefit of ELCA followed by balloon angioplasty.

9. Hoyne J, Mahon DJ, Nakamura S, *et al.*: Intravascular ultrasound imaging after excimer laser angioplasty. *Cathet Cardiovasc Diagn* 1994, 32:213–222.
10. Garcia E, Corcos T, Faverau X, *et al.*: Early deterioration after excimer laser assisted coronary angioplasty: a quantitative angiographic analysis [abstract]. *Circulation* 1994, 90:I-332.
11. Diethrich EB, Hanafy HM, Santiago OJ, Bahadir I: Angioscopy after coronary excimer laser angioplasty. *J Am Coll Cardiol* 1991, 18:643–644.
12. • Hamburger JN, Gijsbers GHM, Verhoofstad Geert GAM, *et al.*: Excimer laser coronary angioplasty: a physical perspective to clinical results. In *Current Review of Interventional Cardiology*, edn 2. Edited by Topol EJ, Serruys PW. Philadelphia: Current Medicine; 1995:159–172.

The first results and potential benefits of homogenized light distribution for ELCA are described.

13. Van Leeuwen TG, Van Erven L, Meertens JH, *et al.*: Origin of arterial wall dissections induced by pulsed excimer and mid-infrared laser ablation in the pig. *J Am Coll Cardiol* 1992, 19:1610–1618.
14. van Leeuwen TG, Meertens JH, Velema E, *et al.*: Intraluminal vapor bubble induced by excimer laser pulse causes microsecond arterial dilation and invagination leading to extensive wall damage in the rabbit. *Circulation* 1993, 87:1285–1263.
15. Baumbach A, Haase KK, Rose C, *et al.*: Formation of pressure waves during in vitro excimer laser irradiation in whole blood and the effect of dilution with contrast media and saline. *Lasers Surg Med* 1994, 14:3–6.

16. Gijsbers GHM: Tissue ablation by CW lasers, and a pulsed XeCl excimer laser a used in excimer laser angioplasty [thesis]. Amsterdam: University of Amsterdam; 1992:107.

17. Appelman YEA, Piek JJ, Verhoofstad G, *et al.*: Tissue ablation and gas formation of two excimer laser systems: an in vitro evaluation on porcine aorta. *Lasers Surg Med* 1996, 18:197–205.

18.• Deckelbaum LI, Natarajan MK, Bittl JA, *et al.*: Effect of intracoronary saline infusion on dissection during excimer laser coronary angioplasty: a randomized trial. *J Am Coll Cardiol* 1995, 26:1264–1269.

In 57 randomized patients, ELCA was performed in either a blood field or in a field where the blood was removed by injection of a saline bolus. This saline flush resulted in a 71% reduction of the incidence of moderate or worse dissections.

Chapter 13

Recent Advances in the Development of Platelet GP IIb/IIIa Receptor Antagonists

Shaker A. Mousa
Eric J. Topol

Aspirin has been and will be the standard reference compound for long-term oral treatment of platelet hyperactivity, most notably in secondary prevention of myocardial infarction (MI). Aspirin is also the basic antiplatelet agent for all kinds of acute interventions that may cause platelet-dependent thrombotic vessel occlusion, including percutaneous transluminal coronary angioplasty (PTCA) or fibrinolytic treatment of acute myocardial infarction (AMI). However, aspirin is neither selective for the platelet nor a potent antiplatelet compound and is unable to interfere to any larger extent with the thrombogenic activity of a pre-existing clot. Thienopyridines, such as ticlopidine and clopidogrel are the current therapeutic alternatives used when there is aspirin intolerance.

Abciximab (c7E3, ReoPro; Centocor, Malvern, PA) and related antagonists of the platelet glycoprotein (GP) IIb/IIIa receptors, a final common pathway for platelet agonists, are the most potent and universal inhibitors of platelet aggregation regardless of the agonist. Currently, their use is restricted to acute, more severe platelet ischemic syndromes and impending arterial platelet thrombus formation such as unstable angina pectoris. Treatment with these drugs has been performed in addition to standard antiplatelet therapy such as aspirin. A number of cyclic peptides, peptidomimetics, and nonpeptide analogues are currently under preclinical and clinical investigations for intravenous and oral uses. Thrombin inhibitors are another potential antiplatelet strategy. Thrombotic diseases in which aspirin is of limited value and better alternatives are required include peripheral arterial occlusive diseases, transient ischemic attacks, noncardiac related strokes, as well as any severe acute syndromes involving intravascular platelet activation.

GP IIb/IIIa Antagonists

Integrins and GP IIb/IIIa (αIIb/β3) Receptors

Integrins are a widely expressed family of cell adhesion receptors by which cells attach to extracellular matrices, to each other, or to different cells. All integrins are composed of $\alpha\beta$ heterodimeric units, which are expressed on a wide variety of cells. Most cells express several integrins. The interaction of integrins with the cytoskeleton and extracellular matrix appears to require the presence of both α and β subunits. The binding of integrins to their ligands is cation-dependent. Integrins appear to recognize specific amino acid sequences in their ligands. The most well studied is the arginine-glycine-aspartic acid (RGD) sequence that is found within a number of matrix proteins, including fibrinogen, vitronectin, fibronectin, thrombospondin, osteopontin, von Willebrand factor, and others. However, other integrins bind to ligands via a non-RGD binding domain such as the $\alpha_4\beta_1$ integrin receptors that bind and recognize the LDV sequence within the CS-1 region of fibronectin. There are at least eight known β subunits and 14 α subunits. Although the association of the eight and 14 different β and α subunits could in theory associate to give rise to more than 100 integrins, the actual diversity is much more restricted (Fig. 13-1, Table 13-1).

Recently, a common pathway for all agonists has been identified, namely the platelet GP IIb/IIIa complex, which is the membrane protein mediating platelet aggregation. GP IIb/IIIa in activated platelets is known to bind four soluble adhesive proteins—fibrinogen, von Willebrand factor, fibronectin, and vitronectin. The binding of fibrinogen and von Willebrand factor to GP IIb/IIIa causes platelets to aggregate. Other plasma adhesive proteins that may mediate platelet aggregation through binding to the GP IIb/IIIa complex are von Willebrand factor, particularly under conditions of high shear stress, and fibronectin. Platelet GP IIb/IIIa is a typical heterodimeric integrin that has been shown to be restricted in its cellular distribution to platelets' surface membrane. There are about 70,000 to 90,000 GP IIb/IIIa molecules per activated platelet. The binding of fibrinogen is mediated in part by the RGD recognition sequence that is common to the adhesive proteins that bind to GP IIb/IIIa. Another distinct amino acid sequence, a dodecapeptide, present in the carboxy terminal of fibrinogen γ chain, also binds to GP IIb/IIIa.

Classes of GP IIb/IIIa Antagonists

There are several classes of GP IIb/IIIa inhibitors, including snake venoms and monoclonal antibodies, most notably chimeric anti-β_3 abciximab. RGD peptides have been synthesized and tested in animals and humans, including cyclic compound (DMP728 [Dupont Merck, Wilmington, DE]; MK-852 [Merck & Co., West Point, PA]; Integrelin [Cor Therapeutics, San Francisco, CA]); lamifiban (RO44-9883; Hoffman-LaRoche, Basel, Switzerland), a pseudopeptide; and tirofiban (MK-383; Merck & Co.), a nonpeptide platelet GP IIb/IIIa antagonist (Fig. 13-2). Platelet GP IIb/IIIa antagonists can be classified on the following basis: chemical nature (*ie*, monoclonal antibody, linear peptide, cyclic peptide, peptidomimetic, and nonpeptide); route of administration (intravenous or oral); or binding kinetics profiles (*K*d) to activated versus unactivated platelets; as well as the differences in the dissociation rate constant (*K* off). A key feature among all small molecule GP IIb/IIIa receptor antagonists is the presence of an anionic carboxy acid terminal (COO-) separated by a spatial chemical moiety and a certain distance from the cationic basic amine terminal (benzamidine, piperidine, guanidine). The distance between the anionic and cationic terminals is very critical for optimal affinity binding (confirmation) and specificity to the platelet GP IIb/IIIa receptors, with minimal to no cross-reactivity with other closely related RGD-dependent integrins such as $\alpha_v\beta_3$, $\alpha_5\beta_1$, and $\alpha_v\beta_1$. See Figure 13-2 for detailed chemical series.

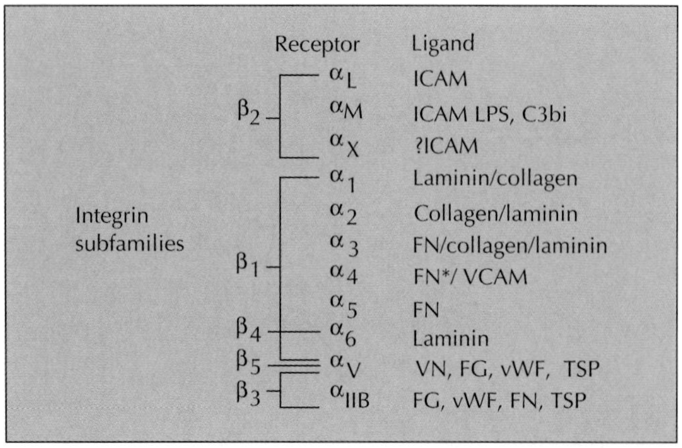

Figure 13-1. The integrin family of CAM consists of multiple heterodimeric forms of alpha and beta subunits associated as shown. The α_4, α_6, α_v subunits can associate with other β subunits such as β_4, β_5, β_6, β_7, and β_8. There are multiple ligands for the different integrins. FG—fibrinogen; FN—fibronectin: ICAM—intracellular adhesion molecule; LPS—lipopolysaccharide; TSPC—thrombospondin; VCAM—vascular cell adhesion molecule; VN—vitronectin; VWF—von Willebrand factor.

The first platelet GP IIb/IIIa antagonists to be developed were murine *monoclonal antibodies*. In vitro, these antibodies completely inhibited platelet aggregation and, in animal models of angioplasty injury and thrombolysis, they prevented rethrombosis post-thrombolysis [1–3]. Because of concerns about their immunogenicity, the derivative product, chimeric monoclonal 7E3 Fab, was created via genetic recombination. This new hybrid molecule consists of the mouse-derived variable regions from the original molecule linked to the constant region derived from human immunoglobulin IgG. Data from various clinical trials indicated the efficacy of c7E3, as is discussed later [4–7,8•].

A series of *synthetic peptides containing the RGD or analogous sequence*, which compete with fibrinogen for the GP IIb/IIIa binding site, have been designed. Several of these peptidomimetics and nonpeptides are now available for clinical studies. The *synthetic antiplatelet peptides*, particularly those that are cyclic and have somewhat rigid confirmations or configurations, are potent antithrombotic agents when tested in platelet-mediated thrombosis in different experimental animals [9,10•,11,12]. Although short cyclic synthetic peptides have a higher potency, they also lack specificity for GP IIb/IIIa and recognize receptors on several integrins [9,10•,11]. Structure-activity studies have revealed a partial dissociation between the inhibition of ex vivo platelet aggregation and bleeding time prolongation and suggest that it might be possible to obtain GP IIb/IIIa antagonists with an optimized antithrombotic versus hemorrhagic ratio [13].

Orally active GP IIb/IIIa antagonists

A high level of platelet antagonism has been required when GP IIb/IIIa antagonists have been employed for acute therapy of coronary arterial disease. However, the requirements for chronic therapy using orally active agents are only now being determined. Interaction with aspirin and other antiplatelet and anticoagulant drugs lead to shifts in the dose-response curves for both efficacy and unwanted side effects, such as increased bleeding time. As we gain experience with this new class of agents, the benefits and pitfalls associated with their use will become clearer. See Table 13-2 for current activities in targeting platelet GP IIb/IIIa integrin [13–17].

Xemlofiban (SC-5468A; Searle, Skokie, IL) is a pro-drug of a nonpeptide mimetic of the tetrapeptide (RGDF). The active metabolite SC-54701A is a potent inhibitor of GP IIb/IIIa and exhibits specificity for this receptor with respect to other integrins [17]. More than 50% of the orally administered pro-drug is absorbed in dogs and half that amount is converted to the active agent [17]. Platelet aggregation is completely inhibited for more than 8 hours after a single oral dose of 2.5 mg/kg. After intravenous administration, the elimination half life of the active moiety is 6.5 hours (4.7 ± 0.1 hours) in dogs and the total plasma clearance is 0.3 L/h/kg. The results of a dose-ranging study show that oral administration of the pro-drug produces a dose-dependent inhibition of platelet aggregation that is maintained during a 14-day administration period in dogs, with no adverse effects. At a dose-inhibiting collagen-induced aggregation by 80%, bleeding time was increased 2.5-fold. Whether these results will translate into less bleeding in a clinical situation upon long-term administration remains to be determined.

Fradafibran (BIBU-104; Karl Thomae, Biberach, Germany) is an orally active pro-drug of the free acid active form, BIBU-52. Escalating single and multiple oral doses between 10 and 100 mg have been investigated in human volunteers and were well tolerated [16]. See Table 13-2 and Figure 13-2 for currently avail-

TABLE 13-1. INTEGRIN FAMILY OF ADHESION RECEPTORS (α AND β SUBUNITS)

	α_1	α_2	α_3	α_4	α_5	α_6	α_M	α_L	α150	αIIb	α_v
β_1	$\alpha_1\beta_1$	$\alpha_2\beta_1$	$\alpha_3\beta_1$	$\alpha_4\beta_1$	$\alpha_5\beta_1$	$\alpha_6\beta_1$					$\alpha_v\beta_1$
β_2							Mac-1	LFA-1	P150		
β_3										$\alpha IIb/\beta_3$	$\alpha_v\beta_3$
β_4						$\alpha_6\beta_4$					
β_5											$\alpha_v\beta_5$
β_6											
β_7				$\alpha_4\beta_7$							
β_8											$\alpha_v\beta_8$

able platelet GP IIb/IIIa antagonists under preclinical or clinical investigations.

The role of platelet integrin GP IIb/IIIa receptor antagonists in the rapid diagnosis of thromboembolic events

Adhesion molecules play a major role in the pathogenesis of many disease states through their cell-matrix interactions. They alter cellular functions upon binding to matrix proteins, which can be regulated by other pathogenic stimuli acting on the cell. Thus, targeting these receptors should be useful in the diagnosis of diseases whose hallmark is cellular injury. In order for an agent to be useful as a diagnostic agent, it must be specific for the disease, as well as possess adequate contrast. Contrast imaging quality is the result of the combination of the rapid clearance of tissue background and the retention at the desired receptor site. The role of the platelet integrin GP IIb/IIIa receptor and its potential utility as a radiodiagnostic agent in the rapid detection of thromboembolic events has been demonstrated [18•].

Comparative Antithrombotic Efficacy

Among the key factors leading to thrombosis are vessel wall injury, platelet activation, and activation of the coagulation cascades. Initially, platelets attach to subendothelial cells and subsequently spread, expressing functional receptors for adhesive molecules. The process of platelet recruitment is mediated by various agonists, including thrombin, generated on phospholipid platelet surfaces; adenosine diphosphate (ADP), secreted from platelet granules; and thromboxane A_2, generated from within the platelets. The recent appreciation of thrombin's key role in promoting platelet-dependent arterial thrombosis suggests the importance of evaluating the antiplatelet effects of thrombin inhibitors compared with platelet GP IIb/IIIa antagonists, which act at the final common pathway for platelet aggregation. We have compared the antiplatelet activity of hirudin; and the 65–amino acid polypeptide, PPACK (phe-pro-arginine-chloromethyl ketone), an irreversible thrombin inhibitor, with the platelet GP IIb/IIIa antagonists 7E3 and DMP728. For this comparison, we have evaluated a number of different platelet functions, including thrombin-induced platelet aggregation, mobilization of intracellular calcium, fibrinogen binding, serotonin and plasminogen activator inhibitor 1 (PAI-1) release. PAI-1 and serotonin secretion were studied because of their possible role in physiological and pathological thromboembolism and vasospastic episodes postthrombolysis. Consequently, the effects of a thrombin inhibitor on platelet PAI-1 and serotonin release may have clinical relevance. Our results revealed specific and potent

Table 13-2. Current Activities in Targeting GP IIa/IIIb Integrin

Drug	Form	Indications	Stage of Development	Manufacturer(s)
7E3 Fab (ReoPro)	IV	Adjunct to angioplasty, antiplatelet	Approved December 1994	Centocor, Eli Lilly
Integrelin	IV	Adjunct to angioplasty, t-PA, antiplatelet	Phase II/III	Cor Therapeutics, Schering-Plough
Xemlofiban (SC-54684A),	Oral	Unstable angina, angioplasty	Phase I/II	Monsanto-Searle
Tirofiban (MK-383)	IV	Unstable angina, adjunct to angioplasty, antiplatelet	Phase III	Merck & Co.
Lamifiban (RO44-9833)	IV	Adjunct to angioplasty, unstable angina, antiplatelet	Phase II/III	Hoffman-LaRoche
Nonpeptide Peptidomimetic	IV, Oral	Antiplatelet	Preclinical or clinical	Karl Thomae, Zeneca, Searle/Daiichi, Searle, Hoffman LaRoche, Hoechst, Takeda, Merck & Co., SmithKline Beecham, Glaxo, Sandoz, Cor Therapeutics,/Eli Lilly

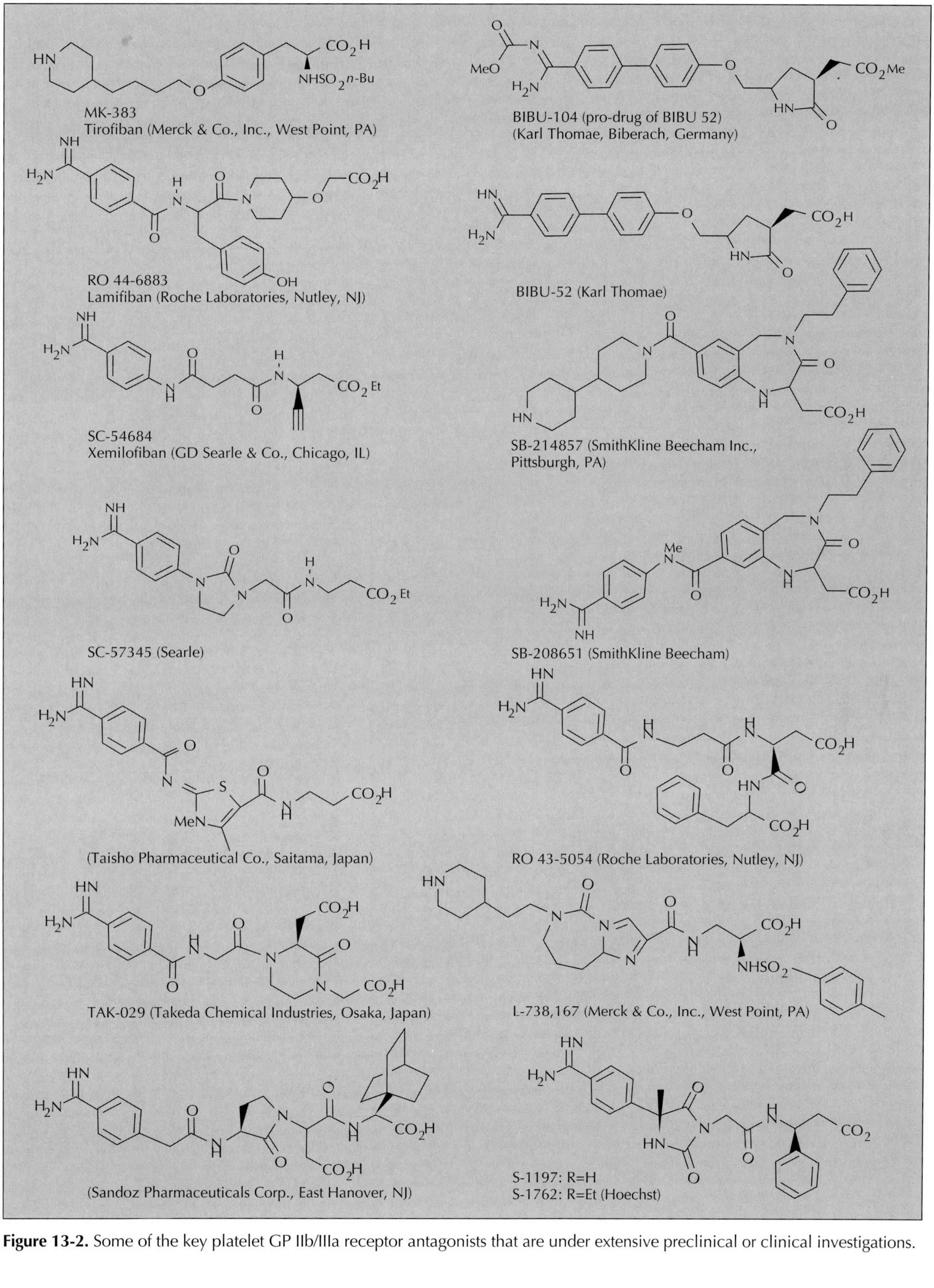

Figure 13-2. Some of the key platelet GP IIb/IIIa receptor antagonists that are under extensive preclinical or clinical investigations.

effects of hirudin and PPACK only against thrombin-induced platelet aggregation and platelet secretion. In contrast, the platelet GP IIb/IIIa antagonists inhibited platelet aggregation against all agonists but not against platelet secretory functions.

Further in vitro and in vivo comparative antithrombotic efficacy for various antiplatelet strategies was carried out using arterial thrombosis models. Both the in vitro and in vivo investigations revealed the superior efficacy of the platelet GP IIb/IIIa receptor antagonists compared with the rest of the other antiplatelet strategies tested (Figs. 13-3 and 13-4). In in vitro antithrombotic efficacy investigations perfusion of human blood through a mechanically injured (external clamping) isolated rabbit aorta was shown to result in cyclic flow reduction (CFR). DMP728 demonstrated total prevention of CFR at 0.1 μm, with no effect on CFR at 0.01 μm. The antithrombotic effects of other standard antiplatelet

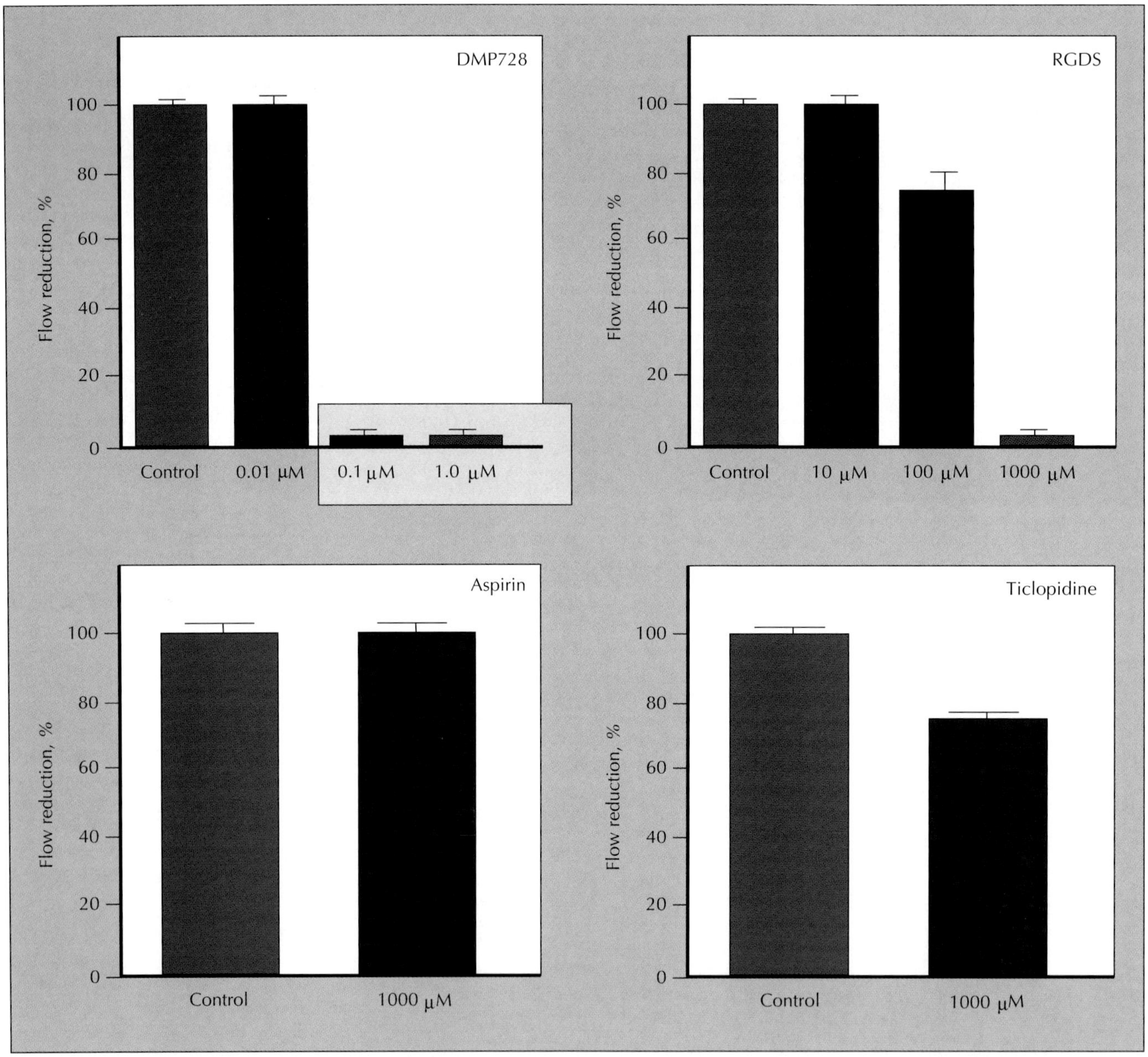

Figure 13-3. Antithrombotic effects of DMP728 in an in vitro arterial thrombosis model. Basal measurements of the frequency of cyclic flow reductions (CFR) were recorded, either saline (control group) or test agent (treated groups) was added at different concentrations to the blood tank, and then the frequency of CFR was monitored throughout the study for up to 3 hours. The effect of DMP728 or arginine-glycine-aspartic acid serine (RGDS) as well as other antiplatelet drugs, including aspirin or ticlopidine, on the frequency of platelet-mediated CFR was evaluated in this model. Data represent mean ± SEM, n = 3 or 4 in each group. (*Adapted from* Mousa and colleagues [9].)

agents, including aspirin and ticlopidine, as well as the GP IIb/IIIa prototype antagonist arginine-glycine-aspartic acid-serine (RGDS) were evaluated. RGDS at 1.0 mm demonstrated 100% antithrombotic efficacy in reducing CFR compared with maximal antithrombotic efficacy with DMP728 at 0.1 µm. In contrast, neither aspirin nor ticlopidine showed any distinct antithrombotic efficacy at concentrations up to 1.0 mm (*see* Fig. 13-3). Additionally, in the same model, but with a balloon-induced intimal wall injury, DMP728 maximally inhibited both platelet deposition and arterial flow reduction at 0.1 to 1.0 µm. DMP728 at 0.01 µm corresponds to 10% to 20% and 0.1 µm corresponds to 100% inhibition of in vitro human platelet aggregation [9].

Additionally, the effects of the direct thrombin inhibitor, hirudin, and the platelet GP IIb/IIIa antagonists, 7E3 and DMP728, on the prevention of thrombosis and rethrombosis after coronary thrombolysis in

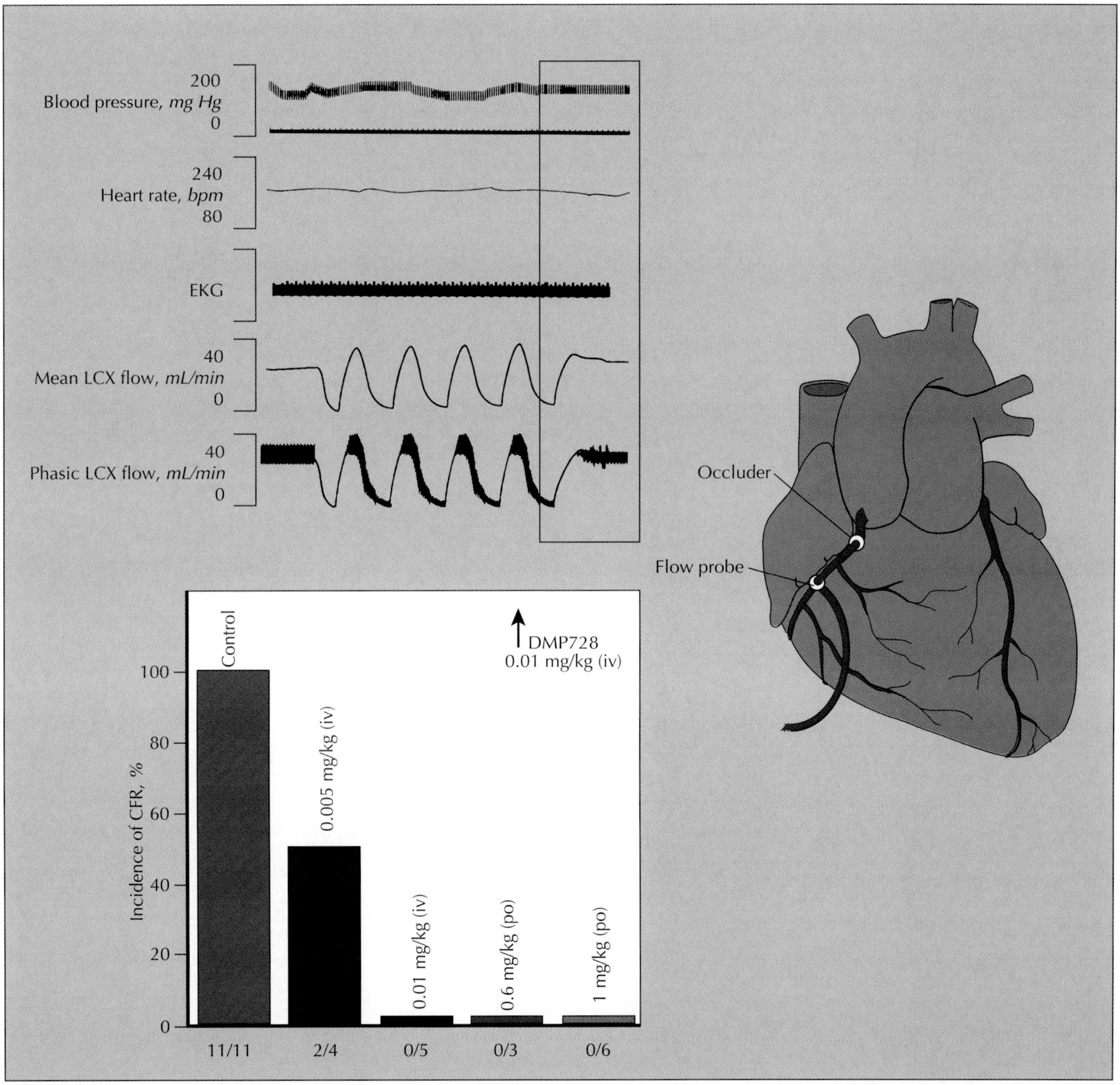

Figure 13-4. DMP728 and arterial thrombosis. Unstable angina, Folts model. CFR—cyclic flow reduction; EKG—electrocardiogram; LCX—left circumflex artery.

a chronic canine model has recently been documented [19,20]. In contrast to the GP IIb/IIIa antagonist tested in this model, which was very effective in preventing thrombosis and rethrombosis, the direct thrombin inhibitor provided less improvement in the incidence of reocclusion and mortality in the same model (Table 13-3). In that study, animals treated with hirudin exhibited rebound reocclusion after the discontinuation of the infusion. Theroux and colleagues [21] recently reported a similar phenomenon with heparin therapy, in which a significant number of patients experienced reactivation of unstable angina episodes. Furthermore, Gold and colleagues [22] reported evidences of rebound coagulation with direct thrombin inhibitor in unstable angina. Also, oscillation in flow or cyclic flow variations occurred in the hirudin-treated animals but not in the 7E3- or DMP728-treated groups. These cyclic flow variations that occur clinically post–tissue plasminogen activator (t-PA) may contribute to myocardial damage, persistent reocclusion, and arrhythmic events. Cyclic flow variations are intensified under stressful conditions associated with catecholamine release, leading to platelet hyperreactivity. Thus, suppressing cyclic flow variations may be as important as the achievement of vessel wall patency. In the Folts model different platelet GP IIb/IIIa antagonists demonstrated maximal efficacy in inhibiting ex vivo platelet aggregation, totally preventing CFR and maintaining coronary flow and coronary arterial patency even upon rechallenge with epinephrine [11,23]. These studies suggest the potential of GP IIb/IIIa antagonists in unstable angina. In contrast, aspirin (0.5–5.0 mg/kg, IV) was shown to be marginally effective in this model and ineffective against epinephrine–re-induced CFR (*see* Figs. 13-3 and 13-4). Hence, it is anticipated that GP IIb/IIIa antagonists might be more effective than aspirin in unstable angina, since platelet activation could be re-induced following elevation of catecholamines, rupture of atherosclerotic plaques, or progression of atherosclerotic lesions. These results suggest greater efficacy for GP IIb/IIIa antagonists compared with aspirin.

It has also been reported that inhibition of thrombin activity alone does not decrease the reocclusion rate following thrombolysis in a coronary artery thrombosis model in dogs with t-PA[23]. It is likely that in most circumstances in which platelet activation occurs thrombin is not the only mediator involved. In experimental models of thrombosis, combined use of thrombin inhibitors with thromboxane A_2 inhibitors or aspirin has been shown to be more effective than either one used alone [24]. A summary of comparative antithrombotic efficacy of direct antithrombin versus GP IIb/IIIa antagonists is shown in Table 13-4. Studies in the dog using everted "inside-out" carotid segments that were inserted into the femoral artery have shown that cyclic flow variation and occlusion rates were significantly reduced with abciximab. Similar results were obtained with another monoclonal antibody, P-37, in the coronary circulation and with DMP728, a cyclic peptide antagonist with a greater than 1000-fold selectivity for GP IIb/IIIa over other RGD-sensitive integrins [9,10•,25]. According to their mechanism of action, thrombolysis-induced platelet activation will be most potently inhibited by GP IIb/IIIa antagonists.

TABLE 13-3. EFFECT OF PLATELET GP IIB/IIIA ANTAGONISTS VERSUS DIRECT THROMBIN INHIBITOR ON INFARCT SIZE AND MORTALITY IN A CHRONIC CORONARY THROMBOSIS MODEL IN DOGS

		GP IIb/IIIa antagonists		Thrombin inhibitor (r-Hirudin)	
Parameters	**Placebo**	**DMP728**	**7E3**	**A***	**B†**
Infarct size, % *LV*	15 ± 2.9	6.6 ± 1.7	10.2 ± 3.3	14.9 ± 2	16 ± 2.6
Mortality < 24 h	6/8	0/8	0/8	3/8	2/6
Mortality < 5 days	6/8	0/8	0/8	4/8	2/6
Oscillatory flow	+	-	-	+	+

**Relatively short-term intravenous infusion.*
†Eleven hours of intravenous infusion.
+ indicates existence of oscillatory flow; - indicates no oscillatory flow.

Several experimental studies have shown that abciximab and peptide inhibitors of GP IIb/IIIa prevent reocclusion after successful lysis and also enhance the effectiveness of fibrinolytic agents [2,10•].

Because the platelet GP IIb/IIIa receptors represent the final common pathway for platelet aggregation, use of a potent and specific GP IIb/IIIa antagonist may prove to be a highly effective antithrombotic strategy (Fig. 13-5). However, the combination of other antiplatelet agents such as a safe and effective thrombin inhibitor or aspirin with a platelet GP IIb/IIIa antagonist may prove to be the ultimate antithrombotic strategy in humans because of the lack of platelet anti-secretory efficacy of GP IIb/IIIa antagonists that could be compensated with other antiplatelet approaches. On the other hand, the lack of effect of a specific GP IIb/IIIa antagonist on platelet functions other than platelet aggregation (*eg*, adhesion) might be an important safety aspect for the maintenance of the hemostatic balance.

Clinical Experiences

GP IIb/IIIa antagonists have so far only been tested in larger clinical trials in severely ill patients, those with unstable angina, MI and lysis, as well as PTCA. Abciximab was found to largely eliminate cyclic flow variations associated with PTCA that could not be prevented by aspirin alone [26]. In most if not all studies, these patients additionally received aspirin, nitrates, and heparin. A bolus injection of 0.25 mg/kg caused an 87% blockade of the platelet GP IIb/IIIa receptor, an 88% inhibition of ADP-induced platelet aggregation and a greater than 30-minute prolonged bleeding time at 2 hours [4–7,8•]. The regular type of treatment (*eg*, EPIC [Evaluation of c7E3 Fab in the Prevention of Ischemic Complications] trial) was bolus injection (0.25 mg/kg) followed by a 12-hour infusion. In patients with unstable angina bolus injection of 7E3 resulted in a dose-dependent prolongation of bleeding time and thrombocytopenia. A marked prolongation of bleeding time (> 30 minutes) was seen if more than 90% of the receptors were blocked. However, there was no spontaneous hemorrhage and the changes were reversible within 24 hours [27–31]. The results of these initial studies have led to various Phase III trials in unstable angina (UA), angioplasty, and AMI, as shown in Table 13-5.

TABLE 13-4. COMPARATIVE ANTITHROMBOTIC EFFECTS OF DIRECT THROMBIN INHIBITOR VERSUS PLATELET GP IIB/IIIA ANTAGONISTS*

Antithrombotic profiles	Thrombin inhibitor	GP IIb/IIIa antagonists	
	Hirudin	7E3	DMP72
Unstable angina–type model (Folts)			
Prevention or reduction of CFR	+++	+++	+++
Prevention or reduction of epinephrine-re-induced CFR	-	+++	+++
Chronic coronary artery electrolytic thrombosis model + t-PA			
Improved artery patency/survival	+	+++	+++
Suppression of cyclic flow variations	-	+++	+++
Prevention of rebound reocclusion	-/+	+++	+++

**The different arterial thrombosis models used were in dogs.*
+++ indicates very effective; + indicates modestly effective; - indicates ineffective.
CFR—cyclic flow reduction; t-PA—tissue plasminogen activator.

Potential Indications for Platelet GP IIb/IIIa Antagonists

Unstable Angina

Patients with unstable angina were actually the first clinical group to receive the platelet fibrinogen receptor antagonist, 7E3 [28]. The clinical efficacy of abciximab in severe unstable angina was studied in a randomized, placebo-controlled trial in 60 patients refractory to conventional medical therapy. There was a significant reduction in events during a hospital stay (death, MI, urgent intervention) and significant angiographic improvement of the lesions. This required a greater than 90% blockade of the GP IIb/IIIa receptors and was associated with a greater than 90% reduction in ex vivo platelet aggregation to ADP and significantly prolonged bleeding time without excess bleeding [29,32,33].

In a Phase II trial with lamifiban, 360 patients with chest pain within the previous 24 hours were randomly assigned to a placebo or one of four escalating doses of lamifiban [14,15]. A significant reduction in death, MI, or need for urgent intervention was demonstrated during the infusion period (≤ 5 days) from 8.2% in the control group to 3.4% in all lamifiban groups ($P \leq 0.046$). At 1-month follow-up, there was also a significant decrease in the incidence of death and MI in the high-dose lamifiban groups. However, there was a trend toward increased bleeding with lamifiban, especially in combination with heparin. Simoons and colleagues [28] performed a pilot study with c7E3 in patients with refractory unstable angina. In this multicenter trial, 60 patients with angina at rest that was unresponsive to maximal drug therapy, and with electrocardiogram (ECG) changes, were randomly assigned to receive a 24-hour infusion of c7E3 or heparin. Patients receiving c7E3 had reduced rates of recurrent ischemia, MI, and need for urgent angioplasty or bypass surgery. The incidence of a composite endpoint of death, MI, or repeat coronary revascularization was reduced from 20% in the placebo group to 3% in the c7E3 group [32–34].

Integrelin use in patients with unstable angina has also yielded positive results [35•]. In a multicenter trial involving 17 centers, 227 patients were randomly assigned to either low- or high-dose Integrelin or an active treatment group (4.1% in the 12-hour infusion group vs 12.2% in the placebo group). The incidence of

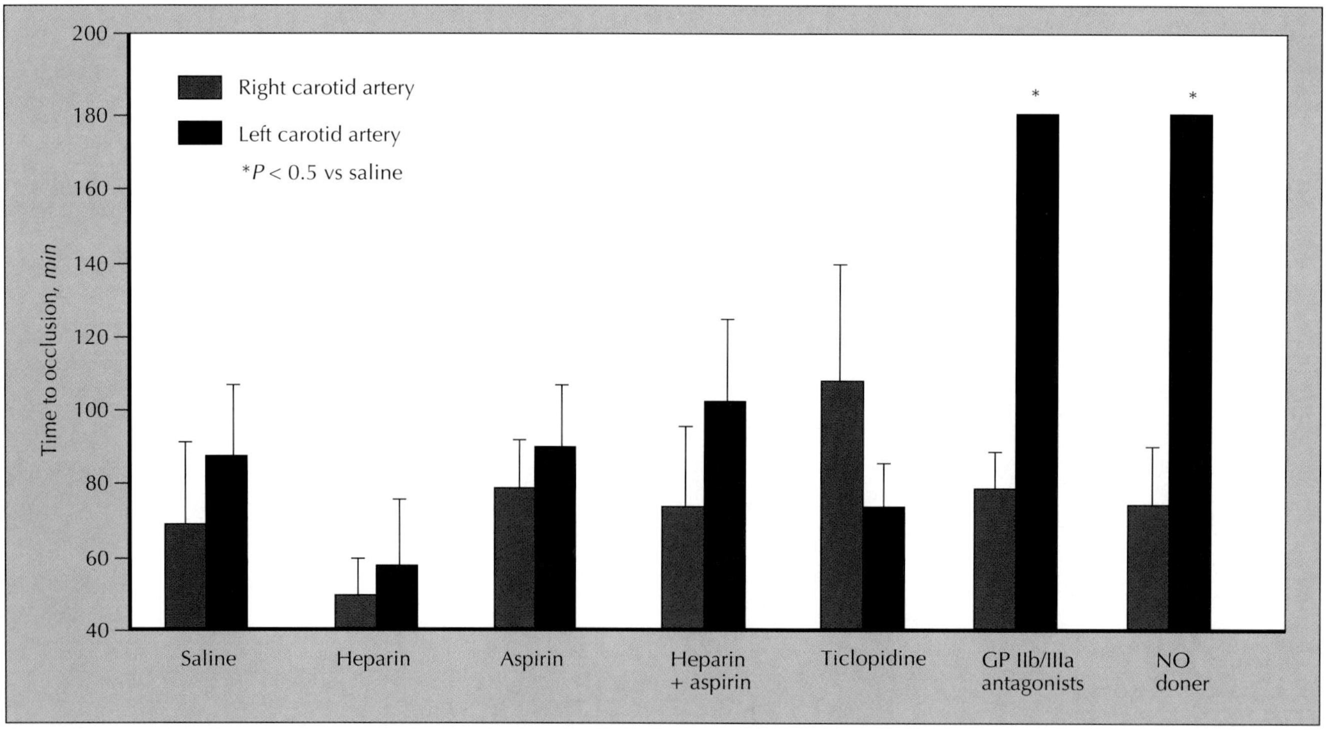

Figure 13-5. Effects of different antiplatelets and anticoagulants on arterial thrombus formation in carotid artery electrolytic injury model in dogs.

bleeding was similar in the placebo and Integrelin groups. Additionally, laboratory evaluation demonstrated profound platelet inhibition that was sustained for the duration of the Integrelin infusion.

Coronary Angioplasty

GP IIb/IIIa inhibitors have been evaluated extensively in the setting of coronary angioplasty. On a mechanistic level, GP IIb/IIIa blockade abolishes cyclic flow variation following angioplasty, which is a marker of platelet thrombus formation and a harbinger of thrombotic occlusion [26]. Early pilot studies with 7E3 also showed a dose-dependent effect on bleeding time, receptor blockade, and platelet aggregation, no major bleeding complications, and a low incidence of abrupt closure and recurrent ischemia [7,32]. These early studies provided the background for the large-scale EPIC trial. This double-blind trial randomly assigned 2099 patients at greater-than-normal risk for ischemic complications to one of three treatment groups: 1) a bolus of c7E3 plus a continuous infusion for 12 hours, 2) c7E3 bolus followed by a placebo infusion, and 3) a placebo bolus followed by a placebo infusion. All patients also received aspirin, and heparin was administered during the procedure to keep the activated clotting time between 300 to 350 seconds. The principal finding of this study was a significant 35% reduction in acute ischemic events in patients receiving the bolus and 12-hour infusion of c7E3 compared with placebo. Chimeric 7E3 was especially effective at reducing the occurrence of MI, and specific patient subsets, including those with unstable angina, those undergoing angioplasty for AMI [33], and those having directional atherectomy, derived particular benefit. However, c7E3's effect was at the cost of an increased rate of bleeding events, which were chiefly related to vascular access sites. Apart from its acute benefits during angioplasty, GP IIb/IIIa inhibition also had an important effect on medium-term clinical outcome in the EPIC trial. At 6 months there was a 23% reduction in the rate of clinical restenosis, defined by the composite endpoint of death, MI, and repeat revascularization, as compared with placebo. In contrast, bolus c7E3 alone had little effect on clinical restenosis. The reduction in clinical restenosis was largely due to a lower incidence of repeat revascularization in patients with initially successful procedures. As a result, this study was the first large-scale randomized trial to show clinically meaningful long-term ischemic outcomes after coronary intervention.

PROLOG trial

The recently completed PROLOG pilot study investigated whether lower doses of heparin could be used in conjunction with GP IIb/IIIa inhibition during coronary angioplasty to help minimize bleeding risk, without a concomitant increase in ischemic events. In this multicenter trial, the weight-adjusted, low-dose heparin group (70 U/kg bolus without any further doses) had a lower incidence of bleeding complications compared with the standard heparin group (100 U/kg bolus plus additional doses to keep activated clotting time over 300 seconds). Although patient numbers were small, there was no apparent increase

TABLE 13-5. GP IIB/IIIA INHIBITORS: RESULTS OF PHASE III CLINICAL TRIALS

Trial	Agent	Population	Sample size	Endpoint
EPIC*	Abciximab	PTCA	2099	Composite†
IMPACT-II*	Integrelin	PTCA	4010	Composite
EPILOG	Abciximab	PTCA	≈ 4500	Composite
RESTORE	Tirofiban	PTCA	2100	Composite
CAPTURE	Abciximab	UA	1100	Composite
PURSUIT	Integrelin	UA	≈ 10,000	Death or MI
PARAGON	Lamifiban	UA	9500	Death or MI
PRIZM	Tirofiban	UA	≈ 3000	Composite
PRIZM-Plus	Tirofiban	UA	1600	Composite

**Trial completed (the others are in progress and paradigm is being planned).*
†Death, myocardial infarction (MI), need for repeat vascularization (percutaneous intervention or coronary artery bypass).
AMI—acute myocardial infarction; PTCA—percutaneous transluminal coronary angioplasty (may also include atherectomy); UA—unstable angina.

in ischemic complications in the low-dose heparin group. Consequently, a low-dose, weight-adjusted heparin strategy is currently being evaluated in the large-scale (4800 patients) trial, which was stopped at 2872 patients (EPILOG [Evaluation of PTCA to Improve Long-term Outcome by c7E3 Glycoprotein Receptor Blockade] trial) (Table 13-6).

IMPACT-I trial

Integrelin was also recently evaluated during coronary angioplasty in the IMPACT (Integrelin to Minimize Platelet Aggregation and Prevent Coronary Thrombosis)-I study. In this pilot trial of 150 patients, 101 were randomly assigned in a double-blind fashion to Integrelin and 49 to placebo. In contrast to the EPIC trial, this study was open to all patients undergoing coronary intervention, yet there still was significant suppression of ischemic events in the placebo. After 24-hour infusion, high-dose Integrelin was found to decrease both the number and duration of ischemic events as detected by continuous ST-segment monitoring, without an excess in bleeding episodes. A pilot study with the nonpeptide agent tirofiban in 71 patients with unstable angina also demonstrated a trend toward a reduction in the incidence of refractory angina [36•]. The consistently beneficial and encouraging results of these pilot trials has led to a number of large-scale clinical trials with these agents in unstable angina.

CAPTURE trial

The CAPTURE (Chimeric 7E3 Antiplatelet Therapy in Unstable Refractory Angina in patients undergoing angioplasty) trial was also stopped early—after 1050 of the planned 1400 patients had been enrolled—because of significant efficacy seen with c7E3. This trial is actually a coronary intervention trial, because all of the patients had to have a screening angiogram to determine their eligibility for angioplasty. Results showed a 30-day event rate of 10.8% in the c7E3 group versus 16.4% with placebo. MI was reduced from 9.4% to 4.5%, and urgent intervention from 10.7% to 6.9%. The combination of death or MI was reduced by 50% (from 10.3% to 5.1%). Bleeding occurred in 9.7% of c7E3 patients, with major bleeding in 2.9% and transfusions in 7%. In patients with placebo bleeding occurred in 5.4% of patients, with major bleeding in 1.7% and transfusions in 3.2%. CAPTURE was designed to enroll 1400 patients with refractory angina who were scheduled to undergo PTCA to receive either c7E3 or placebo during approximately 24 hours preceding the intervention and continuing until 1 hour after the intervention. When the study was stopped, a total of 1266 patients had been enrolled. CAPTURE enrolled patients with refractory unstable angina defined as at least one episode of chest pain with an abnormal ECG compatible with myocardial ischemia and at least one episode with either pain or ECG changes during therapy with aspirin, heparin, and nitroglycerin. This episode should occur within 48 hours of enrollment. A first diagnostic angiogram should be made within 24 hours of enrollment. Subsequently, patients were randomized to receive either c7E3 or placebo during 18 to 24 hours. At this time a second angiogram was performed as well as PTCA of the culprit lesion. Patients in the two treatment groups were balanced for baseline characteristics. The study drug was started within 6 hours after the first angiogram in 73% of the patients. Fifty-nine percent of the patients had at least one episode of ischemia within 12 hours preceding initiation of drug therapy. This confirms that these patients were really very unstable. In patients receiving c7E3 major bleeding occurred in 1.7%, and any bleeding occurred in 5.4% of the patients. In patients receiving a placebo major bleeding occurred in 2.9%, and any bleeding occurred in 9.7%. The primary endpoint of

TABLE 13-6. SUMMARY OF DIFFERENT GP IIB/IIIA ANTAGONISTS: RESULTS IN A CLINICAL SETTING AT 30 DAYS

	Major bleeding complications, %	Death or MI vs placebo, %
IMPACT II Integrelin Phase III angioplasty, %	5.1	7.5 vs 9.3
EPIC ReoPro Phase III angioplasty, %	2.5	7.2 vs 10.3
EPILOG ReoPro Phase IV angioplasty, %	2.6	3.1 vs 8.1
CAPTURE ReoPro Phase III angioplasty, %	2.9	5.4 vs 10.9

MI—myocardial infarction.

death, MI, or urgent re-intervention up to 30 days occurred in 10.8% of patients treated with c7E3 and 16.4% of placebo patients.

RESTORE trial

The RESTORE (Randomized Efficacy Study of Tirofiban for Outcomes and Restenosis) trial had the usual primary endpoint—a composite of death, MI, and urgent intervention at day 30 after angioplasty. Tirofiban reduced the risks for these adverse events from 12.2% to 10.3% (a relative reduction by 16%), but the effect at day 30 was not statistically significant (P = 0.16). Tirofiban's results were better at 48 hours (a reduction by 38%) or 7 days (a reduction of 27%) after angioplasty but diminished over time and lost statistical significance (just as for Integrelin). In the RESTORE study for patients undergoing angioplasty the drug reduced the event rate in the first 7 days, but this beneficial effect was lost by 30 days. It has been suggested that longer administration of the drug may have given better results (tirofiban was given for 36 hours in the study).

The RESTORE study group consisted of 2100 randomized angioplasty patients who had an MI or unstable angina attack within the previous 72 hours before receiving tirofiban or a placebo. All patients received aspirin and heparin. The primary efficacy endpoint was a composite of death, MI, coronary artery bypass (CABG), repeat angioplasty, or stent implantation at 30 days. This endpoint occurred in 10.3% of tirofiban patients versus 12.2% of placebo patients (not statistically significant, P = 0.16). MI occurred in 4.2% of the tirofiban group and 5.7% of the placebo group (P = 0.113). The results were significant at 2 days, with the composite endpoint occurring in 5.4% of tirofiban patients versus 8.7% of those on placebo (P = 0.005), and MI in 2.7% of tirofiban patients and 4.4% of patients receiving placebo (P = 0.039). The results were also significant at 7 days, with the composite endpoint occurring in 7.4% of tirofiban and 10.1% of placebo patients (P = 0.027). There was a slight increase in bleeding with tirofiban, with major bleeding occurring in 6% of the active treatment group versus 4.5% of placebo patients. Transfusions were increased from 2.3% with placebo to 3.9% with tirofiban, but there was no increase in thrombocytopenia (1.5% on tirofiban vs 1.2% on placebo). Tirofiban is also in Phase III trials in unstable angina [37]. In the EPILOG 4000 low-risk angioplasty patients were randomized to placebo or c7E3 with either standard-dose or low-dose heparin. c7E3 was given as a bolus followed by a 12-hour weight-adjusted infusion. The trial was stopped prematurely following an interim analysis of the first 2792 patients because of significant benefits in the c7E3 groups. Data on the first 1500 patients were presented at the American College of Cardiology meeting. The primary endpoint of death, MI, or urgent intervention at 30 days was reduced from 8.1% in the placebo group to 2.6% in the c7E3 plus low-dose heparin group, a 68% reduction (P = 0.0008). The event rate was also significantly reduced in the c7E3 plus standard heparin group (3.6%). The clinical benefit was seen across the full spectrum of patients, with most benefit in patients with unstable angina. Bleeding complications did not increase with c7E3. Major bleeding occurred in 1.8% of patients on c7E3 plus low-dose heparin, 3.5% of those on c7E3 plus standard heparin, and 3.1% of placebo (*see* Table 13-6).

Acute Myocardial Infarction

Although experimental work has supported a beneficial role for potent platelet antagonism as an adjunct to thrombolysis, there have been few clinical trials with simultaneous administration of a thrombolytic and a GP IIb/IIIa inhibitor because of concerns about the potential bleeding hazard. However, the TAMI-8 (Eight Thrombolysis and Myocardial Infarction) project evaluated murine 7E3 Fab use after tissue plasminogen activator thrombolysis. There was evidence of improved vessel patency at 24 hours and a trend toward less recurrent ischemia in the 7E3 groups. The study also demonstrated a consistent, dose-dependent inhibition of platelet aggregation. Bleeding episodes were not increased. Preliminary results of the IMPACT-AMI (Integrelin to Minimize Platelet Aggregation and Prevent Coronary Thrombosis-Acute Myocardial Infarction) trial have shown profound inhibition of platelet aggregation, although high levels of Integrelin are required, suggesting that this patient population is associated with a highly reactive platelet pool. Despite very high doses of Integrelin there has not been a consistent decrease in the time required to achieve coronary thrombolysis. Overall, these findings are promising, and a large-scale trial of Integrelin as an adjunct to thrombolysis is currently nearing completion.

The nonpeptide GP IIb/IIIa antagonist tirofiban was studied in healthy volunteers by intravenous infusion and caused a dose-dependent inhibition of platelet aggregation and prolongation of bleeding time. These effects were 55% to 89% lower about 3 hours after stopping the infusion [36•]. The compound is about four orders of magnitude more selective for GP IIb/IIIa than for vitronectin $\alpha_v\beta_3$ integrin. Similar results were reported for lamifiban, which in an experimental study was found to prevent cyclic flow variations in the injured guinea-pig carotid artery, being more effective than aspirin and hirudin [13–15]. Lamifiban was tested versus aspirin or heparin and reduced the combined event rate from 8.2% to 2.5% at 1 month. Recent data reported at the American College of Cardiology [37] is shown in Table 13-7.

In conclusion, as more data with these agents comes to fruition, we believe these issues will be resolved. Large-scale placebo-controlled studies have unequivocally demonstrated the efficacy of GP IIb/IIIa receptor blockade with c7E3 Fab and to a lesser extent with tirofiban or Integrelin in reducing ischemic complications among a broad spectrum of patients treated with coronary balloon angioplasty or atherectomy. A comparison of all trials with GP IIb/IIIa is denoted in Tables 13-1 through 13-5. It may be anticipated that agents such as c7E3 or Integrelin would be useful in preventing ischemic complications during high-risk stenting procedures and may produce a complementary beneficial effect with stenting on the incidence of restenosis. Important in the debate about optimal timing of drug administration is data from EPIC, EPILOG, and IMPACT II documenting that the majority (65%) of coronary ischemic events occur within the 24 hours of coronary intervention. Although practical experience has indicated that abciximab is a useful adjunct once complications of coronary angioplasty have occurred, large scale studies of the utility of GP IIb/IIIa blockade in the setting of intraprocedural thrombosis and coronary stent implantation remain to be conducted.

Finally, optimal use of the GP IIb/IIIa blockers is currently being defined. Proper patient selection should be based on clinical data and be balanced by both the bleeding potential and the monetary cost of this agent. Continued research will undoubtedly expand indications for use. Today, it appears that the best interventional approach optimizes the mechanical device strategy when appropriate while taking full advantage of the additional benefits of pharmacologic modulation. Justification of the costs associated with this aggressive approach will require demonstration of benefits at both the level of the patient as well as to the overall health care system.

New orally active compounds inhibited human platelet aggregation in vitro at sub-micromolar concentrations. The oral doses ranged from 1 to 7.5 mg/kg and the bioavailability ranged from 5% to 25%, with various duration of antiplatelet effects [17]. Early clinical trials with xemlofiban suggested oral antiplatelet efficacy in humans [38••]. Antagonists of GP IIb/IIIa might have major advantages in comparison with the other antiplatelet agents discussed in terms of efficacy.

Adverse Effects

The major adverse effect is an increased risk for bleeding [30,31]. Because of the risk of bleeding complications and because the study was only in high-risk angioplasty patients, further evaluation is necessary before the treatment can be recommended to other patient groups. In addition, thrombocytopenia may occur. Critical thrombocytopenia, eventually leading to uncontrolled bleeding, has been estimated to be less than 1% with abciximab. There was no significant increase in thrombocytopenia with abciximab in the EPIC trial. Thus, there is a marked inhibition of hemostatic function of the platelet and a substantial bleeding tendency. However, because of the short duration of action, this effect, unlike with aspirin, is rapidly reversible. Further, data of eight trials showed the occurrence of bleeding events cannot be predicted from the prolongation of bleeding time [30]. Although this may become a problem after oral administration, some compounds have only a weak effect on bleeding time. If these actions could be separated, then these compounds may become alternatives to aspirin in secondary prevention and perhaps in primary prevention as well.

Table 13-7. Recent Data from the EPILOG-ReoPro Phase 4 Study (Angioplasty)

Outcomes	Placebo	ReoPro/low-dose heparin	ReoPro/high-dose heparin
Major blood	3.1	1.8	3.5
Minor blood	2.9	3.8	7.6
Death	8.1	2.6	3.0 (P = 0.00008)
Death or myocardial infarction	7.1	2.0	2.6 (> 4 × CPK)

CPK—creatine phosphokinase.

Key Issues

Efficacy

It is not yet clear what level of platelet aggregation inhibition versus which agonist at what concentration or, perhaps more importantly, what level of percentage of receptor occupancy is needed to drive certain clinical benefits in the different subset of coronary artery diseases. Additionally, it is not totally clear how much heparin, if any, is required in conjunction with the GP IIb/IIIa antagonists. Another important and unresolved question is whether all GP IIb/IIIa antagonists are equivalent in terms of expected antiplatelet efficacy or safety (*ie*, small molecules versus c7E3). It is also worth noting that both Integrelin and tirofiban have demonstrated lesser efficacy compared to c7E3 in the same patient population (coronary angioplasty) despite prolonged infusions of 20 hours for Integrelin and 36 hours for tirofiban. It is still unclear if these differences in the outcome (*ie*, greater efficacy of c7E3 vs Integrelin or tirofiban) might be due to the need of either higher doses or longer duration of treatment with either Integrelin or tirofiban to achieve comparable levels of efficacy as c7E3.

Bleeding Risk

The principal and most concerning potential adverse effect of GP IIb/IIIa inhibition is bleeding. In the EPIC trial, there was a doubling of the overall rate of major bleeding in the c7E3 bolus plus infusion group compared with placebo. The rate of blood product transfusion was also significantly higher in patients receiving c7E3. Despite this, the incidence of intracerebral hemorrhage was not increased with c7E3 use, and most of the major bleeding events were related to vascular access sites. Specific patient groups appeared to be at increased risk, including those with lower body weight, those undergoing long (more than 70 minutes) procedures, and women. However, a recent pilot study of c7E3 in conjunction with low-dose heparin during coronary angioplasty suggested that early discontinuation of heparin combined with early sheath removal can reduce the vascular access site bleeding rate associated with GP IIb/IIIa. Nevertheless, bleeding remains a significant limitation to GP IIb/IIIa receptor inhibition and continued attention needs to be directed at minimizing this risk during the ongoing evaluation of these agents.

Integrin Specificity

The GP IIb/IIIa inhibitors are a diverse group of drugs, and it is not known whether differences in pharmacologic properties among the various agents will be reflected in differences in clinical effects. The monoclonal antibody c7E3 stands out as being relatively integrin "nonspecific," interacting with other integrins, including the vitronectin receptor $\alpha_v\beta_3$ integrin. The vitronectin receptor, in particular, is highly expressed on endothelial cells, and it remains possible that at least part of the benefit of c7E3 in preventing clinical restenosis is mediated through blockade of this integrin. In contrast, KGD (lysine-arginine-aspartate) peptides such as Integrelin were designed to be exquisitely specific for the platelet GP IIb/IIIa receptor, with little or no effects on other integrins. Whether these differences in specificity will have any influence on the clinical efficacy of these agents is uncertain, and these issues will need to be addressed in ongoing and future evaluation of these drugs.

Conclusions

This review provided various evidence for the role of platelets in health and diseases and the key role of the platelet membrane GP IIb/IIIa receptors in the mediation of platelet aggregation and thrombosis in various thromboembolic disorders, as demonstrated preclinically and clinically. The clinical evolution of the GP IIb/IIIa inhibitors has reached a crossroads. Clearly, there is an urgent need for more efficacious antiplatelet and antithrombotic drugs that are superior to aspirin or ticlopidine for the prevention and treatment of various cardiovascular and cerebrovascular thromboembolic disorders. The realization that the platelet integrin αIIb/β_3 is the final common pathway for platelet aggregation regardless of the mechanism of activation prompted the development of several small molecule αIIb/β_3 receptor antagonists for intravenous and oral antithrombotic utilities. The platelet αIIb/β_3 receptor blockade represents a very promising therapeutic and diagnostic strategy of thromboembolic disorders, which is yet to be reviewed. Clinical experiences (efficacy and safety) gained with injectable αIIb/β_3 antagonists (c7E3, Integrelin, tirofiban, lamifiban) will provide valuable insights into the potential of long-term chronic usage of oral αIIb/β^3 antagonists that are in early clinical [38••] or late preclinical developments. Various clinical trials have demonstrated the utility of GP IIb/IIIa blockade during coronary angioplasty and in patients with unstable angina. A number of large-scale trials are currently underway to widen the indications and improve efficacy and safety.

References and Recommended Reading

Recently published papers of particular interest have been highlighted as:

- • Of special interest
- •• Of outstanding interest

1. Coller BS, Scudder LE: Inhibition of dog platelet function by in vivo infusion of F(ab')2 fragments of a monoclonal antibody. *Blood* 1985, 66:1456–1460.
2. Cadroy Y, Hanson SR, Kelly AB, *et al.*: Relative antithrombotic effects of monoclonal antibodies targeting different platelet glycoprotein-adhesive molecule interactions in nonhuman primates. *J Clin Invest* 1994, 83:3218–3224.
3. Yasuda T, Gold HK, Fallon JT, *et al.*: Monoclonal antibody against the platelet glycoprotein (GP) IIb/IIIa receptor prevents coronary artery reocclusion after reperfusion with recombinant tissue-type plasminogen activator in dogs. *J Clin Invest* 1988, 81:1284–1291.
4. Tcheng JE, Ellis SG, George BS, *et al.*: Pharmacodynamics of chimeric glycoprotein IIb/IIIa integrin antiplatelet antibody Fab 7E3 in high-risk coronary angioplasty. *Circulation* 1994, 90:1757–1764.
5. Kleiman NS, Ohman E, Califf RM, *et al.*: Profound inhibition of platelet aggregation with monoclonal antibody 73E Fab after thrombolytic therapy: results of the Thrombolysis and Angioplasty in Myocardial Infarction (TAMI) 8 Pilot Study. *J Am Coll Cardiol* 1993, 22:381–389.
6. EPIC Investigators. Use of a monoclonal antibody directed against the platelet glycoprotein IIb/IIIa receptor in high-risk coronary angioplasty. *N Engl J Med* 1994, 330:956–961.
7. Topol EJ, Califf RM, Weisman HF, *et al.*: Randomized trial of coronary intervention with antibody against platelet IIb/IIIa integrin for reduction of clinical restenosis: results at six months. *Lancet* 1994, 343:881–886.
8. • Simoons ML, de Boer MJ, Van den Brand M, *et al.*: Randomized trial of IIb/IIIa platelet receptor blocker in refractory unstable angina. *Circulation* 1994, 89:596–603.

These reports describe the early trials with intravenous platelet GP IIb/IIIa antagonist in high-risk PTCA, MI, and refractory unstable angina.

9. Mousa S, Bozarth J, Forsythe M, *et al.*: Antiplatelet, antithrombotic efficacy of DMP 728, a novel platelet GPIIb/IIIa receptor antagonist. *Circulation* 1994, 89:3–12.
10. • Mousa S, Forsythe M, Diemer M, *et al.*: Thrombolytic antithrombotic, efficacy of the platelet GP IIb/IIIa antagonist DMP 728. *Coronary Artery Diseases* 1994, 5:919–927.

This series of studies was among the first to document potential thrombolytic efficacy of GP IIb/IIIa antagonist alone and the synergy with standard thrombolytics in animal models.

11. Nichols AJ, Ruffolo RR, Huffman WF, *et al.*: Development of GPIIb/IIIa antagonists as antithrombotic drugs. *Trends in Pharmacological Sciences* 1992, 13:413–417.
12. Foster MR, Hornby EJ, Brown S, *et al.*: Improved potency and specificity of Arg-gly-Asp (RGD) containing peptides as fibrinogen receptor blocking drugs. *Thromb Res* 1993, 72:231–245.
13. Cook NS, Kottirsch G, Zerwes H-G: Platelet glycoprotein IIb/IIIa antagonists. *Drugs Future* 1994, 19:135–159.
14. Jones CR, Ambros RJ, Rapold HJ, *et al.*: Ro 44-9883: a novel non-peptide GPIIb/IIIa antagonist in man [abstract]. *Thromb Haemost* 1993, 69:560.
15. Théroux P, Kouz S, Knudtson ML, *et al.*: A randomized double-blind controlled trial with the non-peptide platelet GPIIb/IIIa antagonist RO 44-9883 in unstable angina [abstract]. *Circulation* 1994, 90:I–232.
16. Weisenberger NH, Muller TH, Deichsel G, Krause J: Tolerability and platelet fibrinogen receptor occupancy (FRO) after oral treatment with BIBU 104 XX in healthy volunteers [abstract]. *Thromb Haemost* 1995, 73:1315, 1592.
17. Nicholson NS, Panzer-Knodle SG, Salyers AK, *et al.*: SC-54684: an orally active inhibitor of platelet aggregation. *Circulation* 1995, 91:403–410.
18. • Barrett J, Edward S, Harris T, *et al.*: The development of technetium-99 agent for imaging deep vein thrombosis. In *Chemistry and Nuclear Medicine*. Edited by Nicolini, *et al.* Padova: SG Editorial; 1995, 275–280.
19. Rote W, Mu D-X, Bates ER, *et al.*: Prevention of rethrombosis after coronary thrombolysis in a chronic canine model. I. adjunctive therapy with monoclonal antibody 7E3-F(ab')2. *J Cardiovasc Pharmacol* 1993, 23:194–202.
20. Rote W, Mu D-X, Bates ER, *et al.*: Prevention of rethrombosis after coronary thrombolysis in a chronic canine model. II. adjunctive therapy with r-Hirudin. *J Cardiovasc Pharmacol* 1993, 23:203–211.
21. Theroux P, Waters D, Lam J, *et al.*: Reactivation of unstable angina after discontinuation of heparin. *New Engl J Med* 1992, 327:141–145.
22. Gold HK, Torres FW, Garabedian HD, *et al.*: Evidence of a rebound coagulation phenomenon after cèssation of a 4-hour infusion of a specific thrombin inhibitor in patient with unstable angina. *J Am Coll Cardiol* 1993, 21:1039–1047.
23. Nicolini FA, Rios G, Lee P, *et al.*: Inhibition of thrombin activity alone does not decrease the reocclusion rate following r t-PA-induced thrombolysis in canine coronary artery thrombosis. *Throm Heomost* 1993, 69:992–997.
24. Clarke RJ, Mayo G, Fitzgerald GA, Fitzgerald DJ: Combined administration of aspirin and a specific thrombin inhibitor in man. *Circulation* 1991, 83:1510–1518.
25. Mousa SA, Reilly TM: Antiplatelet effects of direct acting thrombin inhibitors and platelet GPIIb/IIIa antagonists: comparative analysis. *Cardiovascular Disease*, edn 2. Edited by Gallo LL. New York: Plenum Press, 1995: 32:255–268.
26. Anderson HV, Kirkheeide RL, Krishnaswami A, *et al.*: Cyclic flow variations after coronary angioplasty in humans: clinical and angiographic characteristics and elimination with 7E3 monoclonal antiplatelet antibody. *J Am Coll Cardiol* 1994, 23:1031–1037.

27. Gold HK, Gimple LW, Yasuda T, *et al.*: Pharmacodynamic study of F $(ab')_2$ fragments of murine monoclonal antibody 7E3 directed against human platelet glycoprotein IIb/IIIa in patients with unstable angina pectoris. *J Clin Invest* 1990, 86:651–659.

28. Simoons ML, de Boer MJ, van den Brand MJBM, *et al.*: Randomized trial of a GPIIb/IIIa platelet receptor blocker in refractory unstable angina. *Circulation* 1994, 89:596–603.

29. Kleiman N, Ohmann M, Califf R, *et al.*: Profound inhibition of platelet aggregation with monoclonal antibody 7E3Fab after thrombolytic therapy. *J Am Coll Cardiol* 1993, 22:381–389.

30. Bernardi MM, Califf RM, Kleiman N, *et al.*: Prolonged bleeding times do not predict hemorrhagic events in patients receiving the 7E3 glycoprotein IIb/IIIa platelet antibody [abstract]. *Circulation* 1992, 86 (suppl 1):I–260.

31. Ellis SG, Tcheng JE, Navetta FI, *et al.*: Safety and antiplatelet effect of murine monoclonal antibody 7E3 Fab directed against platelet glycoprotein IIb/IIIa in patients undergoing elective coronary angioplasty. *Coronary Artery Dis* 1993, 4:167–175.

32. EPIC Investigators: Use of a monoclonal antibody directed against the platelet glycoprotein IIb/IIIa receptor in high-risk coronary angioplasty. *N Engl J Med* 1994, 330:956–961.

33. Lincoff AM, Califf RM, Anderson K, *et al.* for the EPIC Investigators: Striking clinical benefit with platelet glycoprotein IIb/IIIa inhibition by c7E3 among patients with unstable angina: outcome in the EPIC trial [abstract]. *Circulation* 1994, 90(4 pt 2):I-21.

34. Weisman HF, Califf RM, Topol EJ: Pharmacodynamics of chimeric glycoprotein IIb/IIIa integrelin antiplatelet antibody Fab 7E3 in high-risk coronary angioplasty. *Circulation* 1994, 90:1757–1764.

35.• Horrigan MC, Tcheng JE, Califf RM, *et al.*: Maximal benefit of integrelin antiplatelet GPIIb/IIIa blockade 6–24 hours after therapy: results of the IMPACT-II trial [abstract]. *J Am Coll Cardiol* 1996, 27:536–542.

This trial showed the effect of Integrelin in routine rather than high-risk coronary intervention.

36.• Peerlinck K, De Lepeleire I, Goldberg M, *et al.*: MK-383 (L-700, 462), a selective nonpeptide platelet glycoprotein IIb/IIIa antagonist, is active in man. *Circulation* 1993, 88:1512–1517.

This clinical study showed antiplatelet efficacy and safety of MK-383.

37. Kereiakes DJ, Kleiman NS, Ambrose J, *et al.: Randomized, double-blind, placebo-controlled, dose-ranging study of Tirofiban (MK-383) platelet IIb/IIIa blockade in high-risk patients undergoing coronary angioplasty.* J Am Coll Cardiol *1996, 27:536–542.*

38.•• Simpfendorfer C, Kottke-Marchant K, Topol EJ: First experience with chronic platelet GPIIb/IIIa receptor blockade: a pilot study of Xemlofiban an orally active antagonist in unstable angina patients eligible for PTCA [abstract]. *J Am Coll Cardiol* 1996, 27(suppl A):242.

Review of the first trial using non-peptide orally active GP IIb/IIIa antagonist in unstable angina patients.

Chapter 14

Structure and Function of Platelet GP IIb/IIIa Receptors

Shaker A. Mousa
Joel S. Bennett

The objective of this review is to highlight the role of platelets in primary hemostasis and thrombosis, summarize progress made in understanding platelet function, and describe recent advances in the development of novel platelet glycoprotein (GP) IIb/IIIa antagonists. The ideal antiplatelet agent should specifically block platelet-dependent thrombogenic events in vascular diseases without interfering with the platelet function required for primary hemostasis and wound healing. Moreover, it should have no major side effects, be available for both oral and intravenous routes of administration, and have a duration of action appropriate for its therapeutic effect. As progress in understanding platelet function is made, we are continuously moving closer to achieving these goals.

The maintenance of normal hemostasis and vascular tone are critical components of normal homeostasis. Nevertheless, when these normal physiologic processes are expressed at the site of a ruptured atherosclerotic plaque they can result in thrombosis and often in life-threatening tissue ischemia (Table 14-1). The thrombi that form on the arterial side of the circulation (white thrombi) are composed primarily of platelets [1]. Consequently, the aberrant expression of otherwise normal platelet function is primarily responsible for the acute morbidity and mortality associated with cardiovascular, cerebrovascular, and peripheral arterial diseases (Table 14-2). Platelet function can be divided into four phases—adhesion, aggregation, secretion, and elaboration of procoagulant activity—based on the unique character of each phase and on the existence of congenital disorders of platelet function that are specific for each. Thus, when platelets are exposed to connective tissue components following denudation of the surface of an atherosclerotic plaque or to the thrombogenic contents of the interior of a ruptured plaque, they rapidly adhere to these components and form aggregates. Moreover, as platelets aggregate, they generate arachidonic acid metabolites such as thromboxane A_2 to potentiate the aggregation stimulus [2], secrete the contents of their dense granules such as adenosine diphosphate (ADP) and serotonin to extend the aggregation stimulus to other platelets in the vicinity [3], and provide a phospholipid surface for the assembly of the "tenase" complex that generates activated coagulation factor X and "prothrombinase" complex that generates thrombin [4]. Most therapeutic efforts aimed toward preventing arterial thrombi by modulating platelet function have been directed at impairing platelet stimulation and the resulting platelet aggregation [5]. Thus, aspirin prevents thromboxane A_2 synthesis from arachidonic acid by irreversibly inhibiting platelet cyclooxygenase [6], and ticlopidine interferes with the ability of ADP to stimulate platelets [7]. Nevertheless, although these agents have been shown to be of potential benefit, their efficacy, especially in acute situations, is less than desired.

PLATELET FUNCTION

Platelet Adhesion

Platelets are fragments of the cytoplasm of bone marrow megakaryocytes that are released into the circulation, where they survive for approximately 10 days [8]. The number of circulating platelets is regulated by the hormone thrombopoietin, which influences the proliferation and maturation of megakaryocytes and the rate of platelet release [9]. Platelets circulate in the blood in an inactive state. However, when vascular damage occurs, platelets rapidly adhere to the site of damage and aggregate to fill the breach in the vessel wall [1] (Fig. 14-1). The initial platelet adhesive event involves the interaction of specific receptors on the platelet surface and their cognate proteins in the subendothelial connective tissue matrix. Under low shear conditions, such as those present in the venous circulation, platelets adhere to collagen, fibronectin, or laminin. However, these matrix proteins cannot support platelet adhesion at the high shear forces present in arterioles and the microcirculation, and the protein von Willebrand factor must be present in the subendothelium for platelet adhesion to occur [10]. To complete the hemostatic plug, platelets aggregate to form an occlusive mass. Platelet aggregation is an active metabolic process in which agonist-generated intraplatelet signals induce changes in the conformation and distribution of GP IIb/IIIa complexes on the platelet surface [11]. These changes in GP IIb/IIIa in turn expose its binding site for fibrinogen [12]. Plasma fibrinogen then binds to GP IIb/IIIa on adjacent stimulated platelets, thereby cross-linking the platelets into hemostatic aggregates. Although this process is responsible for normal primary hemostasis, an identical sequence of events can occur on the surface of or within an atherosclerotic plaque, resulting in the formation of an occlusive thrombus, rather than a physiologic hemostatic plug.

Platelets contain two receptors on their surface for von Willebrand factor [13]. One receptor is the GP IIb/IIIa complex, which is capable of binding von Willebrand factor after platelet activation [14] or following the exposure of platelets to very high shear stress [15]. The von Willebrand factor receptor responsible for platelet adherence to subendothelium is the glycoprotein Ib/IX complex [16]. GP Ib/IX is a noncovalent heterodimer consisting of the 170,000 molecular weight GP Ib and the 17,000 molecular weight GP IX [16]. GP Ib itself is a heterodimer consisting of the highly glycosylated 143,000 molecular weight glycoprotein Ibα disulfide-linked to the 23,000 molecular weight glycoprotein Ibβ. There are approximately 25,000 GP Ib/IX complexes per platelet. GP Ib/IX is also noncovalently associated with glycoprotein V [16], but the functional consequences of this association are not clear. There are only half as many GP V molecules per platelet as there are GP Ib/IX complexes. Moreover, although the coexpression of GP Ibα, GP Ibβ, and GP IX is required for the efficient expression of the GP Ib/IX complex on the platelet surface, GP V is not [16]. Nevertheless, platelets from patients with the Bernard-Soulier syndrome lacking GP Ib/IX also lack GP V.

Both GP Ib and GP IX are anchored in the platelet membrane by transmembrane domains, and the cyto-

TABLE 14-1. ROLE OF PLATELETS IN HEALTH AND DISEASE

Physiologic role
Hemostasis balance
Release of coagulation factors
Procoagulant activity
Primary adhesion
Platelet plug formation
Vascular tone
Release of vasodilators/vasoconstrictors
Pathologic role
Thrombosis
Homotypic aggregation
Increased procoagulant activities
Platelet/platelet fibrin network
Cellular recruitment
Release of growth factors, mitogens, and other factors
Secretion of extracellular matrix proteins

plasmic portion of GP Ib is associated with the platelet cytoskeleton through binding to actin-binding protein [17]. By electron microscopy, purified GP Ib/IX appears as a 60-nm rod with globular domains at either end [18]. The larger of the globular domains contains the membrane-associated portion of GP Ibα, GP Ibβ, and GP IX, whereas the rod and smaller globular domain are composed by the amino-terminal portion of GP Ibα. The rod-like portion of GP Iba contains a large number of 0-linked sugars that may be responsible for the extended shape of the molecule. Curiously, GP Ibα, GP Iβ, GP IX, and GP V each contain homologous leucine-rich amino acid stretches [16]. The function of these repeats is not known. Although it is possible that they function as "leucine-zippers" involved in the oligimerization of GP Ib/IX/V, they are not located in regions of the molecules involved in known intermolecular associations.

Although platelets adhere to subendothelial von Willebrand factor at higher shear forces, they do not interact with von Willebrand factor in plasma unless the antibiotic ristocetin [19] or the snake venom protein botrocetin are present [20]. There is no definite explanation for this phenomenon. One possibility is that changes occur in the conformation of von Willebrand factor when it is present in the subendothelial matrix and allow it to interact with GP Ib/IX. In favor of this possibility, both ristocetin and botrocetin bind to von Willebrand factor before it interacts with GP Ib/IX [20]. A second but not mutually exclusive possibility is that shear stress generated in the circulating blood directly induces von Willebrand factor binding to GP Ib/IX by changing the conformation of either GP Ib/IX or von Willebrand factor [21]. The ability of shear stress in vitro to induce von Willebrand factor–dependent platelet aggregation supports this possibility.

Platelet Aggregation

Platelet aggregation requires the presence of functional GP IIb/IIIa complexes on the platelet surface [22]. The GP IIb/IIIa complex is a calcium-dependent heterodimer that dissociates into GP IIb and GP IIIa monomers in the presence of calcium chelators [23]. GP IIb is a two-chain molecule with a molecular weight of 136,000 that dissociates into a 125,000 molecular weight heavy chain (GP IIbα) and 23,000 molecular weight light chain (GP IIbβ) after disulfide bond reduction [23]. GP IIIa is a single-chain protein with an unreduced molecular weight of 90,000 [23]. Following the reduction of its 28 disulfide bonds, its apparent molecular weight increases to 110,000. Normally, there are approximately 50,000 GP IIb/IIIa complexes on the surface of resting platelets [23]. When examined by electron microscopy, detergent-solubilized GP IIb/IIIa appears as a 12 × 8 nm globular head with two 18 nm tails extending from one side [24]. The globular head contains the amino terminal portions of GP IIb and GP IIIa, and each tail contains the carboxyl terminal portion of one subunit. Moreover, the globular head contains the ligand-binding domain of the complex, and the tails anchor the complex in the platelet membrane.

Glycoprotein IIb/IIIa is a member of the widely expressed integrin family of adhesion receptors that mediate either cell-matrix or cell-cell interactions and are involved in processes as diverse as tissue migra-

TABLE 14-2. INCIDENCE OF THROMBOEMBOLIC DISEASE IN THE UNITED STATES*

Thromboembolic disease	Patients per year
Coronary artery disease	
Unstable angina	1,000,000
AMI	1,500,000
Abrupt closure, restenosis	250,000
Cerebrovascular disease	
TIAs	375,000
Stroke	500,000
Peripheral arterial occlusive diseases	2,000,000
DVT	2,000,000
PE	200,000

**Data from National Center for Health Statistics and the American Heart Association. AMI—acute myocardial infarction; DVT—deep vein thrombosis; PE—pulmonary embolism; TIA—transient ischemic attacks.*

tion during embryogenesis, cellular adhesion, cancer metastases, and lymphocyte-helper and killer-cell functions [25]. Like GP IIb/IIIa, integrins are heterodimers composed of α subunits homologous to GP IIb and β subunits homologous to GP IIIa. There are at least eight known β subunits and 14 α subunits. Although the diversity of α and β subunits could give rise to more than 100 different integrins, the number of integrins is limited by restrictions on the ability of the various subunits to interact. Consequently, integrins can be grouped in a number of subfamilies based on the use of a particular β subunit. It is noteworthy that integrins recognize specific amino acid sequences in their potential ligands. The best studied amino acid sequence is arginine-glycine-aspartic acid-X (RGDX), in which X can be any of a number of amino acids, including serine, alanine, or phenylanine [25]. The RGDX sequence is present in a number of matrix proteins, including fibrinogen, vitronectin, fibronectin, thrombospondin, osteopontin, and von Willebrand factor. Integrins can also interact with non-RGDX motifs. For example, the integrin $\alpha_4\beta_1$ recognizes the sequence LDV within the CS-1 region of fibronectin [26].

The principal GP IIb/IIIa ligand fibrinogen contains two RGDX sequences in its Aα chain, one at residues 95-98 (RGDF) and the second at residues 572-575 (RGDS) [27]. Because peptides containing RGDX sequences inhibit platelet aggregation and the interaction of GP IIb/IIIa with fibrinogen [28], it is possible that one of these regions of fibrinogen interacts with GP IIb/IIIa. Moreover, RGD-containing peptides can be cross-linked to GP IIIa between residues 109-171 [29]. On the other hand, peptides corresponding to the carboxyl terminal 10-15 amino acids of the fibrinogen γ chain also inhibit GP IIb/IIIa function [30] and can be cross-linked to GP IIb between residues 294-314 [31]. Because of the topography of the fibrinogen molecule [24], it seems unlikely that α chain and γ chain sequences could bind to GP IIb/IIIa simultaneously. Ultrastructural studies of fibrinogen bound to GP IIb/IIIa [24] and studies using recombinant fibrinogen-containing mutated RGD or γ chain sequences [27] have addressed this issue and indicate that fibrinogen binds to GP IIb/IIIa via its γ chain sequences. Nevertheless, the clinical efficacy of peptides or peptidomimetics based on the RGD sequence as inhibitors of GP IIb/IIIa function is difficult to reconcile with these data [5]. However, competitive binding measurements indicate that γ chain and RGD peptide binding to GP IIb/IIIa is mutually exclusive [32], suggesting that the peptides bind to the same or to an overlapping site. Thus, the ligand-binding site in GP IIb/IIIa may be a surface containing both peptide cross-linking sites and fibrinogen binds to GP IIb/IIIa via γ chain sequences, rather than RGD sequences, because the former are available on the surface of the fibrinogen molecule, whereas the latter are not. As noted above, GP IIb/IIIa can also interact with von Willebrand factor, and in vitro studies indicate that it can interact with fibronectin and vitronectin as well [33]. None of these proteins contains sequences similar to the fibrinogen γ chain, but each contains an RGDX motif. In these cases, it is likely that RGDX mediates ligand binding to GP IIb/IIIa.

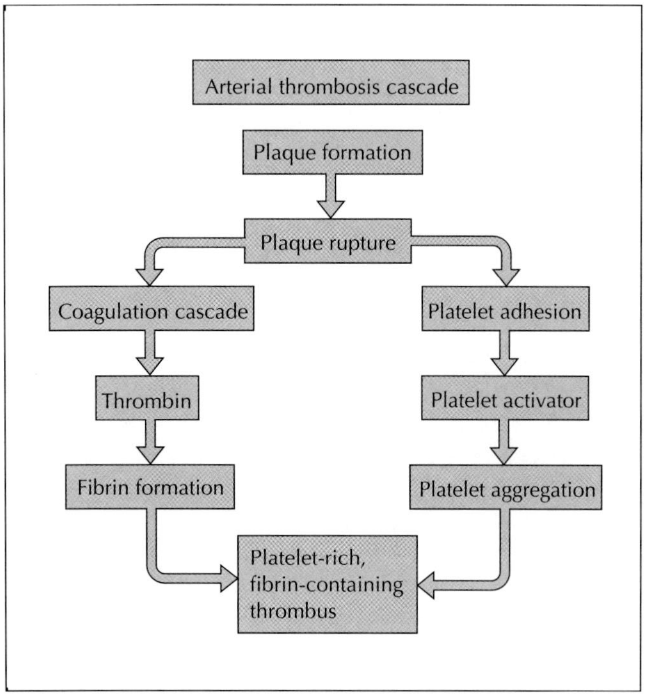

Figure 14-1. Stages in formation of arterial thrombosis.

The GP IIb/IIIa on resting platelets does not interact with fibrinogen or other ligands, but binding rapidly follows platelet stimulation by any of a number of platelet agonists [23]. The process by which intracellular signals initiated by agonists induce ligand binding to GP IIb/IIIa is called "inside-out" signaling [34]. Because this process occurs without an increase in the number of GP IIb/IIIa complexes on the platelet surface, it is assumed to result from a conformational change in GP IIb/IIIa complexes already present on the platelet surface [35]. The "inside-out" signaling pathways that transmit the activation signal to the cytoplasmic portions of GP IIb/IIIa are not known. Most, if not all, agonist receptors on platelets are associated with guanine nucleotide binding or G proteins [36]. G proteins are complexes of α, β, and γ subunits and represent the next level of signal transmission, activating the enzymes phospholipase C and phospholipase A_2 [36]. Phospholipase C hydrolyzes the membrane phospholipid phosphatidylinositol 4,5-bisphosphate into diacylglycerol and soluble inositol

1,4,5-triphosphate (IP_3) [37]. Diacylglycerol in turn activates the enzyme protein kinase C, and IP_3 contributes to an agonist-induced rise in intracellular calcium [38]. Phospholipase A_2 catalyzes the release of arachidonic acid from phospholipids, initiating pathways that result in the synthesis of prostaglandin endoperoxides and thromboxane A_2 [39]. The steps involved in phospholipase C and A_2 activation are not known. Stimulation of platelet protein kinase C by phorbol esters activates GP IIb/IIIa [40], although GP IIb/IIIa itself is not phosphorylated on serine or threonine to a significant extent [41]. Thus, protein kinase C-mediated phosphorylation of other proteins that are not yet identified must be involved in GP IIb/IIIa activation. Platelet stimulation by agonists such as thrombin, ADP, and collagen also results in three waves of tyrosine phosphorylation in platelets [42]. The first wave results in the phosphorylation of pp^{60src}, cortactin, pp^{72syk}, $p^{21ras}GAP$, and proteins with a molecular weight of 59,000 and 68,000 and is independent of GP IIb/IIIa. The second and third waves, however, require occupation of GP IIb/IIIa by ligands. The second wave is associated with the clustering of GP IIb/IIIa and results in phosphorylation of proteins of 140,000 and 50,000 to 68,000 molecular weight and pp^{72syk}. The third wave is a consequence of platelet aggregation and induces the phosphorylation of proteins such as pp^{125FAK} and proteins with a molecular weight of 95,000 to 97,000. Despite the importance of tyrosine phosphorylation in intracellular signal transduction, it has not been possible to directly link tyrosine phosphorylation to the process of GP IIb/IIIa activation.

Platelet Aggregometry

The phenomenon of agonist-induced platelet aggregation has been studied ex vivo using a variety of methods. The most common method, turbidimetric platelet aggregometry described by Born [43], records the increase in light transmittance that occurs as stirred platelets in platelet-rich plasma aggregate. This method is generally adequate for clinical purposes, but is insensitive to the presence of small platelet aggregates and does not record the early stages of aggregation. When platelet aggregation is observed in a turbidimetric aggregometer, the resulting tracings vary according to the nature and concentration of the platelet agonist used. All agonists except epinephrine produce an initial transient decrease in light transmittance that has been attributed to a change in platelet shape from that of a disc to a spiny sphere. Platelet shape change is followed by two "waves" of platelet aggregation. The first wave is reversible and is a direct consequence of agonist stimulation. The second wave is due to the formation of large irreversible aggregates when platelet secretion occurs. Depending on the agonist, the first and second waves may merge into a single continuous tracing.

Low concentrations of ADP (> 1 μm) produce shape change and a reversible first wave of aggregation, whereas higher concentrations produce either two waves of aggregation or a continuous tracing [44]. The second wave of ADP-stimulated aggregation is coincident with platelet secretion, requires the synthesis of thromboxane A_2, and is inhibited by cyclooxygenase inhibitors such as aspirin [44]. Thrombin is the most potent physiologic platelet agonist. At low thrombin concentrations, thrombin-induced aggregation is similar to that induced by ADP. At higher concentrations, either biphasic aggregation or a single continuous tracing is seen. In contrast to ADP, higher thrombin concentrations can overcome the inhibitory effects of cyclooxygenase inhibitors [44]. Collagen-induced aggregation is preceded by a lag period during which collagen polymerizes into fibrils of sufficient size to activate platelets [45]. The lag period is followed by shape change and a continuous wave of aggregation. The aggregation response to low collagen concentrations is inhibited by cyclooxygenase inhibitors, but higher collagen concentrations overcome this inhibition [44].

Turbidimetric platelet aggregometry has been modified to permit the simultaneous measurement of platelet adenosine triphosphate (ATP) secretion by measuring the luminescence generated from the ATP-dependent firefly luciferin-luciferase reaction [46]. Platelet aggregation can also be measured in whole blood, based on the increase in electrical impedance that occurs as platelet aggregates accumulate on a pair of electrodes [47]. Like turbidimetric platelet aggregometry, whole blood aggregometry is insensitive to early events that follow platelet stimulation. The most sensitive method to assess platelet aggregation is based on the disappearance of single platelets following platelet stimulation [48]. Single platelet counting indicates that within 10 seconds of platelet stimulation, 90% of platelets are present in aggregates that may contain up to 100 platelets.

Glanzmann Thrombasthenia

Glanzmann thrombasthenia, a rare congenital hemorrhagic disorder characterized by the absence of platelet aggregation, was originally described by Glanzmann in 1918 [49]. The platelet defect responsible for thrombasthenia is an inherited deficiency or dysfunction of the GP IIb/IIIa complex [50]. The genes for GP IIb and GP IIIa are both present on the proximal portion of the long arm of human chromosome 17 at q21→23 [51] and have been localized to a single 260 kb DNA fragment [52]. Although the genes are in proximity, there is no evidence for the coordinate control of their expression, and studies of GP IIb and GP IIIa biosynthesis indicate that the predominant control of GP IIb/IIIa expression occurs in the endoplasmic reticulum where the assembly of GP IIb/IIIa complexes occurs [53]. Thus, neither GP IIb or GP IIIa appear on the platelet surface unless a complex forms, but the complexes must also be correctly folded to be exported from the endoplasmic reticulum [54].

Thrombasthenia can result from an inadequate number of GP IIb/IIIa complexes on the platelet surface to support platelet aggregation or from the expression of nonfunctional complexes. To date, over 20 mutations that are responsible for the thrombasthenic phenotype have been reported. The majority of these mutations have been complex gene rearrangements, deletions, messenger RNA splicing abnormalities, frameshifts, or missense mutations that have prevented either GP IIb or GP IIIa synthesis. A small number of point mutations, predominantly affecting GP IIb, have also been described that perturb the folding of GP IIb/IIIa in the endoplasmic reticulum enough to prevent its export to the platelet surface [54–56]. Finally, GP IIIa mutations have been reported that involve either its RGD–cross-linking site [57] or its cytoplasmic extension [58] and result in the expression of nonfunctional complexes.

Typically, thrombasthenia presents with mucocutaneous bleeding in the neonatal period or infancy [59]. Spontaneous petechiae are uncommon, and bleeding generally results from a condition that would cause bleeding in an otherwise normal individual. Epistaxis, gingival bleeding, and menorrhagia are frequent. Bleeding at menarche may be severe, and childbirth represents a severe hemorrhagic risk. Nevertheless, the severity of bleeding is unpredictable, even within affected families, and does not correlate with nature or the extent of the GP IIb/IIIa deficiency. Moreover, the severity of thrombasthenia appears to decline with age, probably due to a decrease in the incidence of conditions such as epistaxis.

Antagonists of Platelet Function

The link between platelet function and the clinical manifestations of arteriosclerosis has suggested therapeutic impairment of platelet function as an obvious target for drug discovery and development. The challenge has been and will remain to develop an effective agent with minimal effects on normal hemostasis.

The antiplatelet agents in current clinical use inhibit specific components of the inside-out signaling pathways. Thus, aspirin, by inhibiting platelet cyclooxygenase, prevents the potentiation of platelet aggregation by thromboxane A_2 and ticlopidine interferes with ADP-induced aggregation. Although these agents have proven to be effective in decreasing the incidence of acute occlusive events in patients with established vas-

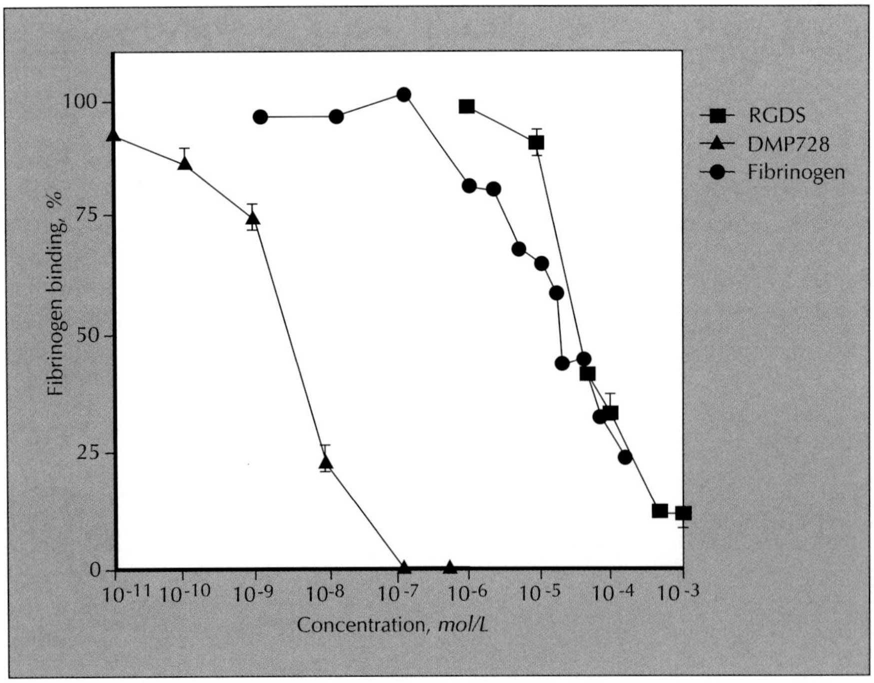

Figure 14-2. The effect of various antiplatelet agents on fibrinogen binding to h-GPP. *T-bars* indicate mean ± SEM. RGDS—arginine-glycine-aspartic acid-serine; DMP728—constrained arginine-glycine-aspartic acid peptides.

cular disease and, in the case of aspirin, in decreasing the incidence of primary acute coronary syndromes, these effects have been relatively small. Moreover, the ability of aspirin to prevent reocclusion after coronary thrombolysis or angioplasty is limited. Consequently, because fibrinogen binding to GP IIb/IIIa is the final common step in the inside-out signaling in platelets and is directly responsible for the formation of platelet aggregates, it is logical to ask whether direct inhibition of this step in platelet function might be more efficacious.

Fibrinogen binding to GP IIb/IIIa can be inhibited by monoclonal antibodies and by RGD-containing peptides in vitro [23–35]. However, the therapeutic utility of peptides has been limited by their low affinity and lack of oral bioavailability, and the one monoclonal antibody in clinical use, 7E3 (ReoPro; Centocor, Malvern, PA) is a chimera of human and murine antibodies and is likely to induce an immune response [23–35].

In contrast to linear RGD-peptides, constrained RGD-peptides (DMP728) inhibit fibrinogen binding to GP IIb/IIIa with considerably higher affinity (Fig. 14-2, Table 14-3). Activation of platelets by agonists causes changes in the number of binding sites or platelets as well as conformational changes to the high affinity state. Additionally, peptides containing the RGD sequence and other ligands for GP IIb/IIIa can induce a conformational change in the receptor, yielding a functional high-affinity binding site known as "ligand-induced binding sites" (LIBS). The association of the GP IIb/IIIa heterodimer via the calcium binding domains is essential for fibrinogen binding and platelet aggregation. Chelation of extracellular calcium can lead to the separation of the heterodimer and hence lack of fibrinogen binding and inhibition of platelet aggregation. Additionally, the discovery of the monoclonal antibody, 7E3, RGD mimetic, as well as the availability of other antithrombotic strategies, should allow for achieving optimal therapeutic strategies (Table 14-4).

TABLE 14-3. ANTI-AGGREGATORY EFFECTS OF DIFFERENT THROMBIN INHIBITORS VERSUS GP IIB//IIIA ANTAGONISTS AGAINST AGONIST-INDUCED HUMAN PLATELET AGGREGATION

	Thrombin inhibitors*		GP IIb/IIIa antagonists*	
	Hirudin	PPACK	DMP728	c7E3
Thrombin†	0.07 + 0.02	0.12 + 0.03	0.049 + 0.020	0.064 + 0.016
ADP‡	—	—	0.026 + 0.004	0.054 + 0.019
TEAC§	—	—	0.037 + 0.009	0.071 + 0.007

**IC50 μm.*
†0.5 IU/mL + 10 μM GPRP.
‡100 μM.
§A mixture of thrombin, 0.001 IU/mL; epinephrine, 100 μM; adenosine diphosphate (ADP), 100 μM; and collagen, 20 μg/mL (inactive at concentrations up to 10 μM).
DMP728—constrained arginine-glycine-aspartic acid peptides;
PPACK—phe-pro-arginine-chloromethyl ketone.

Table 14-4. Antithrombotic Agents Available or Under Clinical Investigation in the United States

Therapeutic class	Agents	Indications
Thrombolytics	Streptokinase Urokinase t-PA	Arterial thrombosis
Anticoagulants	Heparin Warfarin LMWH Hirudin/Hirulog	AMI, PTCA, UA DVT, PE
Antiplatelets	Aspirin Ticlopidine Dipyridamole Hirudin analogues Thromboxane antagonists 7E3 (ReoPro), *MK-383 (Triofiban), Integrelin, RO44-9883 (Lamifiban), Oral GP IIb\IIIa antagonists (SC-5468A, BIBU-104)	AMI, UA, stroke Stroke

**MK-383 (Merck & Co., West Point, PA);*
Integrelin (Cor Therapeutics, San Francisco, CA);
RO44-9883 (Hoffman-LaRoche, Basel, Switzerland);
AMI—acute myocardial infarction; DVT—deep vein thrombosis; LMWH—low molecular weight heparin; PE—pulmonary embolism; PTCA—percutaneous transluminal coronary angioplasty; UA—unstable angina.

References

1. Sixma JJ, Wester J: The hemostatic plug. *Semin Hematol* 1977, 14:265–299.
2. Majerus PW: Arachidonate metabolism in vascular disorders. *J Clin Invest* 1983, 72:1521–1525.
3. Weiss HJ, Lages B: The response of platelets to epinephrine in storage pool deficiency—evidence pertaining to the role of adenosine diphosphate in mediating primary and secondary aggregation. *Blood* 1988, 72:1717–1725.
4. Zwaal RF, Comfurius P, Bevers EM: Platelet procoagulant activity and microvesicle formation. Its putative role in hemostasis and thrombosis. *Biochim Biophys Acta* 1992, 1180:1–8.
5. Lefkovits J, Plow E, Topol E: Platelet glycoprotein IIb/IIIa receptors in cardiovascular medicine. *N Engl J Med* 1995, 332:1553–1559.
6. Roth GJ, Majerus PW: The mechanism of the effect of aspirin on human platelets. I. Acetylation of a particulate fraction protein. *J Clin Invest* 1975, 56:264–260.
7. McTavish D, Faulds D, Goa KL: Ticlopidine. An updated review of its pharmacology and therapeutic use in platelet-dependent disorders. *Drugs* 1992, 40:238–259.
8. Harker LA: Platelet production. *N Engl J Med* 1970, 282:492–494.
9. Foster DC, Sprecher CA, Grant FJ, *et al.*: Human thrombopoietin: gene structure, cDNA sequence, expression, and chromosomal localization. *Proc Natl Acad Sci U S A* 1994, 91:13023–13027.
10. Turrito VT, Weiss HJ, Zimmerman TS, Sussman II: Factor VIII/von Willebrand factor in subendothelium mediates platelet adhesion. *Blood* 1985, 65:823–831.
11. Phillips DR, Charo IF, Scarborough RM: GPIIb-IIIa: the responsive integrin. *Cell* 1991, 65:359–362.
12. Bennett JS, Vilaire G: Exposure of platelet fibrinogen receptors by ADP and epinephrine. *J Clin Invest* 1979, 64:1393–1401.
13. Ruggeri ZM, DeMarco L, Gatti L, *et al.*: Platelets have more than one binding site for von Willebrand factor. *J Clin Invest* 1983; 72:1–12.
14. Ruggeri ZM, Bader R, DeMarco L: Glanzmann thrombasthenia; deficient binding of von Willebrand factor to thrombin-stimulated platelets. *Proc Natl Acad Sci U S A* 1982, 79:6038–6041.
15. Alevriadou BR, Moake JL, Turner NA, *et al.*: Real-time analysis of shear-dependent thrombus formation and its blockade by inhibitors of von Willebrand factor binding to platelets. *Blood* 1993, 81:1263–1276.

16. Lopez JA: The platelet glycoprotein Ib-IX complex. *Blood Coag Fibrinolysis* 1994, 5:97–119.

17. Andrews RK, Fox JEB: Interaction of purified actin-binding protein with the platelet membrane glycoprotein Ib-IX complex. *J Biol Chem* 1991, 266:7144–7147.

18. Fox JEB, Aggerbeck LP, Berndt MC: Structure of the glycoprotein Ib-IX complex from platelet membranes. *J Biol Chem* 1988, 263:4882–4890.

19. Howard MA, Firkin BG: Ristocetin—a new tool in the investigation of platelet aggregation. *Thromb Diath Haemorrh* 1971, 26:362–369.

20. Andrews RK, Booth WJ, Gorman JJ, *et al.*: Purification of botrocetin from *Bothrops jararaca* venom. Analysis of the botrocetin-mediated interaction between von Willebrand factor and the human glycoprotein Ib-IX complex. *Biochemistry* 1989, 28:8317–8326.

21. Roth GJ: Developing relationships: arterial platelet adhesion, glycoprotein Ib, and leucine-rich glycoproteins. *Blood* 1991, 77:5–19.

22. Phillips DR, Charo IF, Parise LV, Fitzgerald LA: The platelet membrane glycoprotein IIb-IIIa complex. *Blood* 1988, 71:831–843.

23. Bennett JS: Structural biology of glycoprotein IIb-IIIa. *Trends Cardiovasc Med* 1996, 16:31–36.

24. Weisel JW, Nagaswami C, Vilaire G, Bennett JS: Examination of the platelet membrane glycoprotein IIb/IIIa complex and its interaction with fibrinogen and other ligands by electron microscopy. *J Biol Chem* 1992, 267:16637–16643.

25. Hynes RO: Integrins: versatility, modulation, and signaling in cell adhesion. *Cell* 1991, 69:11–25.

26. Lobb RR, Hemler ME: The pathophysiologic role of a4 integrins in vivo. *J Clin Invest* 1994, 94:1722–1728.

27. Farrell DH, Thiagarajan P, Chung DW, Davie EW: Role of fibrinogen a and g chain sites in platelet aggregation. *Proc Natl Acad Sci U S A* 1992, 89:10729–10732.

28. Gartner TK, Bennett JS: The tetrapeptide analogue of the cell attachment site of fibronectin inhibits platelet aggregation and fibrinogen binding to activated platelets. *J Biol Chem* 1985, 260:11891–11894.

29. D'Souza SE, Ginsberg MH, Burke TA, *et al.*: Localization of an Arg-Gly-Asp recognition site within an integrin adhesion receptor. *Science* 1988, 242:91–93.

30. Kloczewiak M, Timmons S, Lukas TJ, Hawiger J: Platelet receptor recognition site on human fibrinogen. Synthesis and structure-function relationships of peptides corresponding to the carboxy-terminal segment of the g chain. *Biochemistry* 1984, 23:1767–1774.

31. D'Souza SE, Ginsberg MH, Burke TA, Plow EF: The ligand binding site of the platelet integrin receptor GPIIb-IIIa is proximal to the second calcium binding domain of its a subunit. *J Biol Chem* 1990, 265:3440–3446.

32. Bennett JS, Shattil SJ, Power JW, Gartner TK: Interaction of fibrinogen with its platelet receptor. Differential effects of alpha and gamma chain fibrinogen peptides on the glycoprotein IIb-IIIa complex. *J Biol Chem* 1988, 263:12948–12953.

33. Pytela R, Pierschbacher MD, Ginsberg MH, *et al.*: Platelet membrane glycoprotein IIb/IIIa: member of a family of arg-gly-asp-specific adhesion receptors. *Science* 1986, 231:1559–1562.

34. O'Toole TE, Katagiri Y, Faull RJ, *et al.*: Integrin cytoplasmic domains mediate inside-out signal transduction. *J Cell Biol* 1994, 124:1047–1059.

35. Sims PJ, Ginsberg MH, Plow EF, Shattil SJ: Effect of platelet activation on the conformation of the plasma membrane glycoprotein IIb-IIIa complex. *J Biol Chem* 1991, 266:7345–7352.

36. Brass LF, Manning DR, Shattil SJ: GTP-binding proteins and platelet activation. *Prog Hemostas Thrombos* 1990, 10:127–174.

37. Wilson DB, Neufeld EJ, Majerus PW: Phosphoinositide interconversion in thrombin-stimulated human platelets. *J Biol Chem* 1985, 260:1046–1051.

38. Brass LF, Joseph SK: A role for inositol triphosphate in intracellular Ca^{2+} mobilization and granule secretion in platelets. *J Biol Chem* 1985, 260:15172–15179.

39. Exton JH: Signaling through phosphatidylcholine breakdown. *J Biol Chem* 1990, 265:1–4.

40. Shattil SJ, Brass LF: Induction of the fibrinogen receptor on human platelets by intracellular mediators. *J Biol Chem* 1987, 262:992–1000.

41. Hillery CA, Smyth SS, Parise LV: Phosphorylation of human platelet glycoprotein IIIa (GPIIIa). Dissociation from fibrinogen receptor activation and phosphorylation of GPIIIa in vitro. *J Biol Chem* 1991, 266:14663–14669.

42. Clark EA, Shattil SJ, Brugge JS: Regulation of protein tyrosine kinases in platelets. *Trends Biochem Sci* 1994, 19:464–469.

43. Born GVR: Aggregation of blood platelets by adenosine diphosphate and its reversal. *Nature* 1962, 194:927–929.

44. Charo IF, Feinman RD, Detwiler TC: Interrelations of platelet aggregation and secretion. *J Clin Invest* 1977, 60:866–873.

45. Jaffe R, Deykin D: Evidence for a structural requirement for the aggregation of platelets by collagen. *J Clin Invest* 1974, 53:875–883.

46. Feinman RD, Lubowsky J, Charo I, Zabinski MP: The lumi-aggregometer: a new instrument for simultaneous measurement of secretion and aggregation by platelets. *J Lab Clin Med* 1977, 90:125–129.

47. Ingerman-Wojenski C, Smith JB, Silver MJ: Evaluation of electrical aggregometry: comparison with optical aggregometry, secretion of ATP, and accumulation of radiolabeled platelets. *J Lab Clin Med* 1983, 101:44–52.

48. Gear ARL: Reduction in single platelets during primary and secondary aggregation. *Thrombos Haemostas* 1981, 45:298–301.

49. Glanzmann EL: Hereditäre hämorrhagische Thrombasthenie. Ein Beitrag zur pathologie dur blutplättchen. *J Kinderkr* 1918, 88:1–42.

50. Phillips DR, Agin PP: Platelet membrane defects in Glanzmann's thrombasthenia. *J Clin Invest* 1977, 60:535–545.

51. Sosnoski DM, Emanuel BS, Hawkins AL, *et al.*: Chromosomal localization of the genes for the vitronectin and fibronectin receptors a subunits and for platelet glycoproteins IIb and IIIa. *J Clin Invest* 1988, 81:1993–1998.

52. Bray PR, Barsh G, Rosa J-P, *et al.*: Physical linkage of the genes for platelet membrane glycoproteins IIb and IIIa. *Proc Natl Acad Sci U S A* 1988, 85:8683–8687.

53. Kolodziej MA, Vilaire G, Rifat S, *et al.*: Effect of deletion of glycoprotein IIb exon 28 on the expression of the platelet glycoprotein IIb/IIIa complex. *Blood* 1991, 78:2344–2353.

54. Poncz M, Salahandrin R, Coller BS, *et al.*: Glanzmann thrombasthenia secondary to a Gly273ÆAsp mutation adjacent to the first calcium-binding domain of platelet glycoprotein IIb. *J Clin Invest* 1994, 93:172–179.

55. Wilcox DA, Paddock CM, Lyman S, *et al.*: Glanzmann thrombasthenia resulting from a single amino acid substitution between the second and third calcium-binding domains of GPIIb. Role of the GPIIb amino terminus in integrin subunit association. *J Clin Invest* 1995, 95:1553–1560.

56. Wilcox DA, Wautier JL, Pidard D, Newman PJ: A single amino acid substitution flanking the fourth calcium binding domain of α IIb prevents maturation of the α IIb β 3 integrin complex. *J Biol Chem* 1994, 269:4450–4457.

57. Loftus JC, O'Toole TE, Plow EF, *et al.*: A b3 integrin mutation abolishes ligand binding and alters divalent cation-dependent conformation. *Science* 1990, 249:915–918.

58. Chen Y, Djaffar I, Pidard D, *et al.*: Ser752ÆPro mutation in the cytoplasmic domain of integrin b_3 subunit and defective activation of platelet integrin $^{a}IIb^{b}_{3}$ (glycoprotein IIb-IIIa) in a variant of Glanzmann thrombasthenia. *Proc Natl Acad Sci U S A* 1992; 89:10169-10173.

59. George JN, Caen JP, Nurden AT: Glanzmann's thrombasthenia: the spectrum of clinical disease. *Blood* 1990, 75:1383–1395.

Chapter 15

EPIC, IMPACT II, AND EPILOG TRIALS: PLATELET GP IIB/IIIA INHIBITION FOR PREVENTION OF ISCHEMIC COMPLICATIONS OF PERCUTANEOUS CORONARY INTERVENTION

Victor Guetta
A. Michael Lincoff

Despite significant advances in the technique and equipment for percutaneous transluminal coronary angioplasty (PTCA) and associated improvements in its safety and efficacy, ischemic procedural complications continue to occur in up to 10% to 20% of high-risk patients, and late restenosis develops in at least 30% of these patients within 3 to 6 months [1]. As the pivotal role of platelets in the formation of arterial thrombosis following coronary intervention has been elucidated, aspirin, a weak inhibitor of the cyclooxygenase pathway, has been shown to reduce the risk of ischemic complications by 50% to 70%. However, 10% to 20% of patients continue to suffer coronary occlusion or myocardial infarction (MI) or require emergent repeat revascularization despite the use of aspirin [2]. Although it has been suggested that platelet-rich thrombus formation after vascular injury plays a role in the restenosis process, antiplatelet agents have thus far failed to reduce the incidence of this late complication. It is possible, however, that an inhibitor of platelet aggregation that is more potent than aspirin might further reduce the rate of acute ischemic complications and restenosis after PTCA.

Recent important refinements in our understanding of platelet physiology have focused attention on the platelet glycoprotein (GP) IIb/IIIa integrin, a receptor that mediates the final common pathway of platelet aggregation. Each platelet contains 50,000 to 100,000 GP IIb/IIIa receptors on its surface, which become competent to bind fibrinogen or von Willebrand factor (vWF) when platelets are activated. Each fibrinogen or vWF molecule may bind to GP IIb/IIIa receptors on multiple platelets, thus cross-linking adjacent platelets into an aggregating mass.

Several novel pharmacologic agents that block this final common pathway of platelet aggregation have been developed and tested in clinical trials to determine whether such a strategy might reduce the incidence of acute ischemic complications or restenosis after angioplasty. The first such agent to be developed and the most extensively studied clinically was 7E3, a murine antibody that binds to and blocks the IIb/IIIa receptor [3]. This antibody was modified to a chimeric antibody fragment, which is composed of an antigen-binding fragment with human constant regions and mouse variable regions (c7E3 Fab). Another agent that has been recently investigated in a large-scale clinical trial is Integrelin (Cor Therapeutics, San Francisco, CA), a heptapeptide containing a Lys-Gly-Asp (KGD) sequence that binds selectively to the GP IIb/IIIa receptor.

This chapter discusses the results of three recently completed phase III clinical trials evaluating the efficacy and safety of GP IIb/IIIa blockade in patients undergoing coronary angioplasty.

THE EPIC TRIAL

The EPIC (Evaluation of c7E3 for the Prevention of Ischemic Complications) trial evaluated the efficacy of two dose regimens of c7E3 Fab among patients undergoing high-risk PTCA or directional coronary atherectomy (DCA) [4].

A total of 2099 patients with high-risk characteristics (unstable angina pectoris, acute myocardial infarction [AMI], or adverse angiographic characteristics) were enrolled at 56 clinical sites throughout the United States. Patients were randomly assigned to one of the following three treatment groups in a double-blind design: 1) a c7E3 Fab bolus of 0.25 mg/kg of body weight, followed by a 12-hour infusion of 10 µg per minute; 2) a c7E3 Fab bolus, followed by a 12-hour placebo infusion; or 3) a placebo bolus and placebo infusion. All patients were treated with aspirin (325 mg) and heparin (10,000–12,000 U initial bolus) to achieve an activated clotting time of at least 300 to 350 seconds during the procedure. The primary endpoint of the trial was a composite of any of the following events in the first 30 days postrandomization: death, MI, coronary artery bypass graft (CABG), or repeat percutaneous coronary angioplasty, coronary stent implantation, or insertion of intra-aortic balloon pump for acute ischemia. A secondary clinical endpoint was the composite of death, MI, or the need for a repeat (urgent or elective) revascularization by 6 months follow-up.

Results

Efficacy

The 30-day outcome demonstrated a dose-related effect of c7E3 Fab in the prevention of ischemic complications, with a significant 35% reduction in the incidence of the composite endpoint among the patients receiving the c7E3 Fab bolus and 12-hour infusion compared with the double-placebo group (8.5 vs 12.8%; $P = 0.008$). The bolus only of c7E3 Fab resulted in an intermediate and nonsignificant reduction in this endpoint. A major reduction was observed in the risk of nonfatal MI and the need for urgent revascularization (Table 15-1). The timing of nonfatal postprocedural ischemic events varied among the three treatment groups. Ischemic events occurred more frequently and earlier postintervention in the placebo-treated group compared with the c7E3 Fab–treated groups (Fig. 15-1). When the treatment effect was evaluated according to enrollment criteria (acute ischemic syndromes vs high-risk morphologic features), no significant differences in the magnitude of benefit were noted, and treatment–morphology interactions were not significant [5].

Safety

A significant increase in bleeding complications was observed in the c7E3 Fab–treated groups (Table 15-2). Patients who received c7E3 Fab bolus and infusion experienced substantial increases in the risks of major bleeding (14% compared with 7% in the placebo group; $P < 0.001$) and the need for erythrocyte transfusion (15% compared with 7% in the placebo group; $P < 0.001$), with intermediate increases observed in the group receiving c7E3 Fab bolus only. Major bleeding occurred at sites of femoral vascular access, although treatment with c7E3 Fab was associated with slight increases in spontaneous retroperitoneal or gastrointestinal bleeding as well. There were no differences among groups in the rate of intracranial bleeding or the rate of vascular surgery for bleeding.

An important insight into the safety of c7E3 was offered in the study of patients referred for urgent CABG, which occurred in 33 patients of the c7E3 Fab–treated groups and in 25 patients of the placebo-treated group [6]. There were no significant differences in the incidences of major or minor bleeding among patients who had received c7E3 Fab compared with patients who had been randomly assigned to placebo. Erythrocyte transfusions were required slightly more frequently among patients receiving c7E3 Fab. Platelet transfusions were administered more often as well, but often prophylactically because the EPIC protocol recommended unblinding of the study drug and platelet transfusions in the event of emergency CABG. An unexpected finding was that the incidence of thrombocytopenia after emergency CABG was reduced by more than half in the patients receiving c7E3 Fab compared with those receiving placebo, suggesting a protective effect of c7E3 Fab by preventing the binding of platelet to the cardiopulmonary bypass membranes. Animal data exist to support this concept, demonstrating a reduced incidence of thrombocytopenia and less perioperative blood loss among dogs treated with the GP IIb/IIIa receptor antagonist Integrelin during experimental cardiopulmonary bypass [7].

Several lines of evidence suggest that heparin played a key role in potentiating the bleeding complications related to c7E3 Fab in the EPIC trial. The heparin dose was not adjusted for body weight; thus, the lightest weight patients received the highest dose of heparin per body weight. When bleeding risk was assessed according to body weight, the lightest weight patients had the highest risk of bleeding with c7E3 Fab therapy [8]. Maximum in-laboratory activated clotting time (ACT) also was identified as an independent correlate of bleeding risk. For each of the three treatment groups, there was a clear relationship between increasing maximum ACT and increasing incidence of major bleeding. However, there was no apparent relationship between maximum in-laboratory ACT and the

TABLE 15-1. PRIMARY OUTCOME EVENTS IN VARIOUS TREATMENT GROUPS AT 30 DAYS IN THE EPIC TRIAL

Event	Placebo, *n(%)**	c7E3 Fab bolus, *n(%)*†	c7E3 Fab bolus + infusion, *n(%)*‡	*P* value for dose response§
Primary endpoint	89(12.8)	79(11.4)	59(8.3)	0.009
Death	12(1.7)	9(1.3)	12(1.7)	0.96
Myocardial infarction	60(8.6)	43(6.2)	37(5.2)	0.013
Q-wave	16(2.3)	7(1)	6(0.8)	0.020
Large non–Q-wave	28(4)	19(2.7)	21(3)	0.265
Small non–Q-wave	16(2.3)	17(2.4)	10(1.4)	0.239
Emergency PTCA	31(4.5)	25(3.6)	6(0.8)	< 0.001
Emergency CABG	25(3.6)	16(2.3)	17(2.4)	0.177
Stent placement	4(0.6)	12(1.7)	4(0.6)	0.98
Balloon pump insertion	1(0.1)	1(0.1)	1(0.1)	0.99

**Total number of patients, 696.*
†Total number of patients, 695.
‡Total number of patients, 708.
§P = 0.009 for overall test for trend; P = 0.43 for comparison of placebo group with c7E3 bolus only; and P = 0.008 for comparison of placebo group with c7E3 bolus + infusion.
CABG—coronary artery bypass grafting; PTCA—percutaneous transluminal coronary angioplasty.

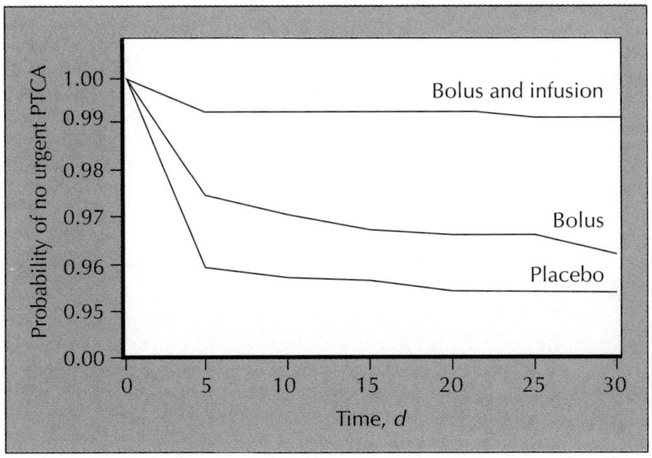

Figure 15-1. Thirty-day EPIC (Evaluation of c7E3 for the Prevention of Ischemic Complications) trial results. Kaplan-Meier curve showing the probability of no urgent repeated percutaneous revascularization procedures in the three treatment groups. Events began to occur shortly after the index procedure in the placebo group, between 6 and 12 hours after the procedure in the group given c7E3 Fab bolus only and even later in the group given c7E3 Fab bolus and infusion. PTCA—percutaneous transluminal coronary angioplasty. (*From* Topol and colleagues [9].)

incidence of ischemic complications for the placebo- or the c7E3 Fab-treated patients. Thus, for both body weight and maximum in-laboratory ACT, there was an apparent dissociation between prevention of ischemic events and bleeding complications. Per the EPIC trial protocol, the arterial sheath was left in place for at least 12 hours following the procedure, which may also have increased the bleeding risk. Thus, with modulation of the heparin dose, adjustment to the patient weight, and early sheath removal, the risk of bleeding complications was decreased.

Six-month follow-up

At 6 months there was a 23% reduction in major ischemic events or elective revascularization in the c73E Fab bolus plus infusion group compared with the placebo group (27% vs 35.1%, respectively; P = 0.001) (Fig. 15-2) [9]. This clinical benefit was mainly due to a significant 26% reduction in the need for repeat target vessel revascularization in the c7E3 Fab bolus plus infusion group (16.4%) compared with the placebo group (22.3%;P = 0.007) (Fig. 15-3). For the patients treated with c7E3 Fab bolus and infusion who had an initially successful coronary intervention (no events in the first 48 hours), there was a significant reduction in the need for repeat PTCA (16.5% to 11.6%; P = 0.01), a reduction in the need for any revascularization (23% to 18%; P = 0.025), and a significant reduction in the composite of death, MI, and any revascularization (25.4% to 19.2%; P = 0.007) compared with the placebo group. Thus, the effect of c7E3 Fab over 6 months in the EPIC trial was not merely a

TABLE 15-2. SAFETY OF TREATMENT IN VARIOUS TREATMENT GROUPS WITH C7E3 FAB IN THE EPIC TRIAL

	c7E3 bolus, %	c7E3 bolus + infusion, %	Placebo, %	*P* value*
Major bleeding	11	14	7	0.001
Stroke	0.1	0.4	0.3	0.98
Blood transfusion	13	15	7	< 0.001

**c7E3 bolus and infusion vs placebo.*

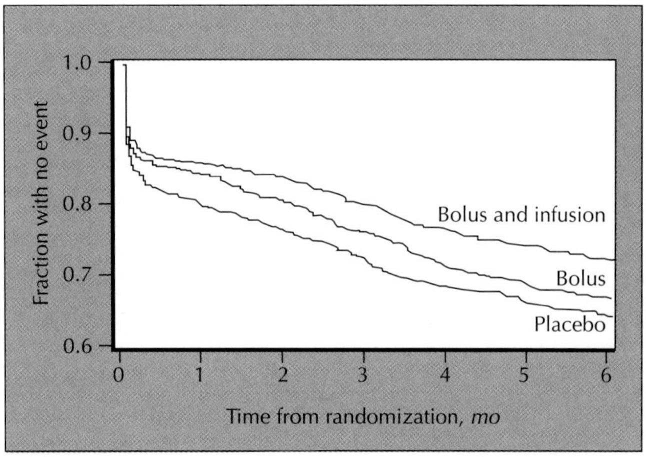

Figure 15-2. Six-month EPIC (Evaluation of c7E3 for the Prevention of Ischemic Complications) trial results. Kaplan-Meier curve of all events (death, myocardial infarction, coronary revascularization) for all patients enrolled. A significant reduction of events occurred in the c7E3 Fab bolus and infusion group compared with the bolus only group and the placebo group (P = 0.001). (*From* Topol and colleagues [9].)

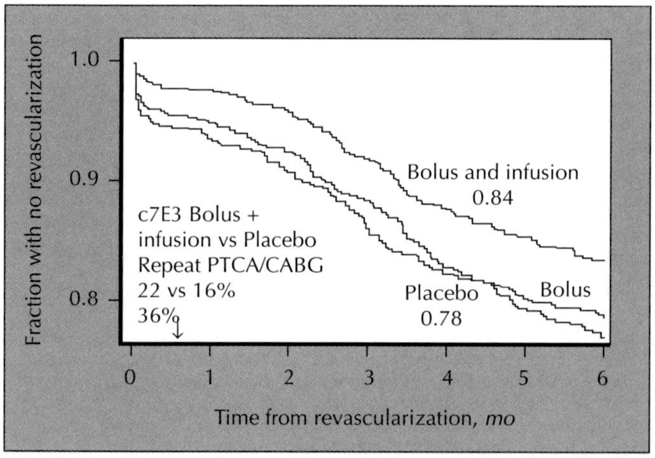

Figure 15-3. Six-month EPIC (Evaluation of c7E3 for the Prevention of Ischemic Complication) trial results. Kaplan-Meier curve of the need for subsequent target vessel revascularization, either by coronary angioplasty or coronary bypass surgery. Repeat revascularization was significantly reduced in the c7E3 Fab bolus and infusion group, compared with that in the placebo group (P = 0.007). CABG—coronary artery bypass grafting; PTCA—percutaneous transluminal coronary angioplasty. (*From* Topol and colleagues [9].)

preservation of acute benefit, but an incremental improvement in clinical outcome. No significant differences in the rate of ischemic events or elective revascularization were found between patients treated with the c7E3 bolus only and placebo.

The EPIC trial was the first large-scale randomized trial in which blinding to treatment allocation was preserved until follow-up was complete in order to demonstrate a clinically important reduction in the need for repeat revascularization, consistent with less restenosis. Systematic 6-month repeat angiography was not used in this trial because the primary endpoint was reduction of acute ischemic events. Thus, although it cannot be determined from EPIC if the long-term clinical benefit is due to reduction in angiographic restenosis, the observed reduction in the need for repeat revascularization was clinically relevant and was not artificially driven by routine protocol angiography. The EPILOG (Evaluation in PTCA to Improve Long-Term Outcome with Reo-Pro Glycoprotein IIb/IIIa Blockage) and IMPACT (Integrelin to Manage Platelet Aggregation to Prevent Coronary Thrombosis) II trials, described later, were designed to include angiographic substudies for detection of 6-month minimal luminal diameter determined by computer-assisted quantitative coronary angiography.

Important Subgroup Analyses

Outcome in patients with acute ischemic syndrome

Patients enrolled in the EPIC trial with unstable angina pectoris experienced an enhanced treatment effect from c7E3 bolus and infusion [10]. Compared with the placebo group, the 30-day incidence of death was reduced from 3.3% to 0.6%, MI from 9.2% to 0.6%, and the need for urgent revascularization from 5.9% to 3.2%. The composite 30-day endpoint was reduced by 70.6% from 13% to 3.8%. At 6 months, the incidences of death and MI remained reduced by nearly 90%, from 6.7% and 11.3%, respectively, in the placebo group, and from 0.7% and 1.3%, respectively, in the c7E3 Fab bolus and infusion group.

Sixty-four patients enrolled in the EPIC trial underwent primary or rescue PTCA for AMI [11]. As in the setting of unstable angina, the treatment effect among patients with AMI appeared to be enhanced. At 30 days, the rates of reinfarction and need for repeat revascularization were both 0% in the c7E3 Fab bolus and infusion group, compared with 8.7% and 17%, respectively, in the placebo group. During the 30-day follow-up, only 4.5% of the patients receiving c7E3 bolus plus infusion experienced an endpoint event (one death), compared with 26% of the patients receiving placebo. During the 6 months follow-up, the composite event rate remained suppressed in patients treated with c7E3 Fab (4.5%), whereas death, MI, or repeat revascularization increased from 26.1% to 47.8% of patients treated with placebo and from 21.1% to 32.3% of patients treated with c7E3 Fab bolus only. These encouraging findings among a small group of patients in the EPIC trial have led to initiation of the RAPPORT (ReoPro in Acute Myocardial Infarction and Primary PTCA Organization and Randomized Trial) study, which will evaluate the role of c7E3 Fab versus placebo among 500 patients undergoing primary PTCA for AMI.

Outcome in patients undergoing atherectomy

Consistent with the finding of CAVEAT (Coronary Angioplasty versus Excisional Atherectomy Trial) the 199 patients who underwent DCA in the EPIC trial experienced a high incidence of non–Q-wave MI: 15.2% compared with 8.1% in the PTCA-treated patients. This excess risk among DCA-treated patients was decreased by treatment with c7E3 bolus and infusion of 4.5% (comparable to the 5% among the PTCA-treated patients), suggesting a platelet-dependent mechanism underlying the occurrence of non–Q-wave MI after coronary atherectomy [12].

The IMPACT II Trial

The pilot trial of IMPACT assessed the efficacy and safety of another GP IIb/IIIa inhibitor, Integrelin, a cyclic heptapeptide with a short circulating half-life [13] and a reversible mechanism of binding. Patients undergoing PTCA were randomly assigned to Integrelin, 90 μg/kg bolus followed by 1.0 μg/kg/min infusion for 4 to 12 hours (101 patients) or to placebo (49 patients). There was a trend toward reduction in the primary endpoint of death, MI, repeat angioplasty, CABG, or stent implantation, from 12.2% in the placebo group to 4.1% ($P = 0.13$) in the 12-hour Integrelin-treated group.

Protocol

IMPACT II was a multicenter, double-blind, placebo-controlled trial of 4010 patients undergoing urgent ("high risk") or elective ("low risk") percutaneous coronary revascularization (paper presented at The European Society of Cardiology Congress, Amsterdam, 1995). Patients were randomly allocated to one of three treatment groups: 1) placebo, 2) Integrelin bolus dose of 135 μg/kg followed by an infusion of 0.5 μg/kg/min for 20 to 24 hours, or 3) Integrelin bolus dose of 135 μg/kg followed by an infusion of 0.75 μg/kg/min for 20 to 24 hours. All patients received aspirin, 325 mg, and weight-adjusted heparin to obtain an ACT above 300 seconds. The primary endpoint was a composite of any of the following events by 30 days: death, MI, urgent repeat angioplasty or CABG, or stent implantation for abrupt vessel closure. A secondary endpoint was the occurrence by month 6 of death, MI, or repeat revascularization (elective or urgent). An angiographic substudy of 928 patients was performed in which systematic follow-up coronary angiography at 6 months was performed to assess the effect of Integrelin on restenosis.

Results

Efficacy

Integrelin was effective in preventing ischemic events during the first 24 hours after coronary angioplasty. The composite endpoint was reduced by 29% in the combined Integrelin groups compared with placebo (6.8% vs 9.6%; $P = 0.002$). There was some erosion of clinical benefit of Integrelin between 24 hours and the primary endpoint period of 30 days.

By 30 days (Table 15-3) the primary composite endpoint was reduced by 19% with the low-dose Integrelin versus placebo (9.2% vs 11.4%; $P = 0.065$) and by 13% with high-dose Integrelin (9.9% vs 11.4%; $P = 0.22$). The difference in outcome was accounted for primarily by reductions in the incidence of MI and the need for stent placement by Integrelin.

Safety

Integrelin appeared to be safe in patients undergoing coronary angioplasty at the dosing regimens studied. No increases in major bleeding events, need for transfusion, or intracranial bleeding were observed among patients receiving Integrelin compared with placebo (Table 15-4).

Six-month follow-up

At 6 months, in the Integrelin high- or low-dose groups compared with the placebo group, there was a preservation of the approximately 2% absolute reduction in the incidence of the composite endpoint seen at 30 days (30.1% or 30.8% vs 32.5%, respectively).

No difference was found in the need for repeat revascularization among patients treated with the Integrelin high- or low-dose compared with placebo (20.4% or 21.7% vs 21.3%, respectively). This clinical finding was concordant with the angiographic substudy that showed no differences in the 6-month minimal luminal diameters (1.14 mm vs 1.26 mm vs 1.33 mm, respectively) or dichotomous restenosis rates (56% vs 48% vs 47%, respectively).

Important Subgroup Analyses

Outcome in patients with acute ischemic syndrome

In contrast to the EPIC trial, patients with AMI or unstable angina pectoris, prospectively stratified as "high risk," paradoxically experienced less of a treatment effect with Integrelin than did the "low risk" elective group. The 30-day composite endpoint was reduced by low-dose Integrelin compared with placebo from 11.5% to 8.7% in the "low risk" patients, but from 11.2% to 10.0% among the "high risk" patients. This finding, along with phase II data indicating that an increased Integrelin dose may be required to achieve complete platelet inhibition in patients with unstable ischemic syndromes, suggested that the Integrelin doses used in IMPACT II may have been inadequate to obtain an optimal clinical benefit [14].

Outcome in patients undergoing atherectomy

The 451 patients treated with DCA in IMPACT II had a higher incidence of large non–Q-wave MI (creatine phosphokinase–MB > 5 × normal) compared with patients treated with PTCA (12% vs 7%, $P = 0.001$). The 30-day composite endpoint was also higher in the

TABLE 15-3. PRIMARY COMPOSITE OUTCOMES AND COMPONENTS FOR VARIOUS TREATMENT GROUPS AT 30 DAYS OF TREATMENT IN THE IMPACT II TRIAL

	Integrelin high dose, *n(%)**	Integrelin low dose, *n(%)*†	Placebo, *n(%)*‡
Composite event	132(9.9)	124(9.2)	151(11.4)
P values vs placebo	0.22	0.063	
Death	11(0.8)	7(0.5)	15(1.1)
Myocardial infarction	92(6.9)	89(6.6)	107(8.1)
Emergency PTCA	38(2.9)	35(2.6)	37(2.8)
Emergency CABG	27(2)	22(1.6)	27(2.8)
Stent placement	7(0.5)	7(0.5)	18(1.4)

**Total number of patients, 1333.*
†Total number of patients, 1349.
‡Total number of patients, 1328.
CABG—coronary artery bypass grafting; PTCA—percutaneous transluminal coronary angioplasty.

DCA than in the non-DCA patients (15% vs 10%; P = 0.002). Unlike the effect of c7E3 Fab observed in the EPIC trial, this difference between DCA and non-DCA patients was not altered by treatment with Integrelin (15% vs 13% vs 16%; P = 0.62 for high-dose Integrelin vs low-dose Integrelin vs placebo, respectively) [15]. In the IMPACT II trial, 371 patients were treated by rotational atherectomy (245 patients in the Integrelin groups and 126 patients in the placebo group). Rotational atherectomy patients suffered non–Q-wave MI at a higher rate than patients treated with PTCA. Integrelin reduced the incidence of non–Q-wave MI by 25.5% in patients undergoing rotational atherectomy (10.8% vs 14.5%, in the Integrelin and placebo groups, respectively; P = 0.386). The 30-day composite endpoint was reduced by 37% by Integrelin (12.5% vs 19.9%; P = 0.059) [14]. This finding suggests the need for further study of the role of potent platelet IIB/IIIa receptor inhibition in the setting of rotational atherectomy.

The EPILOG Trial

A pilot trial, PROLOG, was conducted to determine if bleeding complications associated with use of c7E3 Fab could be diminished by reduction of heparin dosing. The efficacy and safety of c7E3 Fab is combination with two weight-adjusted heparin regimens and two strategies of sheath removal were evaluated. A total of 103 patients undergoing coronary intervention procedures were randomly assigned to receive c7E3 with standard dose (100 U/kg, activated clotting time > 300 seconds) or low-dose (70 U/kg) weight-adjusted heparin, and were further randomly assigned to early or late sheath removal. The results suggest that the low-dose weight-adjusted heparin dose and early sheath removal (~ 6 hours postprocedure) were associated with a reduced risk for bleeding and no apparent increase in ischemic complications.

Protocol

Based on the encouraging results of PROLOG, the EPILOG trial was carried out. A total of 4800 patients undergoing elective or urgent percutaneous coronary intervention were enrolled. Patients with AMI or refractory unstable angina were excluded based on data derived from EPIC suggesting extraordinary clinical benefit from c7E3 Fab therapy in these groups of patients. Planned rotational atherectomy was excluded due to the greater incidence of non–Q-wave MI after this mode of coronary intervention is performed. Patients undergoing elective stent placement were excluded initially because of uncertainties regarding the proper anticoagulation regimen following stent implantation; in the late phase of trial enrollment, patients suitable for elective stent implantation were randomly assigned to stent placement or PTCA.

Patients were randomly assigned in a double-blind design into three treatment arms: 1) bolus administration of heparin 100 U/kg (≤ 10,000 U) to achieve an activated clotting time of 300 seconds or more with c7E3 Fab 0.25 mg/kg bolus and 0.125 µg/kg/min in infusion for 12 hours ≤ 10 µg/min); 2) bolus administration of heparin 70 U/kg (≤ 7000 U) to achieve an activated clotting time of 200 seconds or more with c7E3 Fab 0.25 mg/kg bolus and 0.125 µg/kg/min in infusion for 12 hours (≤ 10 µg/min); or 3) bolus administration of heparin 100 U/kg (≤ 10,000 units) to achieve an ACT of 300 seconds or more with placebo bolus followed by placebo infusion for 12 hours. All patients were treated with aspirin, 325 mg. The primary endpoint of the trial was a composite of any of the following events in the first 30 days postrandomization: death, MI, or severe ischemia requiring urgent intervention. The 6-month clinical endpoint was a composite of death, MI, or the need for a repeat revascularization procedure (urgent or elective). Secondary endpoints of the trial included bleeding events and

Table 15-4. Safety of Treatment with Integrelin for Various Treatment Groups in the IMPACT II Trial

	Integrelin high dose, %	Integrelin low dose, %	Placebo	*P* value*
Major bleeding	5.2	5.1	4.8	0.74
Stroke	0.2	0.1	0.2	0.78
Blood transfusion	5.9	5.6	5.2	0.74

**Low dose vs placebo.*

assessment of angiographic restenosis in a subgroup of 900 randomly assigned patients. Enrollment in EPILOG was stopped after 2792 patients had been entered because the interim analysis of the data on the first 1500 patients had been reviewed by the Data and Safety Monitoring Committee.

Efficacy

There was a highly significant 56% to 68% reduction in the risk of death or MI by 30 days, the prespecified endpoint of the interim analyses, among patients receiving c7E3 Fab with the low-dose or standard-dose weight-adjusted heparin regimens compared with patients receiving placebo (2.6% and 3.6% vs 8.1%, respectively; *P* < 0.0001) (Table 15-5).

Safety

The safety of c7E3 Fab in combination with weight-adjusted heparin was markedly improved compared with the EPIC trial. Clinical benefit from c7E3 Fab was achieved without appreciable increase in bleeding risk. At the interim analyses of 1500 patients, the incidence of major bleeding was only 1.8% and 3.5%, respectively, in the patients treated with c7E3 Fab plus low-dose and standard-dose weight-adjusted heparin compared with 3.1% in the placebo group (*P* = 0.178) (*see* Table 15-5). The risk of intracranial bleeding was slightly, although not significantly, higher in the c7E3 Fab-treated patients (0.2% in both arms vs 0% for placebo).

Conclusions

The EPIC, IMPACT II, and EPILOG study results demonstrated unequivocally that platelet GP IIb/IIIa receptor inhibition during coronary intervention markedly reduces the incidence of postprocedural ischemic events, as summarized in Table 15-6. Although this therapy may carry an increased risk of bleeding complications, such excess hemorrhagic risk

Table 15-5. Interim Analysis of 1500 Patients in the EPILOG Trial

	Placebo, %	c7E3 + low-dose weight-adjusted heparin, %	c7E3 + standard-dose weight-adjusted heparin, %	*P* value (low dose vs placebo)
Death	0.8	0.4	0.4	0.444
Death and MI (> 3 × CPK)	8.1	2.6	3.6	< 0.0001
Major bleeding	3.5	1.8	3.1	0.18
Stroke	0.2	0.2	0	0.99

CPK—creatine phosphokinase; MI—myocardial infarction.

Table 15-6. Efficacy at 30 Days of Treatment with Glycoprotein IIb/IIIa Inhibitors

	EPIC Trial			IMPACT II Trial			EPILOG Trial		
Study	c7E3 bolus + infusion, %	Placebo, %	*P* value	Integrelin low dose, %	Placebo, %	*P* value	c7E3 low-dose heparin, %	Placebo, %	*P* value
Composite endpoint	8.3	12.8	0.008	9.21	11.4	0.063	2.6	8.1	0.0001
Death	1.7	1.7	0.87	0.5	1.1	0.12	0.4	0.8	0.44
MI	5.2	8.6	0.016	6.6	8.1	0.17			
PTCA	0.8	4.5	0.0001	2.6	2.8	0.85			
CABG	2.4	3.6	0.25	1.6	2.8	0.57			

CABG—coronary artery bypass graft; MI—myocardial infarction; PTCA—percutaneous transluminal coronary angioplasty.

can be minimized by preventive strategies such as dose reduction, early sheath removal, and conservative management of the vascular access site. As demonstrated in the EPILOG trial, extraordinary clinical benefit in terms of reduction in ischemic complications after coronary intervention may be achieved with a small increase in bleeding risk.

The diminished effect of Integrelin observed in the IMPACT II trial, as opposed to the profound and sustained effects of c7E3 Fab among patients undergoing coronary intervention, raises interesting questions concerning the clinical importance of different receptor specificities of the various GP IIb/IIIa inhibitors. Integrelin is highly specific for the GP IIb/IIIa receptor, in contrast to c7E3 Fab, which binds not only to the GP IIb/IIIa receptor but also to other integrins, including the vitronectin receptor ($\alpha_V\beta_3$). Whether the long-term effects of c7E3 on the need for target vessel revascularization are mediated more through other integrins than through GP IIb/IIIa receptor inhibition is an issue that remains to be resolved.

The role of platelet GP IIb/IIIa receptor inhibition in the acute coronary syndromes of unstable angina and AMI is an exciting new frontier in ischemic heart disease and is currently under investigation in phase II and large-scale phase III trials. The complementarity of these agents with new devices, such as stents, for coronary revascularization is also the subject of an important new trial (EPILOG Stent). Finally, future studies also will focus on the role of long-term GP IIa/IIIb inhibition with the new generation of orally active agents.

References

1. Ellis SG: Percutaneous coronary intervention in the 1990s: results in patients with single or multivessel disease [review]. *Herz* 1992, 17:18–26.
2. Tenaglia AN, Fortin DF, Califf RM, *et al.*: Predicting the risk of abrupt vessel closure after angioplasty in an individual patient. *J Am Coll Cardiol* 1994, 24:1004–1011.
3. Coller BS: A new murine monoclonal antibody reports an activation-dependent change in the conformation and/or microenvironment of the platelet glycoprotein IIb/IIIa complex. *J Clin Invest* 1985, 76:101–108.
4. The EPIC Investigators: Use of a monoclonal antibody directed against the platelet glycoprotein IIb/IIIa receptor in high-risk coronary angioplasty. *N Engl J Med* 1994, 330:956–961.
5. Ellis SG, Wildermann N, Ivanc TB, *et al.*: Should use of glycoprotein IIb/IIIa inhibitors to prevent ischemic complications of angioplasty be dependent on baseline coronary morphology [abstract]. *Circulation* 1994, 90:I-62.
6. Boehrer JD, Kereiakes DJ, Navetta FI, *et al.*: Effects of profound platelet inhibition with c7E3 before coronary angioplasty on complications of coronary bypass surgery. *Am J Cardiol* 1994, 74:1166–1170.
7. Uthoff K, Zehr KJ, Geerling R, *et al.*: Inhibition of platelet adhesion during cardiopulmonary bypass reduces postoperative bleeding. *Circulation* 1994, 90:II269–II274.
8. Aguirre FV, Topol EJ, Ferguson JJ, *et al.*: Bleeding complications with the chimeric antibody to platelet glycoprotein IIb/IIIa integrin in patients undergoing percutaneous coronary intervention. *Circulation* 1995, 91:2882–2890.
9. Topol EJ, Califf RM, Weisman HF, *et al.*: Randomized trial of coronary intervention with antibody against platelet IIb/IIIa integrin for reduction of clinical restenosis: results at six months. *Lancet* 1994, 343:881–886.
10. Lincoff AM, Califf RM, Anderson K, *et al.*, for the EPIC investigators: Striking clinical benefit with platelet GP IIb/IIIa inhibition by c7E3 among patients with unstable angina [abstract]. *Circulation* 1994, 90:I-2.
11. Lefkovits J, Anderson K, Weisman H, Topol EJ, for the EPIC investigators: Increased risk of non Q MI following DCA: evidence for a platelet dependent mechanism from the EPIC trial [abstract]. *Circulation* 1994, 90:I–214.
12. Lefkovits J, Ivanhoe R, Anderson K, *et al.*, for the EPIC investigators: Platelet IIb/IIIa receptor inhibition during PTCA for acute myocardial infarction: insights from the EPIC trial [abstract]. *Circulation* 1994, 90:I-564.
13. Tcheng JE, Harrington RA, Kottke-Marchant K, *et al.*: Multicenter, randomized, double-blind, placebo-controlled trial of the platelet integrin glycoprotein IIb/IIIa blocker Integrelin in elective coronary intervention. *Circulation* 1995, 91:2151–2157.
14. Harrington RA, Ohman EM, Sigmon KN, *et al.*: Intensity of inhibition of platelet glycoprotein IIb/IIIa receptor differs among disease states [abstract]. *Circulation* 1995, 92:I-488.
15. Teirstein PS, Yakubov SJ, Thel MC, *et al.*: Platelet IIb/IIIa blockade with Integrilin: atherectomy patients [abstract]. *J Am Coll Cardiol* 1996, 27:334.

Chapter 16

NEW THROMBOLYTIC AGENTS

R. David Anderson
Merle Myerson
E. Magnus Ohman

In the past 15 years there has been remarkable progress in our understanding of the role of thrombosis in cardiovascular disease, especially in acute myocardial infarction (AMI), stroke, and pulmonary embolism. It is now well established that the triggering event for a cerebral or myocardial infarction (MI) is not the progression of an atherosclerotic plaque but the cessation of blood flow within an artery due to the formation of thrombus [1,2]. The treatment of patients with these disorders has evolved from the conservative approach of bedrest and watchful waiting with few therapeutic alternatives that was once the norm. Physicians and their patients now have a multitude of options, including pharmacologic agents, noninvasive and invasive methods of risk stratification, revascularization strategies, and cardiac rehabilitation. The growth in our knowledge of these disease entities has been driven not only by an understanding of their pathophysiology, but also by an improvement in statistical methodology and the strict application of these techniques to patients in large clinical trials.

There has probably been no greater advance in the treatment of cardiovascular disease than the recognition of the role of thrombus and the application of drugs with thrombolytic activity to effect its dissolution. Indeed, thrombolytic therapy likely represents the most thoroughly studied pharmacologic agent in the history of medicine. To date, more than 100,000 patients with AMI have been treated with thrombolytic therapy in randomized clinical trials from which we have learned a great deal about the benefits of thrombolysis on infarct-artery patency, left ventricular function, and mortality. We have also found limitations to this modality that have become the impetus for ongoing investigation into newer and more promising approaches to the application of thrombolytic therapy in the treatment of patients with AMI. Cardiovascular disease is still the number one cause of death in the United States. Each year as many as 1.5 million Americans suffer an MI and one-third of them die [3].

This chapter highlights the historical features of thrombolytic therapy as a foundation for current and future work in this field. The limitations of currently available therapy are discussed. The main components of the fibrinolytic system are reviewed and the state of development and testing of the next generation of thrombolytic interventions are presented. The most promising new agents are discussed from the perspectives of both their design and their progress toward clinical availability.

Historical Features

The evolution of thrombolytic therapy to treat patients with AMI began over one century ago. The discovery of the fibrinolytic system and of agents that can cause the dissolution of a blood clot have recently been reviewed in detail [4•,5–7]. The "instability" of blood clots was recognized over 150 years ago [8] but it was late in the nineteenth century when Dastre attributed this phenomenon of spontaneous liquification to fibrinolysis [9]. Only a few years earlier von Brucke [10] had noted the proteolytic activity of human urine and Sahli [11] repeated these experiments observing its specificity for fibrin. The eventual isolation of what is now known as urokinase ultimately did not occur until the mid-twentieth century [12,13].

Perhaps a more seminal discovery was that reported by Tillett and Garner in 1933. They identified the fibrinolytic substance produced by β-hemolytic, group C streptococci, then called "fibrinolysin" and now known as streptokinase [14]. Milstone, one of Tillett's contemporaries, noted in 1941 that the dissolution of fibrin in vitro by fibrinolysin required the presence of a co-factor present only in plasma [15]. He named this co-factor "plasma lysing factor," which was later proven to be plasminogen. The initial use of streptokinase in humans occurred in 1947 for the treatment of empyema and loculated effusions [16]. It was later used in chronic abscess cavities [17]. When intravenous quality streptokinase became available, Sherry, Fletcher, and colleagues were the first to treat patients with AMI in 1958 [18]. In 1979 Rentrop published the first account of the use of intracoronary streptokinase in a patient with an acute occlusion during diagnostic angiography [19]. Over the next two decades, streptokinase was used in many small randomized trials of AMI, but it required meta-analyses to demonstrate its unequivocal benefit in reducing mortality [20,21]. Due to the lack of large clinical trials, concern over the risk of hemorrhagic complications, and general skepticism about the role of thrombus in AMI, thrombolytic therapy was not widely used.

A resurgence of interest in thrombolytic therapy occurred in the late 1970s and early 1980s due principally to three observations. The prognostic significance of limiting infarct size was reported by Sobel and colleagues [22], and Rude and colleagues [23] suggested that interventions early in AMI might limit the size of an infarct. Even though the concept of thrombosis was embodied in Herrick's description of AMI in 1912, it was not until the angiographic evidence of thrombus in a majority of AMI patients (90%) was provided by DeWood [1] in 1980 that the modern era of thrombolytic therapy began. Larger clinical trials of both intracoronary and intravenous streptokinase therapy for AMI soon followed [24–26], leading to Food and Drug Administration (FDA) approval of intracoronary streptokinase in 1982 and intravenous therapy in 1987. The pace of research on other agents also accelerated. The anisoylated plasminogen streptokinase activator complex (APSAC) anistreplase was first used to treat AMI in 1985 [27], and it received FDA approval in 1989. The initial preparation of tissue plasminogen activator (t-PA) from uterine tissue was reported in 1979 [28], and with the use of molecular biology techniques recombinant t-PA from human melanoma cells was expressed by *Escherichia coli* in 1983 [29]. This led to the use of recombinant t-PA in patients in 1984 [30] and to its FDA approval as an intravenous thrombolytic agent for the treatment of AMI in 1987.

Limitations of Thrombolysis

The widespread study and application of thrombolytic therapy has led to extensive knowledge of its benefits and limitations [31–34]. The mortality benefit of thrombolysis has now been documented in many comparative trials. The controversy over the theoretical superiority of fibrin-specific therapy versus nonspecific therapy has been laid to rest by the 41,021 patient GUSTO (Global Utilization of Streptokinase and Tissue Plasminogen Activator for Occluded Arteries)-I trial [35]. The use of fibrin-specific t-PA with immediate intravenous heparin resulted in a 6.3% 30-day mortality versus 7.3% ($P = 0.001$) for streptokinase in patients with acute infarctions. The importance of a patent infarct artery, previously in doubt, was confirmed in the angiographic substudy of the GUSTO-I trial [36] validating the open-artery hypothesis. Those patients with TIMI (Thrombolysis

In Myocardial Infarction) 3 grade flow on a 90-minute angiogram had the lowest 30-day mortality regardless of the therapy received. Patients treated with t-PA had the highest 90-minute patency (TIMI 2 and 3 grade flow, 81%), although TIMI 3 grade flow occurred in only 54% of patients.

In fact, resistance to recanalization remains a serious drawback of therapy and occurs in 15% to 40% of patients treated with thrombolysis [37]. The inability of thrombolytic therapy to maintain coronary patency is another of its potential limitations. Reocclusion following successful thrombolysis has been documented in 5% to 30% of patients [38]. In a review of patients in the TAMI (Thrombolysis and Angioplasty in Myocardial Infarction) studies, reocclusion led to increased morbidity and in-hospital mortality (11.0% vs 4.5%, $P = 0.01$) [39]. The time to reperfusion also remains long, with an average of at least 45 minutes for the restoration of antegrade coronary blood flow [32,33]. If optimal reperfusion is defined as the establishment of early and sustained patency, with TIMI grade 3 flow, the absence of reocclusion, and adequate perfusion at the myocardial tissue level, only about 25% of thrombolytic-treated patients are estimated to achieve it [36].

Other issues sustain the search for improved thrombolytic agents. The bleeding complications associated with therapy, particularly intracerebral hemorrhage that occurs in 0.3% to 0.7% of patients, continue to be significant despite early predictions that fibrin-specific therapy would decrease their incidence [24,25,34]. There are endogenous inhibitors of plasminogen activators, most notably plasminogen activator inhibitor 1 (PAI-1), that attenuate the ability of these agents to promote fibrinolysis. Finally, with the exception of APSAC, the clearance of currently available thrombolytic agents is so rapid that their therapeutic utilization requires continuous intravenous infusion. This contributes to the systemic "lytic state" and adds to the cost of applying this therapy. There are, therefore, significant limitations to the currently available thrombolytic regimens. These fuel the drive to develop more potent plasminogen activators with longer half-lives and greater fibrin specificity, coupled with strategies to reduce resistance to clot lysis, prevent reocclusion, and decrease bleeding complications.

The Fibrinolytic System

Several complete descriptions of the fibrinolytic enzyme system have recently been published [7,40,41,42••]. The primary function of this proteolytic system is the dissolution of fibrin clots in the vascular bed. It is comprised of the inactive proenzyme, plasminogen, which can be converted by different plasminogen activators to the active enzyme, plasmin. Plasmin facilitates the degradation of insoluble fibrin and other extracellular proteins into soluble fibrin degradation products. Inhibition of this mechanism occurs mainly at two levels. Two inhibitors of plasminogen activators, plasminogen activator inhibitor 1 and 2 (PAI-1 and PAI-2), have been identified and characterized. PAI-1 appears to require stabilization by the cell adhesion protein vitronectin. Inhibition at the level of plasmin occurs mainly by the serine proteinase inhibitor α_2-antiplasmin.

Physiologic fibrinolysis is a tightly regulated system of activation and inhibition. Native t-PA is a very weak activator of plasminogen in the absence of fibrin. In the presence of fibrin, the affinity of t-PA for plasminogen is 40 to 400 times greater [41]. The plasminogen structure includes two lysine-binding sites that interact with fibrin. The generation of free plasmin yields a product with a very short half-life that is rapidly degraded by α_2-antiplasmin. Plasmin generated on the surface of fibrin results in occupation of both its lysine-binding sites, and subsequent inactivation by α_2-antiplasmin can occur only slowly. Therefore, plasmin generated on the surface of fibrin is protected from rapid degradation, whereas plasmin released from the fibrin surface would be rapidly inactivated.

The mechanisms described above have important implications for the design of new thrombolytic agents. Thrombolytic drugs are typically classified as either fibrin or nonfibrin specific. Nonfibrin specific agents have no particular affinity for fibrin and activate both free-circulating and clot-associated plasminogen. This results in the formation of plasmin in the bloodstream that is rapidly inactivated by α_2-antiplasmin. It is not until the inhibitors are exhausted that the remaining plasmin can begin clot lysis. This process occurs with the degradation of other plasma proteins as well (fibrinogen, factor V, factor VIII, etc.) leading to an increased risk of bleeding, and occurs only after fibrin-associated plasminogen has been depleted ("plasminogen steal"). Thus, the use of nonfibrin-specific agents requires doses high enough to generate free plasmin, but leads to the so-called "lytic state." Fibrin-specific therapy, on the other hand, is localized to the fibrin surface and activates plasminogen only in situ. This has the theoretical advantage of providing a greater thrombolytic efficacy and contributing less to the lytic state. Concerns about the lower thrombolytic efficacy of nonfibrin-specific agents and their breakdown of the hemostatic system have fueled the search for more efficient and fibrin-specifc pharmacotherapy.

Thrombolytic Agents

Five thrombolytic agents have been studied in clinical trials and are available for use. The characteristics of these five are shown in Table 16-1. A description of their basic structure and function will facilitate an understanding of their limitations as therapeutic agents and also form a basis for the design of newer, more potent and efficient plasminogen activators.

Tissue plasminogen activator is a naturally occurring enzyme produced commercially by the cloning of messenger RNA from the Bowes human melanoma cell line and its expression in *Escherichia coli* [29]. The molecule contains four distinct regional domains: 1) the NH_2-terminal or "finger" F domain that is homologous with the finger domains of fibronectin responsible for fibrin binding; 2) the E domain homologous to human epidermal growth factor and considered important in cellular binding; 3) two regions kringle 1 (K_1) and kringle 2 (K_2) that share an amino acid sequence with the five kringle domains of plasminogen; and 4) the serine protease portion of the structure containing the active site [31,34,40]. Tissue plasminogen activator is synthesized as a single chain but is converted to a two-chain form by plasmin. The binding of t-PA to fibrin increases its plasminogenolytic activity and is thought to be due to the finger and kringle domains.

The other naturally occurring human activator protein is single-chain urokinase plasminogen activator (scu-PA, prourokinase, Saruplase). It is produced mainly by renal and vascular endothelial cells and made commercially available through recombinant technology. Scu-PA contains three domains: 1) an NH_2-terminal epidermal growth factor-like region; 2) a kringle region similar to those in plasminogen and t-PA; 3) a serine protease segment with an active site. The single chain scu-PA activates fibrin-bound plasminogen more efficiently than circulating plasminogen. Upon scu-PA binding to plasminogen, plasmin is produced which then rapidly converts scu-PA to two-chain urokinase plasminogen activator (tcu-PA, urokinase). The two-chain form, being less fibrin specific, activates both free and fibrin-bound plasminogen extensively, leading to α_2-antiplasmin depletion and the lytic state [7,32,40,43].

Streptokinase is still produced by purification from bacterial cultures of β-hemolytic streptococci. Its mechanism of activation is indirect. A streptokinase-plasminogen complex is formed and then converts other plasminogen molecules to plasmin. Streptokinase may be neutralized by pre-existent antibodies. A few days after treatment with streptokinase, antistreptokinase (anti-SK) antibody titers rise dramatically and persist for 4 to 6 months. APSAC is a noncovalent complex of plasminogen and streptokinase with its catalytic site reversibly acylated. Upon introduction to the circulation deacylation occurs, uncovering the active site. APSAC has a half-life determined by its deacylation rate and is more than three times that of streptokinase (*see* Table 16-1). It is, however, also affected by pretreatment anti-SK antibodies and causes a marked increase in post-treatment antibody titers within 2 to 3 weeks [40].

Several approaches to the engineering of new thrombolytic agents have been taken, and agents currently under development are shown in Table 16-2. Increases in thrombolytic potency, efficiency, and resistance to inhibition have been sought by creating mutants of native t-PA by both domain deletion and amino acid substitution techniques. Increased efficacy of some

Table 16-1. Plasminogen Activator Characteristics

	Plasminogen activation	Fibrinogen depletion	Half-life, *min*	Antibody response	Fibrin specific
Streptokinase	Indirect	4+	20	+	-
APSAC	Indirect	3+	70	+	-
scu-PA	Indirect	2+	8, 48*	-	++
tcu-PA	Direct	3+	10	-	+
t-PA	Direct	1–2+	5	-	++

**Biphasic clearance.*

APSAC—anisoylated plasminogen streptokinase activator complex; scu-PA—single-chain urokinase plasminogen activator (prourokinase); tcu-PA—two-chain urokinase plasminogen activator (urokinase); t-PA—tissue plasminogen activator.

mutants has also been realized by choosing variations that exhibit decreased rates of clearance. Plasminogen activator constructs have been made that are chimeric, combining the properties of two distinct activators into a single molecule. The attachment of antibodies to existing plasminogen activators directed either at fibrin or the platelet are also currently being evaluated. The search for activators from other animal and bacterial sources continues. Table 16-3 lists the characteristics of recently developed activators that are in various stages of clinical development, which are discussed in detail below.

VARIANTS OF T-PA

Reteplase (r-PA, K2P, LY210825, BM 06.022)

Reteplase or r-PA is a single chain deletion variant of human t-PA lacking the finger (F), the epidermal growth factor (E), and kringle 1 domains that is expressed in *E. coli*. The active site of r-PA is the same as that of t-PA, although ex-vivo tests have indicated that r-PA has a lower affinity for fibrin, preferentially activating plasminogen bound to fibrin [43]. This is believed to be a result of the lack of the finger domain.

TABLE 16-2. PLASMINOGEN ACTIVATORS UNDER DEVELOPMENT

	Source	Type	Unique feature	Characteristics
r-PA	Recombinant	t-PA DD	Lack of F, E, K_1	Reduced clearance
TNK–t-PA	Recombinant	t-PA AAS	thr^{103} to asp khrr 296-299 aaaa asp^{117} to glu	Reduced clearance Fibrin specific PAI-1 resistance Reduced clearance
E6010	Recombinant	t-PA AAS	cys^{84} to ser	Reduced clearance
bat-PA	Recombinant cDNA clone	Vampire bat salivary gland	Homology to t-PA	Fibrin specific Reduced clearance
Staphylokinase	Recombinant	Bacterial		Fibrin specific
$K_1K_2P_u$	Recombinant	Chimeric	K_1K_2 of t-PA SP of rscu-PA	Retained potency Reduced clearance Bolus injection
FK_2t-PA	Recombinant	Chimeric	F, K_2 of t-PA and SP of rscu-PA	Increased potency
K_2t-PA	Recombinant	Chimeric	K_2 of t-PA and SP of rscu-PA	Increased potency
t-PA-59D8	Recombinant	Antibody conjugate	Antibody to fibrin	Increased potency Less systemic lysis
rscu-PA/MA-15C5	Recombinant	Antibody conjugate	Antibody to fibrin D-dimer	Increased potency Reduced clearance
Urokinase-7E3(Fab′)	Recombinant	Antibody conjugate	Antibody to GP IIb/IIIa	Increased potency Inhibits platelet aggregate

AAS—amino acid substitution; bat-PA—t-PA of salivary gland from bat Desmodus rotundus*; DD—domain deletion; E—epidermal growth factor domain; E6010—monteplase; F—finger domain; GP—glycoprotein; K—kringle domain; K_1—kringle 1; K_2—kringle 2; MA—monoclonal antibody; MA-15C5—monoclonal antibody to fibrin D-domain; PAI-1—plasminogen activator inhibitor 1; Pu—serine protease from rscu-PA; r-PA—reteplase (BM 06.022, K2P, LY210825); rscu-PA—recombinant single chain urokinase plasminogen activator (prourokinase); SP—serine protease domain; TNK–t-PA—T103N, N117Q, KHRR 296-299 AAAA; 59D8—monoclonal antibody to fibrin.*

Inhibition of r-PA and t-PA by PAI-1 was also found to be similar in initial characterization studies, but as a consequence of finger and epidermal growth factor domain deletion, binding of r-PA to endothelial cells and monocytes was reduced. This accounts for the reduced clearance of r-PA and its longer half-life.

In studies comparing r-PA with t-PA in the rabbit jugular vein thrombosis model r-PA was found to be nearly four times more potent than t-PA. There was no difference between agents in their effect on fibrinogen levels. The pharmacokinetic analysis revealed that in the rabbit, the half life of r-PA was 18.9 ± 1.5 minute versus 2.1 ± 0.1 minute for t-PA [44]. The increased potency of r-PA over t-PA was therefore felt to be due to its decreased clearance. In a canine model of coronary thrombosis r-PA was compared with t-PA for its ability to achieve more rapid reperfusion. This work confirmed the longer half-life of r-PA, suggesting it could be administered as an intravenous bolus. It was also shown that the time to reperfusion with r-PA was much shorter than that of t-PA and that r-PA–treated animals had significantly fewer reocclusions [45]. This study was followed by a comparison of r-PA with APSAC in the canine model, both arms using bolus injections, and again the time to reperfusion was significantly shorter with r-PA [46]. It was further found that r-PA had a more modest effect on plasma levels of fibrinogen, plasminogen, and α_2-antiplasmin, suggesting that bleeding complications might be reduced with this agent.

Phase 1 studies of this agent quickly followed and showed that in humans the half-life of r-PA was indeed 14 to 18 minutes [47]. The results of the phase II studies of r-PA in patients with AMI are shown in Table 16-4. The initial dose-finding study of r-PA yielded 90-minute patency rates that were lower than the prespecified goal of 70%, hence the dose was raised to 15 MU. Patency rates for the two regimens were similar at 30 and 60 minutes, but at 90 minutes the 15 MU dose yielded a rate of 75% versus 66% for the lower dose [48]. Reocclusion occurred in 20% of low dose and 15% of higher dose patients, but no increase in bleeding

TABLE 16-3. NOVEL PLASMINOGEN ACTIVATORS UNDER DEVELOPMENT

	Half-life, *min*	Antibody response	Fibrin specific	Development phase
r-PA	15	-	+	III
TNK–t-PA	15	-	++	I/II
E6010	23	-	+	II
bat-PA	17	-	+++	Animal models
Staphylokinase	6, 37*	+	++	I/II

**Biphasic clearance.*
bat-PA—t-PA of salivary gland from bat Desmodus rotundus; *E6010—Monteplase; r-PA—reteplase (K2P, BM 06.022, LY210825); TNK–t-PA—T103N, N117Q, KHRR 296-299 AAAA.*

TABLE 16-4. DOSE-FINDING STUDIES OF R-PA (RETEPLASE) IN PATIENTS WITH ACUTE MYOCARDIAL INFARCTION

	Study design	Patients, *n*	Dose	90-minute patency*, %	90-minute TIMI 3, %
Neuhaus *et al.* [48]	OL, AMI	42	10 MU	66	52
		100	15 MU	75	69
Tebbe *et al.* [49]	OL, AMI	50	10 + 5 MU	78	58

**Patency is in patients with both TIMI grade 2 and 3 flow.*
AMI—acute myocardial infarction; MU—million units; OL—open label; TIMI—Thrombolysis In Myocardial Infarction.

events was noted. The high reocclusion rates prompted a trial using a double bolus technique, the second dose given 30 minutes after the first. The results of this study showed patency rates as seen in Table 16-4, but more importantly, only one patient had angiographically confirmed reocclusion [49].

This led to the RAPID (Reteplase versus Alteplase Patency Investigation During myocardial infarction) patency trials of r-PA compared with standard (3-hour) and accelerated (90-minute) dose t-PA in AMI patients. RAPID-1 studied standard-dose t-PA versus three different r-PA dosing schemes (10 MU, 10 + 5 MU, 10 + 10 MU) in patients with AMI [50]. The results shown in Table 16-5 reveal that both patency and TIMI 3 flow at 90 minutes were highest in the 10 + 10 MU r-PA arm. In addition r-PA patients treated with 10 + 10 MU had significantly higher TIMI 3 flow at 60 and 90 minutes as well as at the time of follow-up. At the time of acute catheterization, r-PA and t-PA patients had similar ejection fractions. At follow-up, however, there was a significant difference favoring r-PA–treated patients (52.9% vs 49%, $P = 0.05$). While not powered for mortality, the 30-day death rate in r-PA patients was half that of t-PA patients (1.9% vs 3.9%).

The RAPID-2 study compared the 10 + 10 MU r-PA dose identified as having the highest patency rates in RAPID-1 with accelerated t-PA. These results are also shown in Table 16-5 [51]. As in RAPID-1, higher patency and TIMI 3 flow rates were seen with r-PA at 60 and 90 minutes. Reocclusion rates, early and follow-up left ventricular function, and the incidence of intracranial hemorrhage were not different between treatments. As in RAPID-1, this study had insufficient power to assess mortality; however, 4.1% of r-PA–treated patients died within 35 days, compared with 8.4% of t-PA–treated patients ($P = 0.11$).

The first large-scale comparison of r-PA occurred in the phase III INJECT (International Joint Efficacy Comparison of Thrombolytics) trial. This study was a double-blind randomized trial of 6010 patients presenting within 12 hours of symptom onset and treated with double-bolus r-PA or streptokinase. The trial was designed to show equivalence, not superiority, to streptokinase. There was no difference in the primary endpoint (*see* Table 16-5) of 35-day mortality (9.02% r-PA vs 9.53% streptokinase, $P = 0.50$), nor at six-month follow-up (11.14% r-PA vs 12.15% streptokinase, $P = 0.23$) [52••]. No differences were noted in bleeding complications and a nonsignificant excess of in-hospital strokes occurred in r-PA patients, mostly due to intracerebral hemorrhages. Other adverse events were found less frequently in r-PA–treated patients, including cardiogenic shock, congestive heart failure, hypotension, and atrial fibrillation (all $P < 0.05$). These data suggested that r-PA was at least as safe and effi-

Table 16-5. Results of Studies of r-PA (Reteplase) in Acute Myocardial Infarction

	Study design	Patients, *n*	Dose	90-minute patency, %	90-minute TIMI 3, %	35-day mortality, %
RAPID-1 [50]	R, OL	146	15 MU	63	41	
		152	10+5 MU	67	46	
		154	10+10 MU	85	63*	
		154	100 mg t-PA standard dose	77	49	
RAPID-2 [51]	R, OL	169	10+10 MU	83	60*	
		155	100 mg t-PA accelerated	73	45*	
INJECT [52]	R, DB	3004				9.02
		3006	10 +10 MU Streptokinase			9.53

$P < 0.05$ vs t-PA.

DB—double blind; INJECT—International Joint Efficacy Comparison of Thrombolytics; MU—million units; OL—open label; R—randomized; RAPID—Reteplase Versus Alteplase Patency Investigation During Myocardial Infarction; t-PA—tissue plasminogen activator.

cacious as streptokinase and that its use may have beneficial effects in reducing in-hospital morbidity.

Reteplase is currently being compared with accelerated t-PA in the ongoing GUSTO-III trial. The study plans to enroll 15,000 patients, its primary endpoint is 30-day mortality, and its expected completion is in 1996.

TNK–t-PA (T103N, N117Q, KHRR 296-299 AAAA)

TNK–t-PA was developed after a series of observations noted the effects of strategic amino acid substitutions on both thrombolytic activity and the clearance rate of native t-PA. TNK–t-PA is, therefore, a substitution mutant of native t-PA rather than a domain deletion mutant. The importance of amino acid residues 296 to 302 of native t-PA in its reaction with PAI-1 led to many attempts at creating mutants with resistance to PAI-1 [53–55]. One such successful mutation by recombinant techniques was the substitution of Lys^{296}-His-Arg-Arg^{299} with four alanine residues (KHRR 296-299 AAAA). This substitution resulted in greater fibrin specificity and increased resistance to PAI-1. It was also noted that the amino acid substitution $threonine^{103}$-asparagine (T103N), producing an extra glycosylation site on the kringle 1 domain, reduced the clearance of t-PA substantially.

Variants of t-PA with T103N and KHRR 296-299 AAAA mutations combined exhibited four- to fivefold slower clearance in rats and rabbits when compared with native t-PA while possessing greater fibrin specificity and PAI-1 resistance [56]. When given as a bolus in a rabbit arteriovenous shunt model of thrombosis, this mutant was found to have sixfold decreased clearance and displayed greater potency on platelet-rich clots (platelet-rich thrombi are high in PAI-1) relative to native t-PA [57]. A third substitution was added, $asparagine^{117}$-glutamine, which deleted a glycosylation site, and the resultant t-PA variant T (T103N) N (N117Q) K (KHHRR 296-299 AAAA) t-PA appeared to display the properties of reduced clearance, maintained thrombolytic activity, resistance to PAI-1, and minimal effects on systemic fibrinogen levels [58].

TNK–t-PA was tested in a canine arterial and venous thrombosis model and compared with native t-PA. Again, when compared with t-PA, TNK–t-PA was more potent and displayed a markedly decreased rate of clearance (240 ± 32 vs 540 ± 49 mL/min, P = 0.002) [59]. Bolus injections of TNK–t-PA were compared with accelerated t-PA in the thrombosed rabbit carotid artery model [60]. At the highest dose used in the study (1.5 mg/kg) TNK–t-PA was shown to have a faster time to reperfusion (11 ± 2 vs 23 ± 7 minutes, $P <$ 0.02) and a longer duration of recanalization (77 ± 9 vs 51 ± 18 minutes, $P < 0.025$) than the highest t-PA dose (9.0 mg/kg front-loaded). The effects on circulating fibrinogen, plasminogen, and α_2-antiplasmin were significantly less with TNK–t-PA and t-PA elicited nearly twice as much peripheral bleeding.

The study of this agent has reached the clinical arena and results of a phase I trial were recently presented. TIMI 10A was an open-label, dose-finding study of TNK–t-PA in 113 patients with AMI. The primary endpoints were 90 minute patency and TIMI 3 flow. Eight doses were administered, ranging from 5 to 50 mg given as a single IV bolus. At a dose of 30 mg, patency was achieved in 81% of patients and TIMI 3 grade flow in 73%. Reductions in circulating fibrinogen or plasminogen were minimal, and the overall bleeding rate was 6.2% without any instances of intracerebral hemorrhage [61]. Thus, TNK–t-PA represents a new pharmacologic agent that appears to be more fibrin-specific, may be administered as a single bolus, and has a potentially improved patency as well as safety profile. Further clinical trials of this agent are ongoing.

E6010 (Monteplase)

E6010 is another amino acid substitution mutant of native t-PA. It contains a single substitution, cysteine ^{84} to serine, in the epidermal growth factor domain. This agent was found to have reduced clearance and to have more potent thrombolytic activity in a canine model of coronary thrombosis [62]. Similar results were found when E6010 was compared with t-PA in a porcine coronary thrombosis model [63]. Both of these studies were carried out with single bolus infusions of E6010. Several other animal studies were performed showing the thrombolytic activity of E6010 to be as good as or superior to t-PA [64,65]. Studies also performed in the canine copper-coil coronary thrombosis model, comparing E6010 against t-PA and urokinase, seemed to suggest that one hour after reperfusion the E6010-treated animals had significantly higher ejection fractions, although the number of animals was small [66].

E6010 has been used in two clinical trials of patients with acute infarctions. The first study was a phase I dose-finding study with patency as the primary endpoint [67]. The second trial was a randomized comparison of E6010 bolus injection with t-PA in AMI also with patency as the primary endpoint [68]. Both of these trials examined 60- rather than 90-minute patency. The t-PA in the second study was administered as a 10% bolus with the remainder infused over 60 minutes. Patency data are shown in Table 16-6. The high rate of patency in the dose-finding study is promising, although at the higher dose, a bleeding complication rate of 18% overall was reported. Despite this, only 3 of 96 patients required a blood transfusion. Perhaps due to concerns about the bleeding risk, an intermediate dose was chosen for the comparison trial. Again, the reported patency rates are promising, and at 60 minutes E6010 achieved significantly higher patency than did t-PA. There were no differences in recurrent infarction and only one intracerebral hemorrhage occurred in the t-PA arm. Interpretation of these results is made difficult by the use of patency at 60 minutes instead of 90 minutes, a time point used in most other patency trials, and by the administration of t-PA in a nonstandard fashion. Despite this, E6010 appears to achieve a high rate of early patency with no apparent increase in bleeding risk.

Other Plasminogen Activators

bat-PA (Vampire Bat Salivary Plasminogen Activator)

The plasminogen activator from the vampire bat, *Desmodus rotundus*, has been found to be highly homologous with human t-PA. It lacks the K_2 domain of t-PA and the plasmin cleavage site that permits conversion to the two-chain form. It has been made available through recombinant techniques by cloning the cDNA obtained from the salivary gland of the host animal. bat-PA has been applied in many animal models of thrombosis, but has not yet been used in humans.

The isolation and characterization of bat-PA were described in 1989 by Gardell and colleagues. They found that bat-PA exhibits a strict requirement for fibrin as a co-factor that is not met by fibrinogen [69]. In a rabbit model of femoral artery thrombosis, bolus injections of bat-PA were compared with t-PA in its ability to reestablish reperfusion and its effects on plasma protein degradation. The highest of four doses of bat-PA (42.0 nmol/kg), given as a bolus, was found to yield a shorter time to reperfusion with a similar incidence of reperfusion when compared with bolus intravenous t-PA (42.0 nmol/kg) [70]. Most notably, there was an absence of fibrinogenolysis and only minimal decreases in plasminogen and α_2-antiplasmin. The clearance of bat-PA was fourfold slower than t-PA with a half-life of 17.1 minutes. Similar work was performed in the canine femoral artery thrombosis model comparing t-PA and bat-PA. bat-PA again yielded shorter reperfusion times and longer times to reocclusion, whereas maximum blood flow reached as a percentage of baseline flow was also significantly higher (80% for bat-PA vs 41% for t-PA, $P < 0.05$) [71]. As in the rabbit model, there was no effect of bat-PA on plasma protein levels. The most recent work with bat-PA was another comparison with t-PA in the canine coronary thrombosis model. Both agents were administered as a bolus and the results duplicate those of the two femoral artery models mentioned above [72].

The potential benefit of a high degree of fibrin specificity is the lack of systemic protein degradation, or the lytic state. This appears to be one of the promising aspects of bat-PA. Further attempts to quantify the bleeding risk with this agent led to work with the rabbit cuticle bleeding time (CBT) model. In this model, using doses identified in the rabbit femoral artery model, small increases in CBT were observed for bat-PA versus large increases for t-PA (1.6 ± 0.4-fold increase over baseline for bat-PA vs 4.2 ± 0.9-fold

Table 16-6. Results of E6010 (Monteplase) Patency Trials

	Study design	Patients, *n*	Dose	30-minute patency, %	45-minute patency, %	60-minute patency, %
Kawai *et al.* [67]	OL	45	0.167 mg/kg	51	63	73
		51	0.333 mg/kg	75	77	84
Kawai *et al.* [68]	R, DB	97	0.22 mg/kg	62*	74*	79**
		102	t-PA	32	50	65

*$P < 0.01$ compared with t-PA.
**$P < 0.05$ compared with t-PA.
DB—double blind; OL—open label; R—randomized; t-PA—tissue plasminogen activator.

increase for t-PA, $P < 0.05$) [73]. The effect of bat-PA on fibrinogen and α_2-antiplasmin levels was a reduction to 88% and 74% (P = not significant and $P < 0.05$ compared with baseline) of baseline values respectively versus 41% and 21% for t-PA ($P < 0.05$ for each compared with baseline).

Taken together, the animal data suggest that bat-PA is a fibrin-specific agent with high reperfusion rates and a potentially reduced risk of bleeding compared with standard thrombolytic agents. What remains to be demonstrated is the effect of this agent on patency, left ventricular function, bleeding complications, and ultimately mortality in patients with AMI.

Recombinant Staphylokinase (STAR)

Staphylokinase is a 136-amino-acid protein that is produced by several strains of *Staphylococcus aureus*. It was shown to have fibrinolytic properties more than four decades ago, but the initial in vitro and in vivo studies were discouraging [74]. In particular, use of the canine model of thrombosis for this particular agent led to excessive bleeding complications that compromised its development potential as a new agent. In retrospect, the dog may in fact be unusually sensitive to systemic fibrinolytic activation by staphylokinase. The gene for staphylokinase was cloned in the 1980s and the availability of the recombinant product (STAR) generated a resurgence of interest in its use.

The fibrin selective mechanism of staphylococcus is unique. Staphylokinase forms a one to one ratio stoichiometric complex with plasminogen, as does streptokinase. The staphylokinase-plasminogen complex, unlike its streptokinase-plasminogen counterpart, is inactive and requires conversion to staphylokinase-plasmin for exposure of the active site. In plasma, in the absence of fibrin, the staphylokinase-plasminogen complex is inhibited by α_2-antiplasmin. In the presence of fibrin, staphylokinase-plasmin formation is facilitated and inhibition at the clot surface is delayed. The staphylokinase-plasmin complex is rapidly inhibited by α_2-antiplasmin, unlike the streptokinase-plasmin complex, but this reaction is reduced by more than 100-fold in the presence of fibrin. Upon inhibition by α_2-antiplasmin, staphylokinase is released from the staphylokinase-plasmin complex and may be recycled to other plasminogen entities. Hence, the activation of the plasminogen by staphylokinase requires the presence of fibrin and the specificity of this reaction is due to the inhibition of the staphylokinase-plasmin complex by α_2-antiplasmin and the reduction of this inhibition at the fibrin surface [75].

Recombinant staphylokinase was compared with streptokinase in a hamster pulmonary embolism model and a rabbit jugular vein thrombosis model. Intravenous STAR was found to have similar thrombolytic potency to streptokinase in the hamster but less so in the rabbit [76]. In another study of pulmonary embolism in the hamster model, human plasma was used to create platelet-poor, platelet-rich, or platelet-enriched clots. STAR was equipotent to streptokinase in lysing the platelet-poor and -rich clots, but was fivefold more potent in lysing the platelet-enriched thrombi [77].

As a step toward human trials, STAR was studied with streptokinase in a primate model of arterial and venous thrombosis [78]. In baboons, using ^{125}I-fibrin-labeled autologous clots in the jugular veins, STAR and streptokinase effected equivalent and dose-dependent lysis without evidence of systemic fibrinogenolysis. The two agents were also compared in the femoral arterial eversion graft model of thrombus, also in the baboon, which represents the platelet-rich clot seen in the coronary arteries of humans with AMI. Infusion of STAR (0.25 mg/kg) resulted in a greater return of baseline blood flow than streptokinase (1.0 mg/kg) with a longer duration ($P = 0.032$). Animals sensitized with streptokinase over a 5-week period were shown to develop significant neutralizing titers and reduced thrombolytic potency in an ex-vivo thrombosis model. Similar experiments carried out with STAR revealed no increase from baseline in neutralizing titers and no loss of thrombolytic activity. These data suggested that STAR might have increased potency toward platelet-rich clots and less immunogenicity than streptokinase, setting the stage for pilot studies in humans.

In two small series and one randomized trial, patients with AMI were treated with STAR to assess its safety and efficacy. The results of these studies are shown in Table 16-7. The first two pilot studies looked at 40- and 20-minute patency, which occurred in 9 of 10 patients [79,80]. In both studies there was no evidence of fibrinogen or α_2-antiplasmin degradation; by 14 to 35 days, however, there was a significant rise in neutralizing titers in nearly all patients and these did not cross-react with streptokinase [81]. In the randomized trial, the primary endpoints of 90-minute patency and TIMI 3 flow were comparable with t-PA (P = not significant for all comparisons) [82]. As in the pilot trials, there was no decrement in the levels of circulating fibrinogen, α_2-antiplasmin, or plasminogen with STAR. In the first week after treatment with STAR, no neutralizing activity could be found, but by days 10 to 14, titers were significant in the majority of patients.

While the patency rates and the lack of a fibrinogenolytic effect with staphylokinase use in humans is promising, the immunologic response to this agent appears to be more problematic than in animal models. A role for this agent could be foreseen if its use were restricted to a single dose; its lack of cross-reactivity with streptokinase should not make the two mutually exclusive. The ultimate therapeutic potential of this agent remains to be defined by further clinical trials.

Chimeric Plasminogen Activators

The concept of a chimeric plasminogen activator arose with the growth of biotechnology. With the molecular engineering ability of recombinant DNA technology it became possible to attempt to combine selective features of different plasminogen activators into a single molecule. Most of these compounds have been a combination of t-PA and scu-PA, but the thrombolytic properties of these novel agents have not proven to be superior to their parent molecules. Several of these agents are shown in Table 16-2 and a few are discussed below.

A variant of t-PA and scu-PA, $K_1K_2P_u$ was constructed using the kringle 1 and 2 regions of native t-PA and the serine protease portion of prourokinase. This entity has delayed plasma clearance and relatively preserved thrombolytic activity. In a pilot study of six patients with AMI, a single 10-mg bolus of $K_1K_2P_u$ in two patients did not result in recanalization of the angiographically documented occlusion [83]. Two of four patients given a second 10-mg bolus 15 minutes after the first achieved recanalization within 30 minutes. None of the patients developed significant decreases in circulating fibrinogen or α_2-antiplasmin. This pilot study suggests that this agent may promote fibrin-specific fibrinolysis when two bolus injections are used.

Two other chimeric molecules have undergone animal testing. FK_2tu-PA contains the finger and kringle 2 domains of native t-PA combined with the serine protease domain of scu-PA. K_2tu-PA is a chimeric that joins only the kringle 2 domain of t-PA with the active site of scu-PA. K_2tu-PA was shown in the rabbit jugular vein thrombosis model to have a higher thrombolytic activity than either t-PA or scu-PA with similar systemic effects [84]. A hybrid of the u-PA growth factor domain and the kringle 2 and serine protease domains of t-PA was also tested in rabbits. It was found to have a prolonged half-life but absent thrombolytic activity [85]. A chimeric activator was formed by the covalent linkage of the fibrin-binding domains of plasminogen with the serine protease domain of native t-PA. It was shown to have reduced clearance and increased potency in the guinea pig pulmonary embolism model, but only when its active site was acylated to prevent inhibition by α_2-antiplasmin [86].

Conjugate Thrombolytic Therapy

A further attempt at increasing the fibrin specificity of thrombolytic agents is by their conjugation to monoclonal antibodies directed at fibrin or the platelet. Several reports of this method of enhancement have

Table 16-7. Results of Recombinant Staphylokinase (STAR) Trials in Patients with Acute Myocardial Infarction

	Study design	Patients, *n*	Dose	Patency	90-minute TIMI 3, %	Antibody response
Collen and Van de Werf [79]	OL	5	10 mg/30 min	4/5*	-	+
Schlott *et al.* [80]	OL	5	10 mg/30 min	5/5**	-	+
STAR Trial [82]	R, OL	25	10 mg/30 min	68%†	50	+
		23	20 mg/30 min	83%†	74	+
		52	100 mg t-PA accelerated	75%†	62	-

**Patency at 40 minutes.*
***Patency at 20 minutes.*
†Patency at 90 minutes.
P = not significant for all comparisons.
OL—open label; R—randomized; t-PA—tissue plasminogen activator.

been published and three such agents are shown in Table 16-2.

The potential to accelerate clot lysis while simultaneously inhibiting platelet aggregation was shown by Bode and colleagues. These investigators covalently linked urokinase to the monoclonal antibody 7E3 Fab′, which is targeted to the platelet glycoprotein (GP) IIb/IIIa receptor. They were able to show in vitro that urokinase-7E3(Fab′) displayed more rapid clot lysis and greater platelet inhibition than either component alone [87].

Conjugates of monoclonal antibodies to fibrin (MA-59D8) or to fibrin D-dimers (MA-15C5) with scu-PA have been tested in hamsters and rabbits [88]. They have been found to have decreased clearance, increasing their thrombolytic potency. These antibodies have also been linked to t-PA. In a rabbit thrombosis model, t-PA-59D8 was three to 10 times more potent than t-PA alone without a prominent systemic lytic effect [89]. A fraction of the scu-PA moiety, scu-PA-33k, has been conjugated with MA-15C5 (anti-fibrin antibody). This molecule has been shown to have a sixfold greater thrombolytic potency than scu-PA in a hamster model of pulmonary embolism.

These agents are the result of advances in biotechnology that allow the manipulation of several different proteins and their combination in an attempt to improve the characteristics of thrombolytic therapy. The clinical role for these novel approaches, however, remains to be elucidated.

Additional Strategies for Improvement

Time to Treatment

While this chapter focuses on new pharmacologic agents for thrombolysis, there are two adjunctive strategies that are relevant to these new compounds. Compelling evidence exists from the large clinical trials that any reduction in mortality with thrombolytic therapy is greatest when patients are treated early. This process may be facilitated by a therapy that could be given as a bolus. In the GISSI (Gruppo Italiano per lo Studio della Streptokinase nell′ infarto miocardico [Effectiveness of intravenous thrombolytic treatment in AMI]) study [25] a 50% mortality reduction was obtained if patients were treated with streptokinase within the first hour. The relative mortality reduction for patients treated with t-PA and intravenous heparin in the GUSTO trial [35] was 14% overall. For those patients randomized within 2 hours of symptom onset, however, the relative mortality reduction was 17% (mortality 5.4% t-PA vs 6.5% streptokinase, [Fig. 16-1]). The concept that early administration decreases mortality has been reinforced by the recent MITI (Myocardial Infarction Triage and Intervention) and EMIP (European Myocardial Infarction Project) trials [90,91]. Early recanalization of the infarct artery remains the goal of thrombolysis. Striving for the shortest time to treatment is a part of that strategy and bolus therapy may offer an advantage over conventional intravenous dosing.

Adjunctive Therapy

The current standard in antithrombotic treatment was established unequivocally in the ISIS-2 (Second International Study of Infarct Survival) trial [26]. Aspirin was shown to decrease 35-day mortality when compared with placebo (9.4% vs 11.8%, odds reduction 23%, $2P < 0.00001$) and resulted in an additive effect when combined with streptokinase (8.0% vs 13.2% for placebo, odds reduction 42%, $2P < 0.00001$). Aspirin may be limited, however, by its effect on only a single pathway of platelet activation. In addition, the other standard antithrombotic therapy, heparin, is limited by its relative lack of specificity for clot-bound thrombin, thought to be a mediator of reocclusion. Furthermore, heparin has been shown to be important when used with fibrin-selective plasminogen activators, but not for the more nonfibrin selective activators [43]. There was no difference in mortality between streptokinase and intravenous or subcutaneous heparin in AMI patients in the GUSTO trial [35]. These limitations have led to the search for more potent and selective platelet and thrombin inhibitors [92].

New approaches to more selective blockade of platelet aggregation include targeting the GP IIb/IIIa

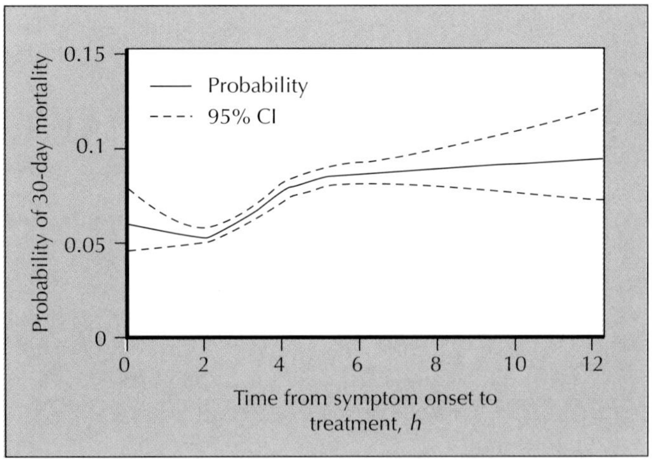

Figure 16-1. The probability for 30-day mortality as a function of time to treatment for all patients in GUSTO (Global Utilization of Streptokinase and t-PA for Occluded Coronary Arteries). CI—confidence interval.

receptor, inhibition of thromboxane synthase, and agents that block the serotonin or endoperoxide receptors [93]. Glycoprotein IIb/IIIa blockade has been facilitated by the use of monoclonal antibodies to the fibrinogen receptor. The murine chimeric monoclonal antibody 7E3 was tested in the pilot TAMI-8 study as an adjunct to therapy with t-PA, aspirin, heparin, and metoprolol [94]. In 60 patients, escalating doses of 7E3 Fab were shown to effectively cause ex vivo platelet inhibition (90% at the highest dose) with no increase in bleeding complications when compared with controls. Infarct-artery patency was increased among treated patients who underwent catheterization at 5 days, and there was a trend toward decreased recurrent ischemia. With the success of c7E3 (abciximab) in patients undergoing high-risk angioplasty [95] larger trials of this therapeutic strategy in patients with AMI are now being planned; concerns remain about the increased bleeding risk.

Other inhibitors of the GP IIb/IIIa receptor include the peptide Integrelin (Cor Therapeutics, San Francisco, CA), containing the arginine-glycine-aspartic acid (RGD) sequence. In a randomized, double-blind, placebo-controlled trial of 106 patients with AMI also receiving aspirin and heparin, Integrelin-treated patients had higher patency and TIMI grade 3 flow rates at 90 minutes. Treated patients had no increase in bleeding complications and experienced less recurrent ischemia [96]. Larger trials of Integrelin in patients with AMI are currently being planned. Several other GP IIb/IIIa inhibitors are under development, including a host of oral agents that offer the promise of easier administration and the potential for more prolonged therapy. Antiplatelet therapy by Ridrogel, a combination of thromboxane A_2 synthase inhibitor and the thromboxane A_2/prostaglandin endoperoxide receptor blocker, has also shown promise in reducing ischemic events after MI [97].

Adjunctive therapy with more selective antithrombins such as hirudin, hirulog, argatroban, and efegatran are currently in various phases of development. The recently completed GUSTO-IIb trial in patients with acute coronary syndromes randomized 12,142 patients to 72 hours of therapy with either hirudin or heparin. A highly significant reduction of death or MI occurred at 24 hours (heparin 2.1% vs hirudin 1.3%, $P = 0.001$) in all patients, but this effect did not persist. The primary endpoint of death or reinfarction at 30 days occurred in 9.8% of heparin- and 8.9% of hirudin-treated patients ($P = 0.058$) [98]. This was mostly due to a reduction in reinfarction (heparin 6.2% vs hirudin 5.4%, $P = 0.046$) that existed in both ST-segment elevation and non-ST–segment elevation strata. While there was no difference in the primary endpoint, the mortality reduction at 24 hours appears to confirm the importance of thrombin inhibition as an adjunct to thrombolytic therapy. Efforts continue to define the role of these new agents.

Two very novel approaches to antithrombotic co-therapy involve recombinant hirudin coupled with an antibody targeted to fibrin or covalently bonded to streptokinase [99,100]. The antibody-mediated hirudin offers the potential for greater thrombin inhibition at 10- to 100-fold lower doses. The combination with streptokinase appears to retain its thrombolytic and antithrombotic activity while having a greater affinity for clot-bound thrombin. All of these therapies offer the potential for improved patency when used as adjuncts to thrombolytic therapy, but their clinical utility and effect on outcome remain to be determined.

Conclusions

The role of thrombus in the pathogenesis of AMI, and the recognition that thrombolytic therapy results in recanalization of the infarct-related artery with preserved left-ventricular function and reduced mortality, have led to a revolution in the development of these agents. Thrombolytic therapy most likely represents one of the most studied pharmacologic treatments in the history of medicine. Despite this scrutiny there remain significant limitations to currently available agents. The incidence of bleeding, reocclusion, and the fact that complete reperfusion is probably uncommon remain significant. The relationship between early infarct-artery patency and outcome has now been confirmed and the search for new pharmacotherapy that will improve current results is intense. The approach to newer thrombolytic therapy should include a continued effort to decrease a patient's time to treatment. An effort to improve adjunctive therapies should also be continued. Many new approaches to thrombolytic agents have been discussed, including mutants of t-PA, new animal or bacterial plasminogen activators, chimeric activators, and conjugate molecules combining site-specific antibodies with available plasminogen activators. Several of these agents are in clinical trials and may become available clinically in the near future. Other thrombolytic possibilities have only begun the evaluation process and will require many more trials before their clinical utility can be defined. It should be remembered that the high patency rates obtained in recent trials may make improvements in therapy more difficult to prove. A continued goal of improved and sustained patency, however, will help reduce morbidity and mortality in patients with AMI.

References and Recommended Reading

Recently published papers of particular interest have been highlighted as:
- • Of special interest
- •• Of outstanding interest

1. DeWood MA, Spores J, Notske R, *et al.*: Prevalence of total coronary occlusion during the early hours of transmural myocardial infarction. *N Engl J Med* 1980, 303:897–902.
2. Mohr JP, Caplan LR, Melski JW, *et al.*: The Harvard cooperative stroke registry: A prospective registry. *Neurology* 1978, 28:754.
3. *Heart and Stroke Facts: 1995 Statistical Supplement.* American Heart Association National Center, Dallas, TX; p. 9.
4.• Mueler RL, Scheidt S: History of drugs for thrombotic disease. Discovery, development, and directions for the future. *Circulation* 1994, 89:432–449.

This report reviews the history of the discovery and development of all classes of antithrombotic drugs. Included is a complete description of the evolution of thrombolytic therapy as well as the development of newer agents.

5. Sherry S, Marder VJ: Thrombosis, fibrinolysis, and thrombolytic therapy: a perspective. *Prog in Cardiovasc Dis* 1991, 34:89–100.
6. Cairns JA: Coronary thrombolysis: history and rationale. *Can J Cardiol* 1993, 9:483–484.
7. Verstraete M: The fibrinolytic system: from petri dishes to genetic engineering. *Thromb Haemost* 1995, 74:25–35.
8. Macfarlane RG, Biggs R: Fibrinolysis. Its mechanism and significance. *Blood* 1948, 3:1167–1187.
9. Dastre A: Fibrinolyse dans le sang. *Arch Norm Pathol* 1893, 5:661–663.
10. von Brucke E: Die verdauende substanz im urin. *SB Akad Wiss (Vienna)* 1861, 43:601–615.
11. Sahli W: Ueber fermente im harn. In *Archiv für die Gesammte Physiologie* 1886; 35–85. Edited by Von Gehrig F. Bonn, Germany: Verlag; 1886:35–85.
12. MacFarlane RG, Pilling J: Fibrinolytic activity in normal urine. *Nature* 1947, 159:779.
13. Williams JRB: The fibrinolytic activity of the urine. *Br J Exp Pathol* 1951, 32:530–537.
14. Tillett WS, Garner RL: The fibrinolytic activity of streptococci. *J Exp Med* 1933, 58:485–502.
15. Milstone H: A factor in normal human blood which participates in streptococcal fibrinolysis. *J Immunol* 1941, 42:109–116.
16. Sherry S: The origin of thrombolytic therapy. *J Am Coll Cardiol* 1989, 14:1085–1092.
17. Tillett WS, Sherry S: The effect in patients of streptococcal fibrinolysin (streptokinase) and streptococcal desoxyribonuclease on fibrinous, purulent, and sanguinous pleural exudations. *J Clin Invest* 1949, 28:173–190.
18. Fletcher AP, Alkjaersig N, Smyrniotis FE, Sherry S: Treatment of patients suffering from early, myocardial infarction with massive and prolonged streptokinase therapy. *Trans Assoc Am Physicians* 1958, 71:287–296.
19. Rentrop KP, Blanke H, Kostering K, Karsh KR: Acute myocardial infarction: intracoronary application of nitroglycerin and streptokinase in combination with transmural recanalization. *Clin Cardiol* 1979, 2:354–363.
20. Stampfer MJ, Goldhaber SZ, Yusuf S, *et al.*: Effects of intravenous streptokinase on acute myocardial infarction: results pooled from randomized trials. *N Engl J Med* 1982, 307:1180–1182.
21. Yusuf S, Collins R, Peto R, *et al.*: Intravenous and intracoronary fibrinolytic therapy in acute myocardial infarction: overview of results on mortality, reinfarction, and side effects from 33 randomized controlled trials. *Eur Heart J* 1985, 6:556–585.
22. Sobel BE, Bresnahan GF, Shell WE, *et al.*: Estimation of infarct size in man and its relation to prognosis. *Circulation* 1972, 46:640–648.
23. Rude RE, Muller JE, Braunwald E: Efforts to limit the size of myocardial infarcts. *Ann Intern Med* 1981, 95:736–761.
24. Ritchie JL, Davis KB, Williams DL, *et al.*: Global and regional left ventricular function and tomographic radionuclide perfusion: the Western Washington Intracoronary Streptokinase in Myocardial Infarction Trial. *Circulation* 1984, 70:867–875.
25. Gruppo Italiano per lo studio della streptokinase nell' infarto miocardico (GISSI): Effectiveness of intravenous thrombolytic treatment in acute myocardial infarction. *Lancet* 1986, i:397–402.
26. ISIS-2 (Second International Study of Infarct Survival) Collaborative Group: Randomized trial of intravenous streptokinase, oral aspirin, both or neither among 17,187 cases of suspected acute myocardial infarction. *Lancet* 1988, ii:349–360.
27. Been M, de Bono DB, Muir AI, *et al.*: Coronary thrombolysis with intravenous APSAC. *Br Heart J* 1985, 53:253–259.
28. Rijken DC, Wijngaards G, Zaal-De Jong M, Welbergen J: Purification and partial characterization of the plasminogen activator from human uterine tissue. *Biochim Biophys Acta* 1979, 580:140–153.
29. Pennica D, Holmes WE, Kohr WJ, *et al.*: Cloning and expression of human tissue-type plasminogen activator cDNA in *E. Coli. Nature* 1983, 301:214–221.
30. Collen D, Topol EJ, Tiefenbrunn AJ, *et al.*: Coronary thrombolysis with recombinant human tissue-type plasminogen activator; a prospective, randomized, placebo-controlled trial. *Circulation* 1984, 69:1012–1017.
31. Bang NU: Tissue-type plasminogen activator mutants. Theoretical and clinical considerations. *Circulation* 1989, 79:1391–1392.
32. Collen D, Lijnen HR, Gold HK: Towards better thrombolytic therapy. *Prog Cardiovasc Dis* 1991, 34:101–112.

33. Collen D, Lijnen HR: On the future of thrombolytic therapy for acute myocardial infarction. *Am J Cardiol* 1993, 72:46G–50G.

34. Collen D: Towards improved thrombolytic therapy. *Lancet* 1993, 342:34–36.

35. The GUSTO Investigators: An international randomized trial comparing four thrombolytic strategies for acute myocardial infarction. *N Engl J Med* 1993, 329:673–682.

36. The GUSTO Angiographic Investigators: The effects of tissue plasminogen activator, streptokinase, or both on coronary-artery patency, ventricular function, and survival after acute myocardial infarction. *N Engl J Med* 1993, 329:1615–1622.

37. Lincoff AM, Topol EJ: Illusion of reperfusion. Does anyone achieve optimal reperfusion during acute myocardial infarction? *Circulation* 1993, 88:1361–1374.

38. Becker RC: Reocclusion following successful thrombolysis. Emerging concepts. *Cardiology* 1993, 82:265–273.

39. Ohman EM, Califf RM, Topol EJ, and the TAMI Study Group: Consequences of reocclusion after successful reperfusion therapy in acute myocardial infarction. *Circulation* 1990, 82:781–791.

40. Collen D, Lijnen HR: Basic and clinical aspects of fibrinolysis and thrombolysis. *Blood* 1991, 78:3114–3124.

41. Collen D, Lijnen HR: Molecular basis of fibrinolysis, as relevant for thrombolytic therapy. *Thromb Haemost* 1995, 74:167–171.

42.•• Collen D: Fibrin-selective thrombolytic therapy for acute myocardial infarction. *Circulation* 1996, 93:857–865.

This report reviews the history of thrombolytic drug development with an emphasis on the evolving understanding of the fibrinolytic system. Emphasis is placed on the discovery and function of native t-PA and recent work with staphylokinase.

43. Bode C, Nordt TK, Runge MS: Thrombolytic therapy in acute myocardial infarction—selected recent developments. *Ann Hematol* 1994, 69(suppl II):S35–S40.

44. Martin U, Fischer S, Kohnert U, *et al.*: Thrombolysis with an Escherichia coli-produced recombinant plasminogen activator (BM 06.022) in the rabbit model of jugular vein thrombosis. *Thromb Haemost* 1991, 65:560–564.

45. Jackson CV, Crowe G, Craft TJ, *et al.*: Thrombolytic activity of a novel plasminogen activator, LY210825, compared with recombinant tissue-type plasminogen activator in a canine model of coronary thrombosis. *Circulation* 1990, 82:930–940.

46. Jackson CV, Frank JD, Craft TJ, *et al.*: Comparison of the thrombolytic activity of the novel plasminogen activator, LY210825, to anisoylated plasminogen-streptokinase activator complex in a canine model of coronary artery thrombosis. *J Pharmacol Exp Ther* 1992, 260:64–70.

47. Martin U, van Mollendorf E, Akpan W, *et al.*: Dose-ranging study of the novel recombinant plasminogen activator BM 06.022 in healthy volunteers. *Clin Pharmacol Ther* 1991, 50:429–436.

48. Neuhaus KL, von Essen R, Vogt A, *et al.*: Dose finding with a novel recombinant plasminogen activator (BM 06.022) in patients with acute myocardial infarction: results of the German Recombinant Plasminogen Activator Study. *J Am Coll Cardiol* 1994, 24:55–60.

49. Tebbe U, von Essen R, Smolarz A, *et al.*: Open, noncontrolled dose-finding study with a novel recombinant plasminogen activator (BM 06.022) given as a double bolus in patients with acute myocardial infarction. *Am J Cardiol* 1993, 72:518–524.

50. Smalling RW, Bode C, Kalbfleisch J, *et al.* for the RAPID Investigators: More rapid, complete, and stable coronary thrombolysis with bolus administration of reteplase compared with alteplase infusion in acute myocardial infarction. *Circulation* 1995, 91:2725–2732.

51. Bode C, Smalling RW, Berg G, *et al.* for the RAPID II Investigators: Randomized comparison of coronary thrombolysis achieved with double bolus reteplase (recombinant plasminogen activator) and front loaded, accelerated alteplase (recombinant tissue plasminogen activator) in patients with acute myocardial infarction. *Circulation* 1996, 94:891–898.

52.•• International Joint Efficacy Comparison of Thrombolytics: Randomized, double-blind comparison of reteplase double-bolus administration with streptokinase in acute myocardial infarction (INJECT): trial to investigate equivalence. *Lancet* 1995, 346:329–336.

This study determined the equivalence of r-PA compared with streptokinase in 6010 patients with AMI. r-PA use also resulted in fewer adverse events. This trial is the basis for the 15,000-patient GUSTO-III trial that is ongoing.

53. Madison EL, Goldsmith EJ, Gerard RD, *et al.*: Amino acid residues that affect interaction of tissue-type plasminogen activator with plasminogen activator inhibitor 1. *Proc Natl Acad Sci* 1990, 87:3530–3533.

54. Paoni NF, Refino CJ, Brady K, *et al.*: Involvement of residues 296-299 in the enzymatic activity of tissue-type plasminogen activator. *Protein Eng* 1992, 5:259–266.

55. Paoni NF, Chow AM, Pena LC, *et al.*: Making tissue-type plasminogen activator more fibrin specific. *Protein Eng* 1993, 6:529–534.

56. Paoni NF, Keyt BA, Refino CJ, *et al.*: A slow clearing, fibrin-specifc, PAI-1 resistant variant of t-PA (T103N, KHRR 296-299 AAAA). *Thromb Haemost* 1993, 70:307–312.

57. Refino CJ, Paoni NF, Keyt BA, *et al.*: A variant of t-PA (T103N, KHRR 296-299 AAAA) that, by bolus, has increased potency and decreased systemic activation of plasminogen. *Thromb Haemost* 1993, 70:313–319.

58. Keyt BA, Paoni NF, Refino CJ, *et al.*: A faster-acting and more potent form of tissue plasminogen activator. *Proc Natl Acad Sci* 1994, 91:3670–3674.

59. Collen D, Stassen JM, Yasuda T, *et al.*: Comparative thrombolytic properties of tissue-type plasminogen activator and of a plasminogen activator inhibitor-1-resistant glycosylation variant, in a combined arterial and venous thrombosis model in the dog. *Thromb Haemost* 1994, 72:98–104.

60. Benedict CR, Refino CJ, Keyt BA, *et al.*: New variant of human tissue plasminogen activator (tPA) with enhanced efficacy and lower incidence of bleeding compared with recombinant human tPA. *Circulation* 1995, 92:3032–3040.

61. Braunwald E: *Thrombolysis In Myocardial Infarction 10A*. Presented at the American Heart Association 68th Scientific Sessions, Anaheim, California, November 13 to 15, 1995.

62. Suzuki S, Saito M, Suzuki N, *et al.*: Thrombolytic properties of a novel modified human tissue-type plasminogen activator (E6010): a bolus injection of E6010 has equivalent potency at lysing young and aged canine coronary thrombi. *J Cardiovasc Pharmacol* 1991, 17:738–746.

63. Adachi H, Nagaoka N, Nomoto K, *et al.*: Thrombolytic effects of a novel modified tissue plasminogen activator, E6010, on coronary thrombosis in the pig. *Jpn J Pharmacol* 1992, 58:309–319.

64. Suzuki S, Saito M, Suzuki N, *et al.*: Intracoronary infusion of E6010 has more potent thrombolytic activity than tissue plasminogen activator (t-PA) in dogs: a higher plasma level of E6010 than t-PA causes potent thrombolytic activity. *J Cardiovasc Pharmacol* 1993, 22:834–840.

65. Suzuki N, Suzuki S, Nagaoka N, *et al.*: Thrombolysis of canine femoral artery thrombus by a novel modified tissue-type plasminogen activator (E6010). *Jpn J Pharmacol* 1994, 65:257–263.

66. Suzuki S, Saito M, Yui Y, Kawai C: A novel modified t-PA, E6010, induces faster recovery of ventricular function after coronary thrombolysis than native t-PA in a canine thrombosis model. *Jpn Circ J* 1995, 59:205–212.

67. Kawai C, Hosoda S, Motomiya T, *et al.* for the E6010 Investigators: Multicenter trial of a novel modified t-PA, E6010, by i.v. bolus injection in patients with acute myocardial infarction (AMI) [abstract]. *Circulation* 1992, 86(suppl):409.

68. Kawai C: *Single Bolus E6010 Injection in the Treatment of Acute MI.* Presented at the American Heart Association 68th Scientific Sessions, Anaheim, California, November 13 to 15, 1995.

69. Gardell SJ, Duong LT, Diehl RE, *et al.*: Isolation, characterization, and cDNA cloning of a vampire bat salivary plasminogen activator. *J Biol Chem* 1989, 264:17947–17952.

70. Gardell SJ, Ramjit BS, Stabilito II, *et al.*: Effective thrombolysis without marked plasminemia after bolus intravenous administration of vampire bat salivary plasminogen activator in rabbits. *Circulation* 1991, 84:244–253.

71. Mellott MJ, Stabilito II, Holahan MA, *et al.*: Vampire bat salivary plasminogen activator promotes rapid and sustained reperfusion without concomitant systemic plasminogen activation in a canine model of arterial thrombosis. *Arterioscler Thromb* 1992, 12:212–221.

72. Witt W, Maass B, Baldus B, *et al.*: Coronary thrombolysis with *Desmodus* salivary plasminogen activators in dogs. Fast and persistent recanalization by intravenous bolus administration. *Circulation* 1994, 90:421–426.

73. Mellott MJ, Ramjit DR, Stabilito II, *et al.*: Vampire bat salivary plasminogen activator evokes minimal bleeding relative to tissue-type plasminogen activator as assessed by a rabbit cuticle bleeding time model. *Thromb Haemost* 1995, 73:478–483.

74. Collen D, Lijnen HR: Staphylokinase, a fibrin-specific plasminogen activator with therapeutic potential? *Blood* 1994, 84:680–686.

75. Collen D, Van Hoef B, Schlott B, *et al.*: Mechanisms of activation of mammalian plasma fibrinolytic systems with streptokinase and with recombinant staphylokinase. *Eur J Biochem* 1993, 216:307–314.

76. Lijnen HR, Stassen JM, Vanlinthout I, *et al.*: Comparative fibrinolytic properties of staphylokinase and streptokinase in animal models of venous thrombosis. *Thromb Haemost* 1991, 66:468–473.

77. Collen D, De Cock F, Vanlinthout I, *et al.*: Comparative thrombolytic and immunogenic properties of staphylokinase and streptokinase. *Fibrinolysis* 1992, 6:232.

78. Collen D, De Cock F, Stassen JM: Comparative immunogenicity and thrombolytic properties toward arterial and venous thrombi of streptokinase and recombinant staphylokinase in baboons. *Circulation* 1993, 87:996–1006.

79. Collen D, Van de Werf F: Coronary thrombolysis with recombinant staphylokinase in patients with evolving myocardial infarction. *Circulation* 1993, 87:1850–1853.

80. Schlott B, Hartmann M, Guhrs KH, *et al.*: High yield production and purification of recombinant staphylokinase for thrombolytic therapy. *Biotechnology* 1994, 12:185.

81. Vanderschueren SMF, Stassen JM, Collen D: On the immunogenicity of recombinant staphylokinase in patients and in animal models. *Thromb Haemost* 1994, 72:297–301.

82. Vanderschueren S, Barrios L, Kerdsinchai P, *et al.*: A randomized trial of recombinant staphylokinase versus alteplase for coronary artery patency in acute myocardial infarction. *Circulation* 1995, 92:2044–2049.

83. Van de Werf F, Lijnen R, Collen D: Coronary thrombolysis with K_1K_2Pu, a chimeric tissue-type and urokinase-type plasminogen activator: a feasibility study in six patients with acute myocardial infarction. *Coron Artery Dis* 1993, 4:929–933.

84. Agnelli G, Pascucci C, Colucci M *et al.*: Thrombolytic activity of two chimeric recombinant plasminogen activators (FK_2tu-PA and K_2tu-PA) in rabbits. *Thromb Haemost* 1992, 68:331–335.

85. Asselbergs FA, Bürgi R, Hamerman J, *et al.*: A hybrid plasminogen activator binds to the u-PA receptor and has a reduced thrombolytic potency in vivo. *Thromb Haemost* 1993, 69:50–55.

86. Robinson JH, Browne MJ, Carey JE, *et al.*: A recombinant, chimeric enzyme with a novel mechanism of action leading to greater potency and selectivity than tissue-type plasminogen activator. *Circulation* 1992, 86:548–552.

87. Bode C, Meinhardt G, Runge MS, *et al.*: Platelet-targeted fibrinolysis enhances clot lysis and inhibits platelet aggregation. *Circulation* 1991, 84:804–813.

88. Holvoet P, Dewerchin M, Stassen JM, *et al.*: Thrombolytic profiles of clot-targeted plasminogen activators. Parameters determining potency and initial and maximal rates. *Circulation* 1993, 87:1007–1016.

89. Runge MS, Bode C, Matsueda GR, Haber E: Antibody-enhanced thrombolysis: targeting of tissue plasminogen activator in vivo. *Proc Natl Acad Sci* 1987, 84:7650–7662.

90. Weaver WD, Cerqueira M, Hallstrom AP, *et al.*: Prehospital-initiated vs hospital-initiated thrombolytic therapy. The Myocardial Infarction Triage and Intervention Trial. *JAMA* 1993, 270:1211–1216.

91. EMIP Group: Prehospital thrombolytic therapy in patients with suspected acute myocardial infarction. *N Engl J Med* 1993, 329:383–389.

92. Sumama MM, Acar J: Thrombolytic therapy: future issues. *Thromb Haemost* 1995, 74:106–110.

93. Collen D, Lijnen HR: New thrombolytic agents and strategies. *Bailliere's Clinical Haematology* 1995, 8:425–435.

94. Kleiman NS, Ohman EM, Califf RM, *et al.*: Profound inhibition of platelet aggregation with monoclonal antibody 7E3 Fab after thrombolytic therapy: Results of the thrombolysis and angioplasty in myocardial infarction (TAMI) 8 pilot study. *J Am Coll Cardiol* 1993, 22:381–389.

95. The EPIC Investigators: Use of a monoclonal antibody directed against the platelet glycoprotein IIb/IIIa receptor in high risk coronary angioplasty. *N Engl J Med* 1993, 330:956–961.

96. Ohman EM, Kleiman NS, Gacioch G: Simultaneous platelet glycoprotein IIb/IIIa integrin blockade and front-loaded tissue plasminogen activator in acute myocardial infarction: results from a randomized trial [abstract]. *J Am Coll Cardiol* 1996, 27:167A.

97. The RAPT Investigators: Randomized trial of Ridrogel, a combined thromboxane A_2, synthase inhibitor and thromboxane A_2/prostaglandin endoperoxide receptor antagonist, versus aspirin as adjunct to thrombolysis in patients with acute myocardial infarction. The Ridrogel versus aspirin patency trial. *Circulation* 1994, 89:588–595.

98. The Global Use of Strategies to Open Occluded Coronary Arteries (GUSTO) IIb Investigators: A comparison of recombinant hirudin with heparin for the treatment of acute coronary syndromes. *N Engl J Med* 1996, 335:775–782.

99. Bode C, Hudelmayer M, Mehwals P, *et al.*: Fibrin-targeted recombinant hirudin inhibits fibrin deposition on experimental clots more efficiently than recombinant hirudin. *Circulation* 1994, 90:1956–1963.

100. Phaneuf MD, Ozaki CK, J MT, *et al.*: Covalent linkage of streptokinase to recombinant hirudin: a novel thrombolytic agent with antithrombotic properties. *Thromb Haemost* 1994, 71:481–487.

Clinical Trials and Future Directions of Thrombolytic Agents

Chapter 17

Stephen L. Kopecky

Myocardial infarction (MI) most commonly results from total or near-complete obstruction of an epicardial artery by a thrombus that is formed on a ruptured atherosclerotic plaque. The subsequent reduction in blood flow results in cell death. Animal studies show that the development of cell death is time-dependent and is related to the severity of the ischemia. Dog myocytes begin to die as early as 20 minutes after abrupt coronary occlusion, but subtotal occlusion may be tolerated for much longer periods. Current treatment of patients with acute myocardial infarction (AMI) should include aggressive attempts to restore coronary blood flow. Thrombolytic therapy is the primary mechanism for accomplishing reperfusion in the great majority of patients with MI because it is readily available, whereas primary angioplasty is not. Reperfusion should minimize infarct size and reduce the clinical sequelae of myocardial injury when given early, preferably in the first 6 hours after obstruction of blood flow. Timely pharmacologic dissolution of blood clots can abort an infarct and preserve myocardium, with subsequent reduction in overall patient mortality.

Thrombolysis can be achieved with intravenous infusion of plasminogen activators [1], which convert plasminogen, the proenzyme of the fibrinolytic system, to the fibrinolytic enzyme plasmin. Plasminogen is converted to plasmin by cleavage of the peptide bond by plasminogen activators. Plasmin digest fibrin to soluble degradation product. Inhibition of the fibrinolytic system occurs both at the level of plasminogen and at the level of the plasmin.

There are three drugs currently used predominantly in the United States for thrombolysis: streptokinase, tissue plasminogen activator (t-PA), and anisoylated plasminogen streptokinase activator complex (APSAC).

Streptokinase

Streptokinase is produced by group C strains of β hemolytic streptococci. Streptokinase is converted spontaneously in the bloodstream to streptokinase-plasmin complex, which is an efficient activator of plasminogen. The streptokinase-plasmin complexes consist of both circulating and fibrin-bound plasminogen, which is converted to plasmin. Circulating plasmin is neutralized by α-antiplasmin, and the result is plasmin that exerts its fibrinolytic effect on plasma coagulation proteins, including fibrinogen and factors V and VIII. The consumption of fibrinogen and the coagulation factors leads to the bleeding risk of streptokinase. This risk is potentiated when it is combined with heparin or other antithrombins in high doses [2]. Streptokinase is much less expensive than t-PA or urokinase, but it is antigenic and may produce fever, urticaria, or rash in less than 5% of the patients. Anaphylaxis is extremely uncommon and occurs in 0.01% of patients [3]. Human plasma contains antibodies directed against streptokinase but the number of allergic reactions occurring in the United States annually is low and use of prophylactic antihistamines or steroid therapy is not indicated. Streptokinase-binding antibodies titers vary among individuals and the streptokinase dose necessary to overcome the immunologic inhibition is also variable, with 350,000 U of streptokinase being adequate to overcome the antibodies in 95% of patients [4].

Tissue Plasminogen Activator

Tissue plasminogen activator is produced by recombinant DNA technology (rt-PA). In the absence of fibrin, t-PA is a poor plasminogen activator, but in the presence of fibrin it activates plasminogen several hundred times more rapidly. The accelerated administration of t-PA (Table 17-1) along with aspirin and intravenous heparin maximizes coronary patency at 90 minutes and has been shown to reduce mortality in left ventricular dysfunction relative to streptokinase [5,6]. This accelerated dosing regimen of t-PA and heparin resulted in coronary artery patency with normal flow at 90 minutes in 54% of patients compared with approximately 30% in the streptokinase-treated groups in GUSTO (Global Utilization of Streptokinase and t-PA for Occluded Coronary Arteries)-1.

Anisoylated Plasminogen Streptokinase Complex

APSAC is a complex of human lys-plasminogen and streptokinase. This combination renders a longer half-life at 90 minutes compared with only 25 to 30 minutes for streptokinase and approximately 10 minutes for t-PA. The 3-minute, 30-U injection does not cause hypotension.

Recent studies and overview analyses have shown that thrombolysis reduces mortality between 25% and 30% when administered within 6 to 12 hours of the onset of pain of an MI [7•]. Patients treated with thrombolysis, compared with those untreated, also have improved left ventricular function, higher coronary artery patency rates, and lower long-term morbidity and disability. All patients with ST segment elevation MI and a small group of those with ST segment depression (Table 17-2) appear to benefit from thrombolysis regardless of age, infarct location, gender, baseline heart rate, or duration of pain of up to 12 hours before treatment.

The optimal thrombolytic agent is controversial in more than just the medical arena. This is also becoming a debated issue among pharmacists and hospital administrators because of the differing costs involved. Currently, in the United States, streptokinase costs approximately $250; APSAC, $1800; and t-PA, $2300.

Table 17-1. Standard Currently Used Dosages of Tissue Plasminogen Activator* and Streptokinase† in Most Current Randomized Trials

Indications	Relative Contraindications
Typical chest pain > 30 min	History of stroke
but < 12 hours unrelieved with NTG SL	Active bleeding
ST ↑ in ≥ 2 contiguous leads	BP > 180 systolic
≥ 1 mm in limb leads	Major surgery trauma in last 3 mo
≥ 2 mm in chest leads ***or***	Recent noncompressible vascular puncture
ST ↓ in V_2 and V_2 ≥ 2 mm ***or***	Possible intracranial event or unclear mental status
New LBBB	Pregnancy

**15-mg bolus then 0.75 mg/kg over 30 min (not > 50 mg) then 0.5 mg/kg over 60 min (not > 35 mg). Total dose ≤ 100 mg.*
†Intravenous SK 1.5 MU infused over 60 min.
NTG SL—nitroglycerin sublingual; LBBB—left bundle branch block.

Many large-scale studies have been completed recently to establish the most appropriate fibrinolytic therapy treatment regimen. Three of the largest trials, GISSI (Gruppo Italiano per lo Studio della Sopravivenza nell'infarto Miocardio)-2 [8], ISIS (International Study of Infarct Survival)-3 [9], and GUSTO-1 [10••] enrolled over 100,000 patients and have been instrumental in developing a scientific and rational approach to choice of thrombolytic agents based on efficacy and safety issues.

The GISSI-2 is the first head-to-head large trial comparing streptokinase and t-PA. The 20,891 AMI patients were randomly assigned to either streptokinase, 1.5 MU over 30 to 60 minutes, or t-PA (alteplase), 100 mg over 3 hours. Patients also randomly received either subcutaneous heparin, 12,000 U twice a day, versus no heparin: all patients received aspirin, 325 mg, at the time of randomization and daily for 30 days. The GISSI-2 study showed no significant mortality at 35 days, with a death rate of 9.6% among t-PA–treated patients and 9.2% among streptokinase-treated patients . There was also a difference between the subcutaneous heparin group at 9.3% and the no-heparin group at 9.4%. In GISSI-2, patients receiving t-PA had a slightly higher incidence of total stroke, which was statistically significant due to an increase in cerebral hemorrhages. There was no significant difference between the groups in long-term morbidity or mortality.

In ISIS-3, AMI patients were randomly assigned to t-PA, streptokinase, or APSAC (30 U over 3 minutes) with or without subcutaneous heparin. In addition, all patients received daily aspirin. In this double-blinded trial of 41,299 patients, there was no difference in mortality among the three thrombolytic regimens. At 35 days the streptokinase mortality was 10.6%, t-PA 10.3%, and APSAC 10.5%, of which there is no statistical significance among the three groups. Morbidity rates including shock, heart failure requiring treatment, cardiac rupture, and ventricular fibrillation were also of no difference. The stroke rate, however, was higher with t-PA (1.4%) and APSAC (1.3%) than with streptokinase (1%) ($P < 0.0001$). These findings were similar to those of GISSI-2. These two trials (GISSI-2 and ISIS-3) taken together suggest that there is no difference in the mortality rate between the thrombolytic regimens when subcutaneous heparin is used, and that the use of streptokinase resulted in a lower stroke rate. However, it was also shown that there was a higher stroke rate and major hemorrhage rate in patients receiving subcutaneous heparin compared with those on no heparin.

The GUSTO-1 study found a statistically significant but small difference in the mortality among over 41,000 patients. In this study, patients were randomly assigned to 1) streptokinase with subcutaneous heparin; 2) streptokinase with intravenous heparin; 3) front-load t-PA given over 90 minutes, or 4) combination of t-PA and streptokinase with intravenous heparin. This has been the most influential of all the mega trials because it had more of a Unites States presence than the above two trials and because it used intravenous heparin, which is a more commonly used regimen in the United States. Scientifically, intra-

Table 17-2. Various Factors to Consider When Choosing a Thrombolytic

	t-PA	t-PA or SK	SK
Location	Anterior	Nonanterior MI	
Risk*	High†	Intermediate‡	Low§
Patient age	< 75 y		> 75 y
Complication	Complicated inferior MI		Killip class 4 (consider PTCA)
History	Prior CABG		
	Prior SK		

Risk factors for cardiovascular death at 6 weeks post-MI (from TIMI II): at initial history, factors include female gender, diabetes, age ≥ 70, prior MI; at initial exam/ECG, factors include hypotension (< 1 00 mm HG) + tachycardia (> 100), atrial fibrillation, anterior MI, rales > 1/3.

†*Number of factors, ≤ 1; 6-wk mortality, < 3%.*

‡*Number of risk factors, 2–3; 6-wk mortality, 13%.*

§*Number of risk factors, ≥ 4; 6-wk mortality, 17%.*

CABG—coronary artery bypass graft; MI—myocardial infarction; PTCA—percutaneous transluminal coronary angioplasty; SK—streptokinase; TIMI—Thrombosis In Myocardial Infarction; t-PA—tissue plasminogen activator.

venous heparin is believed to be required to prevent reocclusion with t-PA, due to the short half-life of t-PA. The GUSTO-1 trial showed that streptokinase with subcutaneous heparin was superior to streptokinase with intravenous heparin regarding mortality, reinfarction, bleeding complications, and stroke. This finding is important when considering heparin regimen choices with streptokinase (Fig. 17-1). These findings indicate the possibility of benefit for streptokinase and aspirin given alone without heparin. Streptokinase with subcutaneous heparin was found to be more effective than streptokinase with intravenous heparin in GUSTO, and increased stroke rates and intracranial hemorrhage rates were shown with the streptokinase subcutaneous heparin combination in GISSI-2 and ISIS-3 when compared with streptokinase without heparin.

Overall, the GUSTO-1 data showed a 0.9% difference in mortality with front-loaded t-PA with intravenous heparin compared with the streptokinase or subcutaneous heparin regimen. In GUSTO-1, t-PA had a slightly higher rate of stroke and intracranial hemorrhage than streptokinase, which is consistent with the GISSI-2 and ISIS-3 findings. The risk of stroke was highest among older individuals and those with hypertension, which has led to the suggestion of using different thrombolytic regimens when treating different subgroups of patients [11].

There was no significant difference in mortality between t-PA and streptokinase patients who had an inferior MI, who were over 75 years of age, or who had the treatment more than 4 hours after the onset of symptoms (Fig. 17-2). Currently in the United States, the average time to treatment after the onset of symptoms is slightly over 4 hours. It is believed that t-PA is more beneficial early in MI, but because of a high incidence of myocardial cell necrosis in the later hours of the infarction, the mortality benefit seen with t-PA is lessened. These data must be combined with the stroke incidence data in which the patients over 75 years of age receiving t-PA had a 1% higher incidence of stroke. Table 17-2 takes into the account the differential benefit to risk ratio among different patient subgroups and the benefit that may be achieved in these patients. In general, among younger patients who do not have risk factors for intracranial hemorrhage or stroke, t-PA may be a better choice, whereas those patients over age 75 at high risk for intracranial hemorrhage may be better treated with streptokinase. In theory, patients with larger clot burdens may have a more beneficial response to t-PA, although this has not been found in all the larger randomized trials. Patients who have received prior streptokinase, certainly in the past 6 to 12 months, should receive t-PA if a thrombolytic regimen is to be given again. Large anterior MIs or complicated inferior MIs may benefit from t-PA; of interest, however, is that patients who were hemodynamically unstable (Killip class 4) did better with streptokinase in the GUSTO-1 trial, although this group may benefit most from percutaneous transluminal coronary angioplasty (PTCA) when available. However, if immediate angioplasty is not available, thrombolytics should be administered until PTCA can be accomplished. Regardless of the thrombolytic regimen used, it is clear that the more rapidly patients with a thrombolysis are treated, the more the mortality is reduced. The time to treatment has repeatedly been a significant predictor of reduction in mortality.

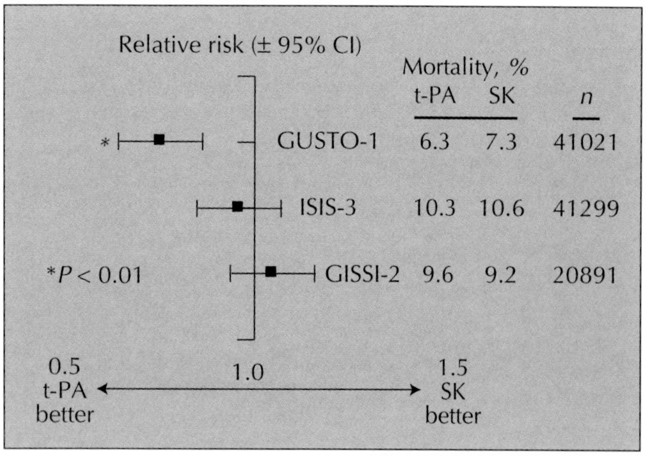

Figure 17-1. Comparative mortality data in acute myocardial infarction. SK—streptokinase; t-PA—tissue plasminogen activator.

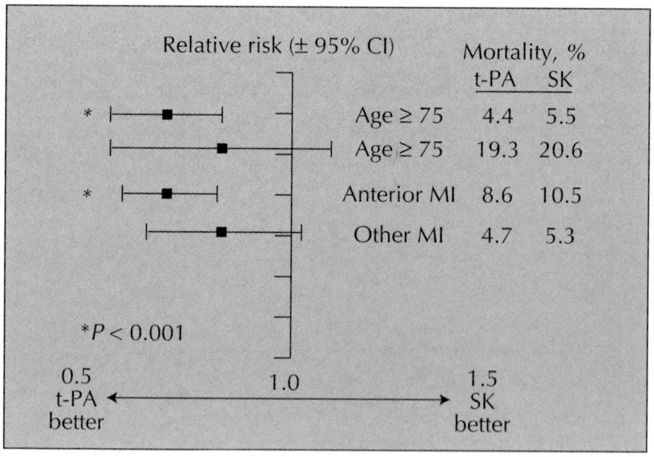

Figure 17-2. Differential effects of streptokinase (SK) and tissue plasminogen activator (t-PA) by patient variable in acute myocardial infarction (MI). Demonstrates subgroup analysis of the relative benefit (relative risk reduction with 95% CI bars) of the use of t-PA versus SK in different settings of acute MI from the GUSTO-1 trial.

In the MITI (Myocardial Infarction Triage and Intervention) trial [12••], patients treated within 70 minutes of their MI chest pain had a mortality of approximately 1% compared with 10% in those patients treated later.

The GUSTO-1 angiographic substudy gave significant insights into the mechanism of the reduction mortality among thrombolytic regimens. Although there was a higher TIMI (Thrombolysis In Myocardial Infarction) 3 flow rate in the 90-minute angiograms among patients receiving t-PA versus streptokinase, there was no significant difference in patency at the 180-minute post-thrombolysis angiogram. This lack of difference persisted throughout the remainder of the angiographic substudy time intervals and there was no difference in the reocclusion rates between the streptokinase/subcutaneous heparin or t-PA/intravenous heparin groups [13•].

Future Directions of Thrombolytic Regimens

Attempts to improve treatments for AMI are ongoing. Recently, the COMPASS (Comparative Trial of Saruplase versus Streptokinase) trial presented results of 3089 patients randomly assigned to saruplase or streptokinase [14]. The 30-day mortality rate was 5.7% in the saruplase-treated group versus 6.7% in the streptokinase-treated group ($P < 0.001$). The overall stroke rates were similar. The IMPACT-AMI (Integrelin to Minimize Platelet Aggregation and Prevent Coronary Thrombosis-Acute Myocardial Infarction) group studied a combination of the platelet glycoprotein IIB/IIIa receptor blocker Integrelin (Cor Therapeutics, San Francisco, CA) in combination with accelerated t-PA in patients with AMI [15]. The combination has been shown to have a dose-dependent effect on ex vivo platelet aggregation when measured by adenosine diphosphate and thrombin receptor–activating peptide (TRAP). A total of 106 patients were randomly assigned to either intravenous t-PA, heparin, and oral aspirin or the same regimen with the addition of intravenous Integrelin. The Integrelin infusion was continued for 24 hours and all patients were studied with 90-minute post-treatment angiograms. The bleeding rates were similar in the placebo versus the Integrelin patients (4% vs 5%) and blood transfusions were similar at 16% versus 18%. The TIMI grade 3 flow was 66% in the t-PA/Integrelin group versus 39% in the t-PA/placebo group ($P = 0.006$), indicating more effective thrombolysis when IIb/IIa inhibitor is added. Whether these beneficial effects can be achieved without increased bleeding risks await further studies such as PARADIGM (Platelet Aggregation Receptor Antagonist Dose Investigation for Reperfusion Gain in Myocardial Infarction), in which lamifiban, a IIb/IIa inhibitor, will be given with streptokinase or t-PA for AMI.

References and Recommended Reading

Recently published papers of particular interest have been highlighted as:
- • Of special interest
- •• Of outstanding interest

1. Vrstrate M, Collen D: Thrombolytic agents. In *Thrombosis in Cardiovascular Disorders.* Edited by Fuster V, Vrstrate M. Philadelphia: WB Saunders Co.; 1992:175–189.

2. Levine MN, Hirsh J, Salzman EW: Side effects of antithrombotic therapy. In *Hemostasis and Thrombosis, Basic Principles and Clinical Practice,* edn. 3. Edited by Coleman RW, Hirsh J, and Marder BJ, *et al.* Philadelphia: JB Lippincott Co.; 1994:936–955.

3. Zoldhelyi P, Fuster V, Chesebro JH: Antithrombins as conjunctive therapy in arterial thrombolysis. *Coronary Artery Disease* 1992, 3:1003–1009.

4. Johnson AJ, McCarthy WR: The lysis of artificially induced intravascular clots in man by intravenous infusions of streptokinases. *J Clin Invest* 1959, 38:1627–1643.

5. Neuhaus KL, vonEssen R, Tebbe U, *et al.*: Improved thrombolysis in acute myocardial infarction with front loaded administration of alteplase: results of the RT-PA-APSAC patency studies (TAPS). *J Am Coll Cardiol* 1992, 19:885–891.

6. GUSTO Investigators: The effects of tissue plasminogen activator, streptokinase or both on coronary artery patency, ventricular function, and survival after acute myocardial infarction. *N Engl J Med* 1993, 329:1615–1622.

7.• Fibrinolytic Therapy Trialists' (FTT) Collaborative Group: Indications for fibrinolytic therapy in suspected acute myocardial infarction: collaborative overview of early mortality in major morbidity results from all randomized trials of more than 1,000 patients. *Lancet* 343:311–322, 1994.

Summary of all major clinical trials of thrombolytic therapy showing the clear benefit for ST elevation infarct and lack of benefit in patients with no ST elevation myocardial infarction.

8. Gruppo Italiano per lo Studio della Sopravivenza nell'Infarto Miocardico (GISSI): GISSI-2: a factorial randomised trial of alteplase versus streptokinase and heparin versus no heparin among 12,490 patients with acute myocardial infarction. *Lancet* 1990, 336:65–71.

9. ISIS-3 (Third International Study of Infarct Survival Collaborative Group): ISIS-3: a randomised comparison of streptokinase vs tissue plasminogen activator vs anistreplase and of aspirin and heparin vs heparin alone among 41,299 cases of suspected acute myocardial infarction. *Lancet* 1992, 339:753–770.

10.•• The GUSTO Investigators: An international randomized trial comparing four thrombolytic strategies for acute myocardial infarction. *N Engl J Med* 1993, 329:673–682.

Direct comparison of t-PA and streptokinase for ST elevation myocardial infarction. There was a small but significantly increased survival rate in patients receiving t-PA with intravenous heparin.

11. Fuster V: Coronary thrombolysis: a prospective for the practicing physician. *N Engl J Med* 1993, 329:723–725.

12.•• Weaver WD, Cerqueira M, Hallstrom AP, *et al.* for the Myocardial Infarct Triage and Intervention and Project Group: Prehospital-initiated thrombolytic therapy. *JAMA* 1993, 270:1211–1216.

Excellent study showing remarkable reduction in mortality when patients were treated with thrombolysis very early after the onset of ST elevation

13.• The GUSTO Angiographic Investigators: The effects of tissue plasminogen activator, streptokinase, or both on coronary artery patency, ventricular function, and survival after acute myocardial infarction. *N Engl J Med* 1993, 329:1615–1622.

Trial showing that the mortality benefits with t-PA were directly related to the improved coronary arterial patency and blood flow down the coronary artery.

14. Tebbe U, Michels R, Adgey J, *et al.*: Thrombolysis with saruplase is at least as effective in acute MI as streptokinase: COMPASS double-blind study in 3,089 patients [abstract]. *JACC* 1996, 27(suppl A):166.

15. Ohman E, Kleiman NS, Gacioch G, *et al*: Simultaneous platelet glycoprotein IIb/IIIa integrin blockade and front-loaded tissue plasminogen activator in acute myocardial infarction: results from a randomized trial [abstract]. *J Am Coll Cardiol* 1996, 27(suppl A):167.

Chapter 18

THE CURRENT ROLE OF ANTITHROMBINS IN INTERVENTIONAL CARDIOLOGY

Jean-Paul R. Herrman
Patrick W. Serruys

Despite developments in technology and increased knowledge of mechanism of action and pathophysiology of intracoronary angioplasty procedures, the high initial success rates of percutaneous transluminal coronary angioplasties (PTCAs) remain hampered by early and late reocclusion [1]. The introduction of adjunctive devices in interventional cardiology has augmented indications for angioplasty in patients, which are expected to result in a higher complication rate. Several randomized pharmacologic multicenter trials have been designed to diminish the rate of reocclusion, but until now no benefit is detected from the variety of drugs tested.

It is evident that thrombin plays an unequivocal detrimental role in the vascular wall injury resulting from angioplasty procedures. Pharmacologic research currently concentrates on inhibition of prothrombin conversion and thrombus formation. Animal experimental work in this field is encouraging, and results of clinical trials will elucidate important questions about safety, efficacy, and immunoallergic potential of modern antithrombins.

THROMBIN

Thrombin is the most potent known platelet activator and interacts with a variety of immunomodulatory cells and hematologic factors. Its action includes a stimulation in the endothelial layer of platelet-derived growth factor production, prostacyclin secretion, platelet-activating factor, and plasminogen activator-inhibitor. In vivo, thrombin receptor expression was demonstrated by endothelial cells in intact vessel walls, macrophages, and vascular smooth muscle cells in atherosclerotic lesions and in endarterectomy specimens [2]. Selectin formation at the endothelial cell surface is stimulated by thrombin and plays a role in the incursion of monocytes and neutrophils to an injured vessel wall. In addition to this, thrombin has a direct chemotactic effect on monocytes [3], and has apparent mitogenic effects on lymphocytes [4] and vascular smooth muscle cells [5] (Fig. 18-1).

The transmembrane thrombin receptor exposes an amino terminal extension that bares two thrombin binding sites: the thrombin cleavage site and a hirudin-like domain [6]. The identification of the thrombin receptor has enabled sophisticated designs of molecules that fit exactly into those sites. In case of deep endothelial injury (as with a successful angioplasty), blood is exposed to collagen and other substances of the subintima, which are potent stimuli for platelet aggregation mediated by the release of adenosine diphosphate (ADP); serotonin; thromboxane A_2 (TXA_2); and the adhesive molecules fibrinogen, fibronectin, thrombospondin, and von Willebrand factor. These substances, including thrombin, activate neighboring platelets by way of different metabolic pathways (TXA_2, ADP, and a platelet-activating factor) and promote intramural thrombus formation, which could cause restenosis [7]. In addition, several growth factors, important ingredients of the platelet granulae, are released during activation. Receptors for these factors are expressed in mesenchymal cells such as the smooth muscle cells and play a prominent role in late restenosis.

Limitations of Available Antithrombotic Drugs

Currently, substantial research is focused on the antithrombotic and antithrombin approach. Until now, no major breakthrough has been reported [8,9], although a clear progression in the understanding and interfering of the mechanism has occurred. The limitations of several antithrombin agents have been determined. Warfarin's action does not block thrombin's extrinsic pathway but does hinder the action of several commonly used drugs. Another weakness of warfarin is the delay between administration and therapeutic effect, as is the case with ticlopidine.

Aspirin has the ability to inhibit platelet TXA_2 synthetase and subsequent platelet activation by irreversibly blocking the enzyme cyclooxygenase that is responsible for the conversion of arachidonic acid to prostaglandin G_2 (PGG_2). This intermediate prostaglandin can be transformed in the metabolic pathway to TXA_2 and thromboxane B_2. Aspirin results in a decreased production of this substance in platelets. It also results in cyclooxygenase blockade in the endothelial cell [10], which is responsible for the conversion of arachidonic acid to prostaglandin I_2 (PGI_2). TXA_2 is a powerful platelet aggregator and vasoconstrictor, but because the biologic actions of TXA_2 and PGI_2 are opposing, acetylsalicylic acid is an antagonist of itself. In addition, it only partially inhibits platelet aggregation induced by ADP, serotonin, epinephrine, collagen, or thrombin.

The effectiveness of heparin is limited in patients having insufficient antithrombin III levels. Another major issue is the limited ability of the large heparin–antithrombin III complex to gain access to clot-bound thrombin or factor Xa in the prothrombinase complex. Furthermore, heparin action is inhibited by fibrin II monomers, thrombospondin, and platelet

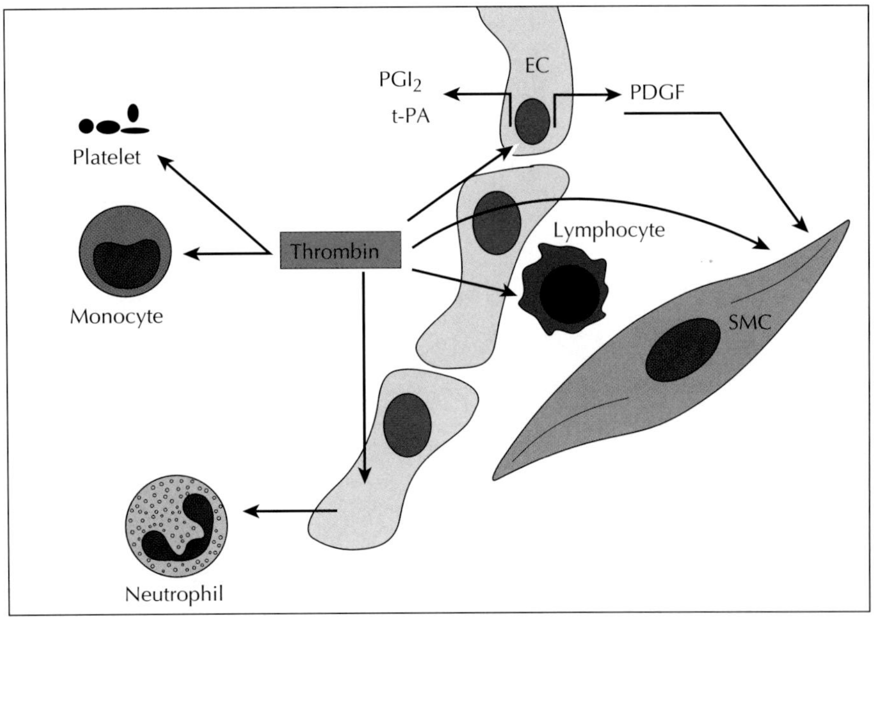

Figure 18-1. The central role of thrombin in platelet aggregation and activation, chemotaxis, and mitogenesis for immunomodulatory and mesenchmyal cells, including vascular endothelial cells. EC—endothelial cell; PDGF—platelet derived growth factor; PGI_2—prostaglandin I_2; SMC—smooth muscle cell; t-PA—tissue plasminogen activator.

factor 4, which is present in the platelet-rich thrombus. The dose-effect response is poor and relatively unpredictable.

The action of low-molecular-weight heparin (LMWH) in factor X inhibition is hampered by the limited ability of the antithrombin III–LMWH complex to block phospholipid membrane-bound factor Xa; also, LMWH shares the limitations of heparin in gaining access to clot-bound thrombin and in functioning effectively under conditions of insufficient antithrombin levels. As is true of heparin, LMWH is a widely varied mixture of sizes of depolymerized heparin molecules and therefore is subject to variety in effectiveness from lot to lot. Both heparin and LMWH have effects on platelets that may manifest as thrombocytopenia.

The potential advantages of specific antithrombins lie in the fact that they overcome the limitations of conventional treatment. The ideal antithrombin drug is a small-sized molecule, able to penetrate the thrombotic material. It is synthetic and therefore has no natural inhibitors, does not need any cofactor, and does not express any antigenic properties. The dose-response relation is predictable. An important support to the success of such a drug is the development of local drug delivery systems, enabling the interventional cardiologist to block thrombin's action entirely at exactly the right spot, not affecting systemic hemostasis levels.

Animal Experimental Work and Human Studies

Heparins

Heparin is currently the most widely used anticoagulant drug in the management of acute thrombotic syndromes. It is a heterogeneous mixture of glycosaminoglycans with a molecular weight ranging from 2000 to 40,000 daltons. The antithrombotic capacities are achieved by the reversible binding with the natural circulating anticoagulant antithrombin III. The binding is responsible for a 1000-fold acceleration of antithrombin III–heparin binding to factor IIa. This complex also involves activated coagulation proteins (factors X, IX, XI, and XII).

Heparin and its low-molecular-weight derivatives have been shown to reduce smooth muscle cell proliferation [11], inhibit smooth muscle cell migration [11], and decrease the number of cells transformed from a contractile to a synthetic phenotype [12]. The antiproliferative actions of the heparins appear not to be related to anticoagulant properties because particular heparin subfractions retain their antiproliferative effects despite their lack of anticoagulant properties. Smooth muscle cell–bound heparin can be internalized, affecting the cell cycle with a consequent reduction in DNA and RNA synthesis by mechanisms unrelated to oncogene expression [13]. The effect on restenosis of various heparin doses and administration schedules has been investigated using regular heparin samples [14–17]. So far, no beneficial influence on the restenosis rate has been detected. Synthetic heparins and LMWH fractions, lacking the heterogeneous nature, are now the subject of research [18–22]. The clinically used LMWH mixtures diverge in molecular weight from 1 to 10 kD. Where heparin operates as a template to link thrombin and antithrombin III, the heparins with a molecular weight of less than 5400 daltons are too small to bind these proteins synchronously, but nonetheless are able to accomplish the binding of antithrombin to activated factor Xa. Inhibition of this central protease results in reduced thrombin generation. In animal experiments using LMWH, significant effects were detected on intimal hypertrophy or diameter reduction [23–25]. Heras and colleagues [26] analyzed the inhibition of thrombus formation using four doses (100, 200, 400, and 500 U/kg) of LMWH (CY 216) in comparison with unfractionated heparin (100 U/kg) and placebo in deep carotid artery injury in pigs. Examination of the treated vessels after 1 hour showed platelet deposition of 22, 29, 9, 9, 11, and 42 $\times$ $10^6/cm^2$. For fibrinogen deposition, the numbers in the groups were 19, 19, 21, 14, 12 ($P < 0.05$), and 35 molecules $\times$ $10^{12}/cm^2$. Thus, the predominantly anti–factor X activity does not clearly inhibit the deposition of thrombotic material after deep arterial injury, when compared to unfractionated heparin.

A group in Tübingen [27] reported the results of 400 anti-Xa units/kg/day administration in 55 rabbits who underwent balloon angioplasty of an electrically induced lesion of the carotid artery. The LMWH (LU 47311, mean molecular weight 3.9 kD) was subcutaneously given from day 1 to day 7 after intervention. Observation period was 3, 7, 14, and 28 days. At the end of the study period, intimal wall thickness in the LMWH-treated rabbits increased from 13 (preangioplasty control group) to 20 cell layers in the treated animals ($P < 0.05$ vs nonangioplasty control group) and from 13 to 35 cell layers in controls ($P < 0.01$ vs nonangioplasty control group). The proliferative response of smooth muscle cells was evaluated by quantification of cells undergoing DNA synthesis. In controls, this showed an increase in S-phase cells in the intima from 0.7% cells before dilatation to 10.2% and 7.7% 3 and 7 days after angioplasty. A mild increase in DNA synthesizing cells was observed in the treatment group (2.7% at 3 days, $P < 0.01$, and 1.9% at 7 days, $P < 0.01$). Normalization of proliferation 14 and 28 days after dilatation occurred in both groups.

Other Factor Xa Inhibitors

Antistasin (r-ATS) is a 15-kD peptide isolated from the salivary glands of the Mexican leech [28]. It is a tight-binding and specific long-acting factor Xa inhibitor. It has been studied in a variety of thrombosis models and found superior to heparin in preventing platelet-rich thrombi in dacron-grafted arteriovenous femoral grafts [29] and as an adjunct to alteplase in a canine model of femoral arterial thrombosis [30]. It was found as effective as heparin in suppressing fibrinopeptide A (FPA) levels in a rhesus monkey disseminated intravascular coagulation model [31]. Because of the apparently strong immunogenicity of antistasin, however, further clinical development in its current configuration is unlikely [32•].

Tick anticoagulant peptide (TAP), is a short-acting inhibitor of factor Xa, originally isolated from the soft tick *Ornithodoros moubata* [33]. Both r-ATS and TAP were tested in New Zealand rabbits during balloon angioplasty, followed by 2 hours of infusion [34]. The reduction in luminal diameter as measured at 28-day follow-up angiography was significantly less in the r-ATS and TAP groups compared to the control group, which received heparin (-0.17 ± 0.11 mm, -0.26 ± 0.22 mm, vs 0.66 ± 0.58 mm, $P \leq 0.02$).

Hirudin

Hirudin is a specific and direct thrombin blocker. This anticoagulant drug is originally extracted from the salivary gland of the leech (*Hirudo medicinalis*). It is a 7-kD protein, composed of 65 amino acids. Thrombin has an active site pocket that can be blocked by the N-terminal three amino acids of hirudin, whereas hirudin's carboxyl tail forms several ionic and hydrophobic complexes with the fibrinogen anion-binding site, thus blocking thrombin-catalyzed fibrinogen cleavage. The fortitude of hirudin in comparison to other serine protease inhibitors is in its potency to block thrombin instantaneously and irreversibly at multiple sites [35] without the need for circulating antithrombin III. Hirudin, because of its small volume, is able to inhibit thrombin tied to thrombus and to restrict further thrombus formation also where the thrombin is clot bound or when thrombolysis takes place [36]. The recombinant configuration differs from the native hirudin by the absence of a sulfate group in the Tyr-63 position [37]. For this reason, the recombinant variant is also called desulfatohirudin or desirudin. The terminal half-life of desirudin in healthy, young volunteers is 50 to 65 minutes [38], with a half-life of its effect on the activated partial thromboplastin time (aPTT) of about 2 hours [39,40]. There is no specific antidote available for reversing the effects of hirudin.

The effects of recombinant hirudin on the restenosing process after balloon-caused arterial injury are intensively studied in animal models. A significantly reduced platelet deposition to only one single layer was found using high-dose hirudin (1.0 mg/kg bolus plus intravenous infusion for 1 hour) [41], and a significantly inhibited restenosis response as assessed by quantitative angiography and quantitative histopathology [42] was found after hirudin administration. The group of Buchwald and colleagues [43] observed the significant effect of hirudin on platelet accumulation and fibrin deposition in stented minipigs. The effect of recombinant hirudin was evaluated in patients undergoing angioplasty for stable angina pectoris in a multicenter, double-blind pilot study [44]. A total of 113 patients were randomized in a 2:1 fashion, receiving either 20 mg hirudin before angioplasty followed by a 24-hour infusion of 0.16 mg/kg/h, or 10,000 IU of heparin followed by a 12 IU/kg/h infusion for 24 hours. At the end of this infusion period, angiography was performed to assess vessel patency and to obtain quantitative measurements. Coagulation parameters were frequently measured. In the heparin-treated group (39 patients), 4 patients experienced a periprocedural myocardial infarction (MI) or emergency coronary artery bypass graft (CABG), compared to only one emergency CABG and one elective CABG 3 weeks after PTCA in the hirudin-allocated group (74 patients). Hemorrhage at the arterial puncture site was seen in four hirudin-treated patients, for which they needed blood transfusion, whereas in the heparin-allocated group one patient experienced visual impairment because of a cerebral infarction. Follow-up angiography at 24 hours revealed a complete perfusion in all the patients from the hirudin-treated group, compared to 92% in the heparin-treated group. Visual assessment furthermore showed one case of intracoronary thrombus in each group. Concentrations of prothrombin fragment 1 and 2 (F_{1+2}) appeared to be somewhat higher in the hirudin group directly and 6 hours after angioplasty (a median of 1.015 vs 0.795 nmol/L and 0.95 vs 0.8 nmol/L), indicating a slightly diminished thrombin inactivation. It was concluded that safety and tolerance for hirudin is similar to that for heparin [44,45], and it can be administered in patients undergoing balloon angioplasty for stable angina pectoris. This study surveyed only the short-term effects of thrombin antagonism, but it was followed by a multicenter, randomized, double-blind, heparin-controlled study, aimed at the prevention of restenosis [46•].

Reports on clinical trials in the setting of acute myocardial infarction (AMI) (thrombolytics and concomitant aspirin) suggest a narrower safety window with recombinant hirudin than initially anticipated. Extremely high rates of intracranial bleeding were encountered with streptokinase in GUSTO-IIA (Global Utilization of Strategies to Open Occluded Coronary Arteries) (with heparin 2.7% and with hirudin 3.2%) [47], or with alteplase in TIMI 9A (Thrombolysis in Myocardial Infarction) (with heparin 1.9% and with hirudin 1.7%) [48], and HIT-III (r[recombinant]Hirudin for Improvement of Thrombolysis) (none with heparin and with hirudin 3.4%) [49]. A baseline creatinine of greater than 1.5 mg/dL, older age, lower body weight, and higher aPTT levels (100 vs 86 seconds in nonstroke patients) were associated with bleeding in desirudin-treated patients.

Hirudin-Derived Drugs

The N-terminal three amino acids of hirudin block the thrombin active site pocket, while the C-terminal site form complexes with the fibrinogen anion-binding site, thus blocking thrombin-catalyzed fibrinogen cleavage. Structure of the latter peptide domain is mimicked in the synthetic peptide hirugen (Fig. 18-2), the potency of which is about 50 times less in comparison with the activity of hirudin. The antithrombin activity of this dodecapeptide is solely due to the blockade of the fibrinogenolytic site and therefore especially valuable in preventing fibrin-dependent thrombosis [50].

X-ray crystallographic analysis enables assembling of highly specific compounds especially designed to inhibit thrombin. Extremely detailed three-dimensional reconstruction of the amino-binding and carboxyl-binding groups has enabled complex technology to link an inhibitor of the active site pocket (D-Phe-Pro-Arg-Pro) to hirugen with optimal positions (at distances of 20 Å) of both of the binding sequences opposite to their target molecules [51]. This drug called hirulog (*see* Fig. 18-2) has been administered safely to healthy human volunteers [52]. Hirulog induces a dose-dependent prolongation of all coagulation parameters, with a half-life of 40 minutes [53]. A dose-escalating multicenter study [54] evaluated this drug in the setting of intracoronary interventions. In the latter, 291 patients received a bolus dose of 0.15, 0.25, 0.35, 0.45, or 0.55 mg/kg (group 1 to 5 encompassing 54, 53, 44, 74, and 54 patients), followed by a 4-hour infusion of 0.60, 1.00, 1.40, 1.80, or 2.20 mg/kg/h. All patients were concomitantly pretreated with 325 mg aspirin. A rapid onset and dose-dependent increase in aPTT and activated coagulation time values at doses of 1.80 and 2.20 mg/kg/h resulted in a sufficient anticoagulant state and reduced abrupt vessel closure within the first 24 hours of the start of the procedure to less than 4% (5 out of 128 patients) versus 11.3% (17 vessels closed in 151 treated patients) in the other three treatment groups. In this study, there was no control group treated with conventional anticoagulant drugs, but the results encouraged a double-blind, randomized clinical trial [55•].

Synthetic Thrombin Inhibitors

PPACK is the abbreviation of D-phenylanalyl-L-prolyl-L-arginyl-chloromethyl ketone. This peptide sequence binds to the active site of thrombin. The effect of this substance, in combination and in comparison with 7E3,

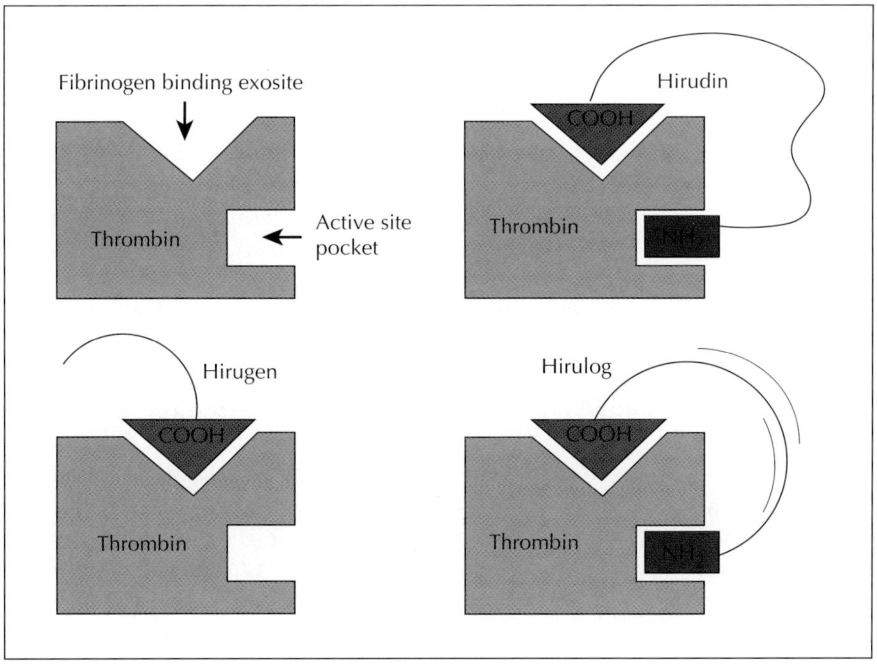

Figure 18-2. Schematic presentation of thrombin inhibition by hirudin, hirugen, and hirulog. COOH—carboxyl group; NH_2—amino group.

on platelet deposition was tested at the site of balloon angioplasty in an ex vivo whole artery perfusion model [56]. Perfusion of the arterial segments with PPACK (10^{-5} M) reduced platelet deposition for 47% (n = 4, P<0.04) with the use of this new antithrombin agent compared with the heparin model (2 U/mL).

Argatroban ((2R,4R)-4-methyl-1-[N^2-((3-methyl-1,2,3,4-tetrahydro-8-quinolonyl)sulfonyl)-arginyl]-2-piperidine carboxylic acid) is an arginine derivative that binds competitively to thrombin [57]. It is shown in animal experimental work that argatroban can prevent coronary thrombosis more effectively than heparin in models of coronary thrombolysis and vessel wall injury [58,59]. This highly specific thrombin inhibitor was infused during 4 hours in patients with unstable angina pectoris [60]. Infusion of the drug (0.5 to 5.0 µg/kg/min) increased the aPTT in a dose-related fashion and was effective against recurrence of ischemic episodes, but remarkably 9 of the 43 patients experienced an episode of unstable angina shortly after termination of the drug. These patients in whom angina reoccurred received significantly higher doses of argatroban during infusion (P = 0.007) and greater elongation of the aPTT (52 ± 12 seconds in the nonangina group vs 66 ± 15 in the nine patients with angina within 24 hours). The authors describe this phenomenon as a rebound effect.

Fitzgerald (not published) treated 12 angioplasty patients, randomizing them either to a bolus of 30 µg/kg argatroban, followed by an intravenous infusion of 2 µg/kg/min during 2 hours, or to a bolus injection of 10,000 IU of heparin plus a 4-hour infusion of 1000 IU/h. These results initiated the so-called pre-Argaplasty trial, a dose verification study, assessing safety and feasibility in patients undergoing balloon angioplasty for either stable or unstable angina. A total of 30 patients were included at four dose levels, the highest being an intravenous bolus injection of 250 µg/kg, followed by a 4-hour infusion of 15 µg/kg/min. At 4 hours, the infusion rate was lowered to 3.8 µg/kg/min and continued for 68 hours. At this level, aPTT was approximately two times normal value, and the sheath was removed without infusion adjustment. Hemostatic, clinical, and angiographic data indicate that argatroban infusion in coronary angioplasty patients can be administered safely and results in an adequate, predictable level of anticoagulation. The clear correlation between plasma levels and anticoagulant effect is demonstrated in Figure 18-3.

New antithrombins under development are aptamers (synthetic oligonucleotides that, similar to hirugen, bind only to the exosite of thrombin [61]). Among those low-weight thrombin inhibitors are SDZ-217766 [62] and RWJ-27755, which binds to only the catalytic site of thrombin [63,64]. The alkylating properties of the latter compound have, however, considerably tempered the enthusiasm for its clinical development [32•]. DUP-714 is a boroarginine tripeptide [65]; its anticipated potential for oral administration has not yet resulted in human studies [32].

Other antithrombins still in development are the thrombin receptor antagonist peptides [66] and the hirudisins—hirudin derivatives combining IIb/IIIa receptor and thrombin inhibition. In the hirudisins, residues from 32 to 35 of hirudin have been replaced by the integrin motif RGDS and KGDS [67]. In addition to inhibiting glycoprotein (GP) IIb/IIIa receptor-dependent platelet interactions, the platelet-binding integrin motif is expected to target the antithrombin action of hirudin to platelets, possibly allowing lower and safer doses of hirudin in the treatment of thrombotic disease [68].

Experimental and Clinical Application of Locally Delivered Antithrombin Into the Vessel Wall

Many reasons for the discrepancy between results from animal models and human trials have been proposed. One explanation has been that doses used in the animal studies were in most instances at least an order of magnitude higher than the highest tolerable doses in humans. It has also been suggested that difficulties in the sustained administration of certain compounds in humans for adequate periods of time to achieve measurable effects may have accounted for the failure of many of the pharmacologic therapies. Finally, the prevention of restenosis judged by histologic measurements in animal models may not translate to angiographic changes in humans [69]. In response to these limitations, the idea of local drug delivery techniques for the administration of pharmacologic compounds at the site of coronary interventions has evolved [70]. Conceptually, local delivery techniques allow for high site-specific concentrations of therapeutic compounds without the complication of systemic side effects.

Administration of heparin using a porous balloon catheter was first accomplished by Wolinsky and Thung [70]. Using catheter-based percutaneous transluminal administration, high concentrations of fluoresceinated heparin within the media could be detected up to 48 hours after infusion. It has been shown that locally delivered heparin can reduce the thrombogenicity of the vessel wall in the acutely injured pig carotid artery model [71]. Site-specific administration of PPACK by way of a porous balloon catheter in an ex vivo model of arterial damage has been shown to reduce platelet deposition at the site of balloon injury [72]. In addition, Nunes and associates [73] have demonstrated decreased platelet deposition on dacron grafts after local treatment with PPACK. Dispensed from a hydrogel-coated angioplasty balloon, PPACK showed considerable local effects without causing a prolongation of the coagulation parameters [73]. A similar reduction in platelet deposition was shown after the local administration of the thrombin inhibitor r-hirudin in a porcine carotid artery model of vascular injury [74]. Using a double-balloon perfusion catheter, high local concentrations of r-hirudin were maintained for 60 minutes without the device causing additional vascular injury.

Since the initial reports of the effectiveness of locally administered heparin [75] and LMWH [76,77] to inhibition of smooth muscle cell proliferation, initial results of long-term studies using site-specific administration of many different drug classes are encouraging. The steady advances made toward the development of clinically applicable atraumatic delivery modalities have allowed the transition from the animal laboratory to human applications.

Preliminary data indicate the technique to be safe for use in human coronary arteries, at diverse anatomic sites [78]. The feasibility of local drug delivery using the Dispatch delivery catheter, a nondilatational infusion-perfusion catheter, has been evaluated in humans [79]. Successful local delivery of heparin in humans was demonstrated for the first time using this device. A delivery efficacy of 1% to 8% with a retention time

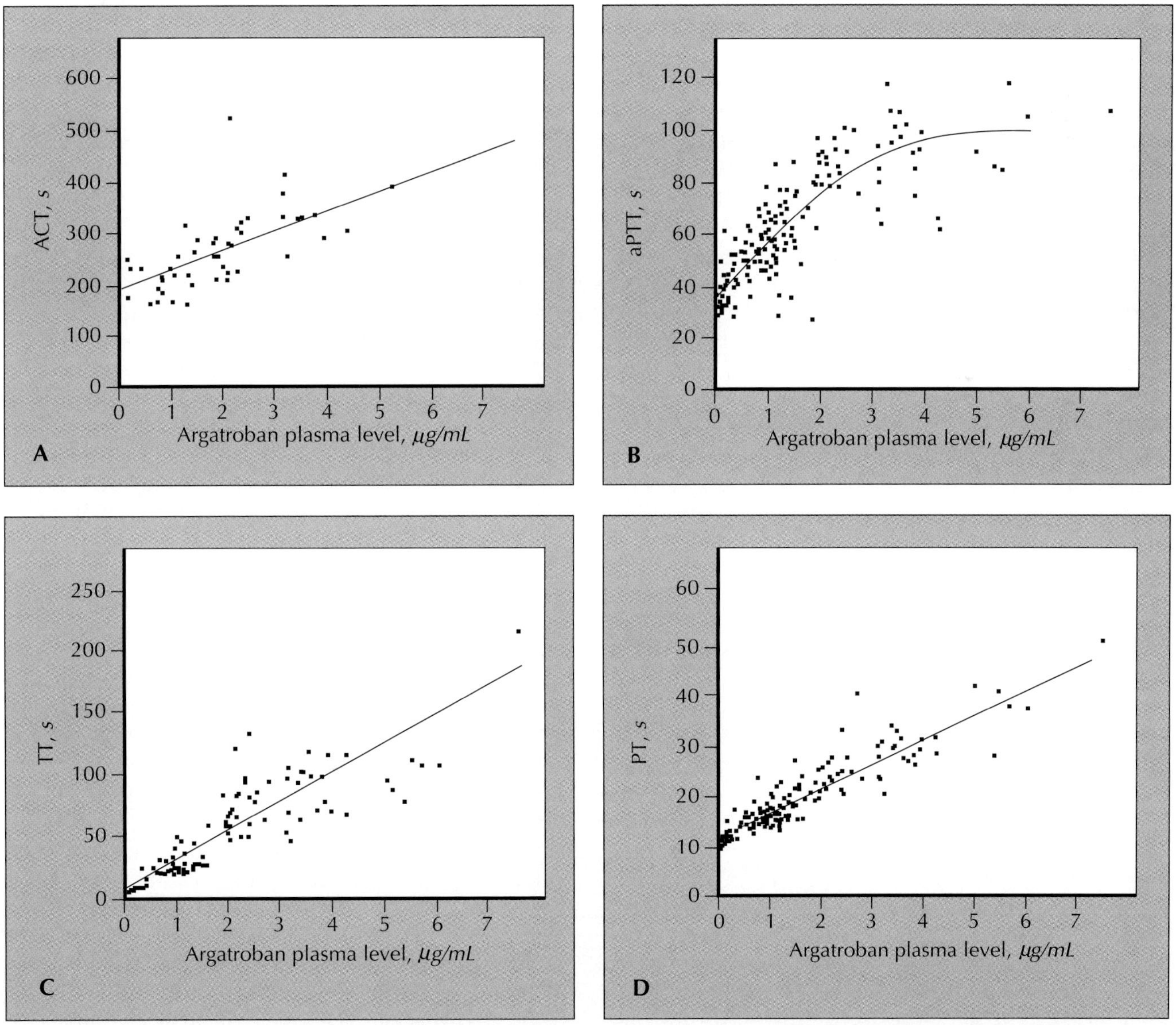

Figure 18-3. A–B, The relationship between argatroban plasma level and the result of coagulation tests. ACT—activated clotting time; aPTT—activated partial thromboplastin time; PT—prothrombin time; TT—thrombin time.

up to 14 hours was shown [80]. Preliminary long-term results of the initial patients treated with locally administered heparin at the time of angioplasty using this device are encouraging, showing a reduction in the need for re-intervention and in the degree of angiographically defined restenosis [79,81–83]. Definitive long-term results are forthcoming.

A group in Tübingen delivered 1500 anti-Xa units LMWH reviparin locally using a porous balloon, besides 24 hours intravenous and 28 days subcutaneous administration of the compound [84]. No major complication occurred during the 28-day follow-up period in the 15 treated patients. Data on restenosis will be available shortly.

With the increased use of percutaneously introduced stents for the treatment of primary and recurrent coronary stenosis, the possibility of using coated or eluting stents as local drug delivery devices is currently being tested. There have been two reports of reduction of subacute stent thrombosis in the rabbit carotid [85], and in stented pig coronary arteries [86] using heparin-coated stents. The pilot study of the BENESTENT II (Belgium Netherlands Stent Trial) has shown that deployment of the Palmaz-Schatz heparin-coated stent was possible with a reduced anticoagulation regimen [87]. Furthermore, the long-term results seem encouraging with an expected restenosis rate lower than those reported in BENESTENT I (13% in the BENESTENT II pilot study compared with 20% in the BENESTENT I) [88••,89]. The dilemma that the inflammatory response of the coating can exceed the beneficial effect of the eluted material is an obstacle that must be overcome [90].

Phase III Restenosis Prevention Studies

The ERA (Enoxaparin Restenosis) trial [91] conducted a study comparing enoxaparin (40 mg every day subcutaneously) to placebo, administered for 28 days, starting within 2 hours of the sheath removal in the prevention of restenosis. A total of 459 patients were enrolled and 86% completed the study protocol, including angiographic follow-up. Treatment comparison resulted in an insignificant difference between the two groups (51% restenosis in the placebo group vs 52% in the treated group, odds ratio [OR] 1.07, $P = 0.63$). Analysis of demographic data and the use of other angiographic restenosis definitions could not reveal any difference in the two groups.

The REDUCE (Restenosis prevention after PTCA, Early administration of LMWH (LU 47-311), Double-blind, Unfractionated heparin and placebo-Controlled Evaluation) study is a double-blind, randomized multicenter trial comparing standard therapy (10,000 IU intravenous bolus unfractionated heparin before PTCA, followed by 24,000 IU over 16 ± 4 hours and placebo subcutaneously twice a day for a further 4 weeks, beginning the evening after angioplasty) with a high-dose regimen of reviparin (7000 IU intravenous bolus before PTCA, followed by 10,500 IU over 16 ± 4 hours, and 3500 subcutaneously twice a day for a further 4 weeks, beginning the evening after angioplasty) in patients undergoing angioplasty for a single de novo lesion. Concomitant aspirin was given. A total of 612 patients were recruited, of whom 306 patients received reviparin. The primary clinical endpoint was the event-free (freedom from death, nonfatal MI, and revascularization) survival within 30 weeks following angioplasty. The primary angiographic endpoint was defined in terms of absolute loss in minimal lumen diameter at the dilated site. Restenosis was defined as loss of more than 50% of the initial gain of PTCA, according to the National Heart Lung Blood Institute (NHLBI) IV definition. Long-term clinical outcome was similar in both treatment groups (33.3% in the reviparin-treated patients, 32.0% in the control group [relative risk (RR) 1.04, 95% CI 0.83 to 1.31, $P = 0.71$]). The absolute loss in lumen diameter was 0.29 and 0.25 mm (analysis of covariance $P = 0.59$). The incidence of bleeding occurred with a similar frequency in the two treatment groups (2.3% in the reviparin group and 2.6% in the heparin control group [RR 0.88, 95% CI 0.32 to 2.41, $P = 0.8$]); however acute events within 24 hours occurred in 3.9% of the reviparin group and in 8.2% of the control group (RR 0.49, 95% CI 0.26 to 0.92, $P = 0.027$) [92]. The authors suggest that the lack of effect in this trial may be due to insufficient local drug concentrations, which might be resolved by local drug delivery techniques, or that the lack in effect in primates [93] might reflect the presence of a heparin-insensitive pathway of smooth muscle cell activation.

The HELVETICA (Hirudin in a European Trial versus Heparin in the Prevention of Restenosis after percutaneous transluminal coronary angiography [PTCA]) trial is a multicenter, double-blind, randomized heparin-controlled study evaluating the clinical efficacy and safety of two hirudin dose regimens in 1154 angioplasty patients [46•]. The primary endpoint was event-free survival 30 weeks after angioplasty. Patients received one of the following treatments: unfractionated heparin (an intravenous bolus injection of 10,000 IU of heparin followed by a continuous intravenous infusion of 15 IU/kg/h of heparin for 24 hours, with placebo given subcutaneously twice daily for 3 consecutive days), intravenous hirudin (an intravenous bolus injection of 40 mg of hirudin followed by a continuous intravenous infusion of 0.2 mg/kg/h hirudin for 24 hours, with placebo given subcutaneously twice a day for 3 consecutive days), or intravenous and subcutaneous hirudin (an intravenous bolus injection of 40 mg of hirudin followed by a continuous intravenous infusion of 0.2 mg/kg/h of hirudin for 24 hours, with 40 mg of hirudin given subcutaneously twice a day for 3 consecutive days). A concomitant dose of aspirin (100 to 500 mg once daily) was given on the day of angioplasty and continued for at least 14 days. To provoke a more distinct outcome, this study included only patients suffering unstable angina because this group of patients is known to have higher restenosis rates [94–96].

The study population was not only limited to balloon angioplasty patients, but also techniques, as laser, directional, and rotational atherectomy were allowed per protocol. Because at the time of design of this trial the anticoagulant drug strategies following stenting were strict and subject to investigation, elective stent implantation was not allowed, and bail-out stenting resulted in discontinuation of the study drug. The event-free survival curve did not demonstrate differences among the treatment groups (Kruskal-Wallis test, $P = 0.61$). Early events (those in the first 96 hours after angioplasty) occurred in 7.9%, 5.6%, and 11.0% in the hirudin intravenous and subcutaneous, the hirudin intravenous and the heparin group (relative risk of hirudin vs heparin 0.37, 95% CI 0.19 to 0.70 $P = 0.007$). The incidence of clinical events and angina at 30 weeks was not significantly different in the three groups ($P = 0.61$). An angiographic follow-up in 86.4% of the population was available and demonstrated an equal distribution of angiographic baseline and postangioplasty parameters as well as the loss in lumen diameter at follow-up. In patients receiving heparin pretreatment, early outcome was significantly superior in the hirudin-treated patients (combined relative risk with hirudin 0.37, 95% CI 0.19 to 0.70, $P = 0.0016$). Because these results suggested a particular benefit of hirudin in the most unstable patients (Braunwald class III), an additional analysis was performed in 236 patients with angina at rest in the 48 hours before randomization. The event rate in this subgroup of patients was 21.6% in the heparin group versus 5.3% and 12.3% in the hirudin intravenous and hirudin intravenous and subcutaneous groups (combined relative risk with hirudin 0.41, 95% CI 0.21 to 0.78, $P = 0.006$). The event-free 7-month survival in the heparin-pretreated or Braunwald class III subgroup of patients demonstrated no effect over the long-term (Fig. 18-4).

The results of prothrombin fragment one and two assays immediately after angioplasty suggest that the thrombin generation in both hirudin groups was unsatisfactorily inhibited, whereas the dosage of heparin used in this trial resulted in an appropriate decrease of prothrombin fragment one and two at 6 hours after the intracoronary intervention. The authors suggest that the adjustment in infusion rate from 0.16 mg/kg/h in the pilot study [44] with stable patients to 0.20 mg/kg/h in the current trial of unstable patients with presumably higher levels of thrombin generation was a too cautious change in dosage. Zoldhelyi and

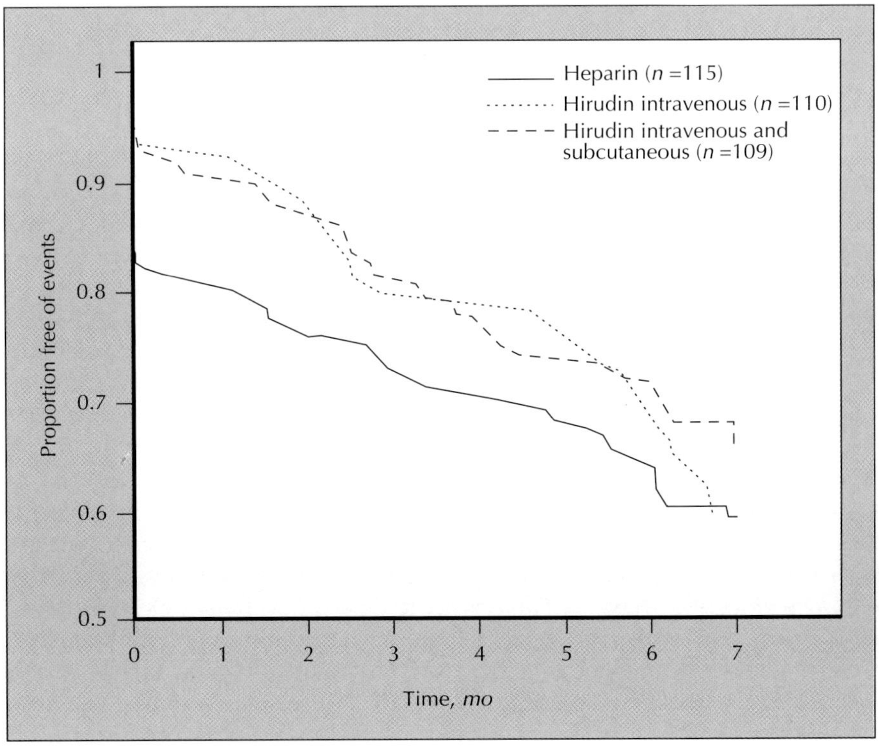

Figure 18-4. Event-free distribution (Kaplan Meier) in the intention-to-treat population of the patients receiving heparin treatment at the time of randomization ($n = 324$). At 4 days there is a remarkable beneficial effect in the hirudin-treated patients (relative risk of hirudin vs heparin 0.37, 95% CI 0.19–0.70, $P = 0.007$). Comparison of the treatment groups at 7 months by the Kruskal-Wallis test reveals a nonsignificant effect ($P = 0.61$).

colleagues [97] reported the failure to block thrombin generation in patients, despite a 10,000-fold molar excess of free hirudin over thrombin-hirudin complex. Infusion rates of hirudin in animal experiments were up to five times higher than those currently used, and this might explain the lack of long-term effect in the present study [41,42].

Another putative explanation for the apparent paradox in improved early outcome despite less appropriate thrombin control might be that the dosage used was insufficient to reach an adequate level of anticoagulation but sufficient to limit thrombin-mediated platelet aggregation and activation, thereby exhibiting effects similar to those observed acutely in the EPIC (Evaluation of c7E3 for the Prevention of Ischemic Complications) trial [98•,99].

In the hirulog angioplasty study [55•], 4312 patients suffering from unstable or postinfarction angina pectoris and scheduled for angioplasty were assigned to receive a body weight–adjusted dosage regimen of either heparin or hirulog and concomitant aspirin (300 to 325 mg). The heparin-allocated patients (n = 2039) received a bolus dose of 175 IU/kg followed by an 18- to 24-hour infusion at a rate of 15 IU/kg/h. Hirulog-treated patients (2059 in total) were given a bolus dose of 1.0 mg/kg, followed by a 4-hour infusion at a rate of 2.5 mg/kg/h and a 14- to 20-hour infusion at a rate of 0.2 mg/kg. Primary endpoint was the in-hospital occurrence of death; MI; abrupt vessel closure; or need for CABG, intra-aortic balloon counterpulsation, or repeat coronary angioplasty. Bivalirudin compared with heparin treatment was not able to lower the incidence of in-hospital cardiac events in the cohort of 4098 treated patients (11.4% vs 12.2%, OR 0.9, 95% CI 0.8 to 1.1, P = 0.44); however, results were positive in the subgroup of patients with postinfarction angina (9.1% vs 14.2%, OR 0.6, 95% CI 0.4 to 0.9, P = 0.04). At 6 months follow-up, the cumulative incidence of cardiac events was similar in the two treatment groups (25.7% vs 26.6%, OR 1.0, 95% CI 0.8 to 1.1, P = 0.54). There was no control angiography included in this study. The level of clinical restenosis, as measured by the incidence of any complication after discharge, was also similar in the two treatment groups (21.0% vs 21.3% OR 1.0, 95% CI not reported, P = 0.85). The incidence of bleeding in the bivalirudin-treated patients was significantly lower as compared to the heparin control subjects (3.8% vs 9.8%, OR 0.4, 95% CI 0.3 to 0.5, $P < 0.001$). The latter was reflected by the lower levels of systemic anticoagulation in the bivalirudin-treated group, as assessed by the measurement of activated clotting times. The authors raise the probability that equivalent rates of ischemic complications may be the result of equivalent degrees of localized thrombin inhibition achieved at lower levels of systemic anticoagulation as reflected by the markedly lower incidence of bleeding. This raised the question whether the preference for the chosen dosage regimen was too low. Supporting arguments for that were a significantly lower activated clotting time just before the coronary intervention in the hirulog-treated patients, and thus conclusions of the hirulog study are based on nonequivalent anticoagulant doses. Because of the different properties of bivalirudin, however, in particular the activity against clot-bound thrombin, absence of natural inhibitors, and more predictable and less variable levels of anticoagulation, it was not a goal to achieve identical activated clotting times with the two agents. Moreover, a recent publication describes the absence of association between major bleeding and activated clotting times [100]. The experiences in both the hirulog and the hirudin trial emphasize the vital importance of critical investigation of dose finding studies for each subset of patients and clinical indication. Although the EPIC trial probably benefited from an initially too potent combination of c7E3 and heparin, the dramatic reduction in clinical events appeared at the cost of bleeding. The reduction in clinical events justified further development and adjustment of the (heparin) dosage regimen to the narrow therapeutic window.

At least four other trials using specific antithrombotic drugs have demonstrated beneficial effects on the acute complications of coronary angioplasty without favorably influencing long-term clinical outcomes [92,101–103]. This is in contradistinction with the EPIC trial [98•,99], which showed a reduction in early cardiac events that was maintained at long-term follow-up. The study was not designed to detect angiographic restenosis; however the evident decrease in revascularization procedures and MI may reflect the effect on the restenosis process. In the EPIC study, the event-free survival curve demonstrates a significant initial difference in clinical outcome, which is even more distinct during 6 months' follow-up as shown by the manifest divergence of the survival curves. It has been speculated that interaction of the compound with vitronectin results in an antiproliferative effect, which might explain the latter finding. The significant surplus of major bleeding complications in the EPIC trial (14.0% vs 6.6%, P = 0.001) emerged as a major drawback for the monoclonal antibody. To investigate the effect of c7E3 on angiographic restenosis, the EPILOG (Evaluation of PTCA to Improve Long-term Outcome by c7E3 Glycoprotein Receptor) trial was designed testing two c7E3 Fab arms versus placebo in a planned 4800 patients. To control bleeding complications, the heparin regimens in the treatment arms (standard and low-dose heparin) were adjusted for weight. This change resulted in a reduction of bleeding rates to that of the same order as placebo. Inclusion was stopped following recruitment of 2792 patients, when interim analysis on 1500 patients revealed that the 30-day incidence of combined death and MI was reduced from 8.1% in the control arm to 2.6% and 3.6% in the low-dose and standard heparin dose [104]. Compared with EPIC and because of the low bleeding rates, more patients received their complete c7E3 treatment, and differences in primary endpoint rates were therefore more distinct, despite the effect that in EPILOG patients with less complex lesions and patients suffering stable angina were randomized. Whether these results will translate into a significant reduction in angiographically assessed restenosis awaits adjudication.

Conclusions

The majority of clinical investigations with thrombin inhibitors has been in coronary artery disease. Despite the evident limitations of heparin and aspirin, their role in interventional cardiology is currently not replaced by a specific thrombin inhibitor. Thrombin antagonists represent a promising class of antithrombotic agents that overcome the pharmacokinetic and pharmacodynamic restrictions of heparin and aspirin and appear safe for clinical application. The lack of specific antidotes with narrow therapeutic windows leaves a risk for overdosing, especially in the context of combined use with thrombolytics and impaired renal clearance, but the anticipated increase in bleeding complications in intracoronary intervention studies is controlled. Notwithstanding all the theoretical advantages, this class embodies, including the established significantly superior acute clinical outcome in various restenosis prevention trials, phase III evaluation has not achieved a convincing improvement of the long-term outcome. Numerous reasons have been proposed to explain this phenomenon, which is not yet clearly understood. Direct thrombin inhibitors at the currently administered dosage regimens do not block thrombin generation completely, as demonstrated by thrombin-antithrombin complex and prothrombin fragment 1 and 2 measurements, and enable some thrombin molecules to escape. Local drug delivery devices may be of critical importance in further attempts to restrict thrombin's action. All large-scale and Food and Drug Administration–approved restenosis prevention trials examining antithrombins used only aspirin as the concomitant drug, without investigating the potential of (weight-adjusted) concomitant heparin therapy as in the thrombolysis studies. Furthermore, there is much left to be learned from optimal dosing in specific conditions and indications, and finally, the discrepancy between animal experimental work and human surveys may suggest a drug-independent or thrombin-independent pathway of smooth muscle cell activation.

References and Recommended Reading

Recently published papers of particular interest have been highlighted as:

- • Of special interest
- •• Of outstanding interest

1. Roux S, Ludin E: Effects of aspirin on coronary reocclusion and recurrent ischemia after thrombolysis: A meta-analysis. *J Am Coll Cardiol* 1992, 19:671–677.
2. Nelken NA, Soifer SJ, O'Keefe J, *et al.*: Thrombin receptor expression in normal and atherosclerotic human arteries. *J Clin Invest* 1992, 90:1614–1621.
3. Bar-Shavit R, Kahn A, Wilner GD, Fenton JW: Monocyte chemotaxis: Stimulation by specific exosite region in thrombin. *Science* 1983, 220:728–731.
4. Chen LB, Teng NNH, Buchanan JM: Mitogenic activity of thrombin and surface alterations on mouse splenocytes. *Exp Cell Res* 1976, 101:41–46.
5. McNamara CA, Sarembock IJ, Gimple LW, *et al.*: Thrombin stimulates smooth muscle cell proliferation by a proteolytic, receptor mediated mechanism. *J Clin Invest* 1993, 91:94–98
6. Vu T-KH, Hung DT, Wheaton VI, Coughlin SR: Molecular cloning of a functional thrombin receptor reveals a novel proteolytic mechanism of receptor activation. *Cell* 1991, 64:1057–1068.
7. Coller BS: Platelets and thrombolytic therapy. *N Engl J Med* 1990, 322:33–42.
8. Herrman J-PR, Hermans WRM, Vos J, Serruys PW: Pharmacological approaches to the prevention of restenosis following angioplasty: the search for the holy grail? Part 1. *Drugs* 1993, 46:18–52.
9. Herrman J-PR, Hermans WRM, Vos J, Serruys PW: Pharmacological approaches to the prevention of restenosis following angioplasty: the search for the holy grail? Part 2. *Drugs* 1993, 46:249–262.
10. Clarke RJ, Mayo G, Price P, Fitzgerald A: Suppression of thromboxane A_2 but not of systemic prostacyclin by controlled-release aspirin. *N Engl J Med* 1991, 325:1137–1141.
11. Guyton JR, Rosenburg RD, Clowes AW, Karnovsky MJ: Inhibition of rat arterial smooth muscle cell proliferation by heparin: in vivo studies with anticoagulant and nonanticoagulant heparin. *Circ Res* 1980, 46:625–634.

12. Clowes AW, Clowes MM: Kinetics of cellular proliferation after arterial injury: inhibition of smooth muscle cell growth by heparin. *Lab Invest* 1985, 52:611–616.

13. Hamon M, Bauters C, Wernert N, *et al.*: Heparin does not inhibit oncogene induction in rabbit aorta following balloon denudation. *Cardiovasc Res* 1993, 27:1209–1213.

14. Lehmann K, Doris RJ, Feuer JM, *et al.*: Paradoxical increase in restenosis rate with chronic heparin use: final results of a randomized trial [abstract]. *J Am Coll Cardiol* 1991, 17:181A.

15. De Vries CJ, Michels HR, Emanuelson M, El Gamal MIH: Does administration of low molecular weight heparin after angioplasty affect restenosis? [abstract]. *Eur Heart J* 1991, 12:386.

16. Wallford GD, Midei MM, Aversano TR, *et al.*: Heparin after PTCA: increased early complications and no clinical benefit [abstract]. *Circulation* 1991, 84(suppl II):592.

17. Perin EC, Turner SA, Ferguson JJ: Relationship between the response to heparin and restenosis following PTCA [abstract]. *Circulation* 1990, 82:III-497.

18. Herrmann HC, LeVeen RF, Tomaszewski JE, *et al.*: Experimental angioplasty restenosis is inhibited by oral administration of cyclodextrin tetradecasulfate [abstract]. *Circulation* 1991, 84(suppl II):296.

19. Timms ID, Shlansky-Goldberg RD, Healey HM, *et al.*: A novel form of nonanticoagulant heparin reduces restenosis following angioplasty in the atherosclerotic rabbit [abstract 2800]. *Circulation* 1992, 86(suppl I):703.

20. Dubé GP, Yan SB, Kurtz WL, *et al.*: Inhibition of intimal thickening by subcutaneous native and novel low anticoagulant heparin (GM 1077) following balloon injury [abstract]. *Circulation* 1992, 86(suppl I):168.

21. Meuleman DG: Orgaran (Org 10172): Its pharmacological profile in experimental models. *Haemostasis* 1992, 22:58–65.

22. Zammit A, Dawes J: Low-affinity material does not contribute to the antithrombotic activity of Orgaran (Org 10172) in human plasma. *Thromb Haemost* 1994, 71:759–767.

23. Oda Y, Asahara T, Usui M, *et al.*: Low molecular weight heparin fails to limit smooth muscle cell proliferation in hyperlipidemic rabbit in experimental balloon injury model for long term observation [abstract 3373]. *Circulation* 1992, 86(suppl 1):847.

24. Buchwald AB, Unterberg C, Nebendahl K, *et al.*: Low molecular weight heparin reduces neointimal proliferation after coronary stent implantation in hypercholesterolemic minipigs. *Circulation* 1992, 86:531–537.

25. Currier JW, Pow TK, Haudenschild CC, *et al.*: Low molecular weight heparin (Enoxaparin) reduces restenosis after iliac angioplasty in the hypercholesterolemic rabbit. *J Am Coll Cardiol* 1991, 17:118B–125B.

26. Heras M, Chesebro JH, Webster MWI, *et al.*: Antithrombotic efficacy of low molecular weight heparin in deep arterial injury. *Arterioscler Thromb* 1992, 12:250–255.

27. Hanke H, Oberhoff M, Hanke S, *et al.*: Inhibition of cellular proliferation after experimental balloon angioplasty by low molecular weight heparin. *Circulation* 1992, 85:1548–1556.

28. Dunwiddie CT, Waxman L, Vlasuk GP, *et al.*: Purification and characterization of inhibitors of blood coagulation factors Xa from hematophageous organisms. *Methods Enzymol* 1993, 223:291–312.

29. Schaffer LW, Davidson JT, Vlasuk GP, *et al.*: Selective factor Xa inhibition by recombinant antistasin prevents vascular graft thrombosis in baboons. *Arterioscler Thromb* 1992, 12:879–885.

30. Melloty MJ, Holahan MA, Lynch JJ, *et al.*: Acceleration of recombinant tissue-type plasminogen-activator induced reperfusion and prevention of reocclusion by recombinant antistasin, a selective factor Xa inhibitor, in a canine model of femoral arterial thrombosis. *Circ Res* 1992, 70:1152–1160.

31. Dunwiddie CT, Nutt EM, Vlasuk GP, *et al.*: Anticoagulant efficacy and immunogenicity of the selective factor Xa inhibitor antistasin following subcutaneous administration in the rhesus monkey. *Thromb Haemost* 1992, 67:371–376.

32.• Verstraete M, Zoldhelyi P: Novel antithrombotic drugs in development. *Drugs* 1995, 49:856–884.

Excellent review manuscript.

33. Waxman L, Smith DE, Arcuri KE, Vlasuk GP: Tick anticoagulant peptide (TAP) is a novel inhibitor of blood coagulation factor Xa. *Science* 1990, 248:593–596.

34. Ragosta M, Gimple LW, Haber HL, *et al.*: Effectiveness of specific factor Xa inhibition on restenosis following balloon angioplasty in rabbits. *J Am Coll Cardiol* 1992, 19:164A.

35. Grütter MG, Priestle JP, Rahuel J, *et al.*: Crystal structure of the thrombin-hirudin complex: a novel mode of serine protease inhibition. *EMBO J* 1990, 8:2361–2365.

36. Weitz JI, Hudoba M, Massel D, *et al.*: Clot bound thrombin is protected from inhibition by heparin-antithrombin III but is susceptible to inactivation by antithrombin III-independent inhibitors. *J Clin Invest* 1990, 86:385–391.

37. Stringer KA, Lindenfeld JA: Hirudins: Anticoagulants. *Ann Pharmacother* 1992, 26:1535–1540.

38. Bichler J, Fichtl B, Siebeck M, Fritz H: Pharmacokinetics and pharmacodynamics of hirudin in man after single subcutaneous and intravenous bolus administration. *Drug Res* 1988, 38:704–710.

39. Talbot MD, Ambler J, Butler KD, *et al.*: Recombinant desulphatohirudin (CGP 39 393) anticoagulant and antithrombotic properties in vivo. *Thromb Haemost* 1991, 61:77–80.

40. Marbet GA, Verstraete M, Kienast J, *et al.*: Clinical pharmacology of intravenously administered recombinant desulphatohirudin (CGP 39 393) in healthy volunteers. *J Cardiovasc Pharmacol* 1993, 22:364–372.

41. Heras M, Chesebro JH, Webster MWI, *et al.*: Hirudin, heparin and placebo during deep arterial injury in the pig: the in vivo role of thrombosis in platelet-mediated thrombosis. *Circulation* 1990, 82:1476–1484.

42. Sarembock IJ, Gertz SD, Gimple LW, *et al.*: Effectiveness of recombinant desulphato hirudin in reducing restenosis after balloon angioplasty of atherosclerotic femoral arteries in rabbits. *Circulation* 1991, 84:232–243.

43. Buchwald AB, Sandrock D, Unterberg C, *et al.*: Platelet and fibrin deposition on coronary stents in minipigs: Effect of hirudin versus heparin. *J Am Coll Cardiol* 1993, 21:249–254.

44. van der Bos AA, Deckers JW, Heyndrickx GR, *et al.*: Safety and efficacy of recombinant hirudin (CGP 39393) versus heparin in patients with stable angina undergoing coronary angioplasty. *Circulation* 1993, 88:2058–2066.

45. Close P, Bichler J, Kerry R, *et al.*: Weak allergenicity of recombinant hirudin CGP 39 393 (REVASC) in immunocompetent volunteers. *Coron Artery Dis* 1994, 5:943–949.

46.• Serruys PW, Herrman J-PR, Simon R, *et al.* for the HELVETICA investigators: a comparison of hirudin with heparin in the prevention of restenosis after coronary angioplasty. *N Engl J Med* 1995, 333:757–763.

Important clinical trial exploring the role of recombinant hirudin in restenosis prevention.

47. The global use of strategies to open occluded coronary arteries (GUSTO) IIa investigators: Randomized trial of intravenous heparin versus recombinant hirudin for acute coronary syndromes. *Circulation* 1994, 90:1631–1637.

48. Antman E for the TIMI-9A investigators: Hirudin in myocardial infarction: safety report from the thrombolysis and thrombin inhibition in myocardial infarction (TIMI-9A) trial. *Circulation* 1994, 90:1624–1630.

49. Neuhaus KL, Essen RV, Tebbe U, *et al.*: Safety observations from the pilot phase of the randomized r-hirudin for improvement of thrombolysis (HIT-III) study. *Circulation* 1994, 90:1638–1642.

50. Cadroy Y, Maraganore JM, Hanson SR, Harker LA: Selective inhibition by a synthetic hirudin peptide of fibrin-dependent thrombosis in baboons. *Proc Natl Acad Sci USA* 1991, 88:1177–1181.

51. Bourdon P, Fenton JW, Maraganore JM: Affinity labeling of lysine-149 in the anion-binding exosite of human alpha-thrombin with an N alpha-(dinitrofluorobenzyl)hirudin C-terminal peptide. *Biochem* 1990, 29:6379–6384.

52. Dawson A, Loynds P, Findlen K, *et al.*: Hirulog-1: a bivalent thrombin inhibitor with potent anticoagulant properties in humans [abstract]. *Thromb Haemost* 1991, 65:830.

53. Fox I, Dawson A, Loynds P, *et al.*: Anticoagulant activity of hirulog, a direct thrombin inhibitor in humans. *Thromb Haemost* 1993, 69:157–163.

54. Topol EJ, Bonan R, Jewitt D, *et al.*: Use of a direct antithrombin, hirulog, in place of heparin during coronary angioplasty. *Circulation* 1993, 87:1622–1629.

55.• Bittl JA, Strony J, Brinker JA, *et al.* for the hirulog angioplasty study investigators: treatment with bivalirudin (hirulog) as compared with heparin during coronary angioplasty for unstable or postinfarction angina. *N Engl J Med* 1995, 333:764–769.

Important clinical trial exploring the role of hirulog in restenosis prevention.

56. Kaplan AV, Leung LLK, Leung WH, *et al.* Roles of thrombin and platelet membrane glycoprotein IIb/IIIa in platelet subendothelial deposition after angioplasty in an ex vivo whole artery model. *Circulation* 1991, 84:1279–1288.

57. Kikumoto R, Tamao Y, Tezuka T, *et al.*: Selective inhibition of thrombin by (2R,4R)-4-methyl-1-[N^2-((3-methyl-1,2,3,4-tetrahydro-8-quinolonyl)sulfonyl)-arginyl]-2-piperidine carboxylic acid. *Biochemistry* 1984, 23:85–90.

58. Jang IK, Gold HK, Zisking AA, *et al.*: Prevention of platelet-rich arterial thrombosis by selective thrombin inhibition. *Circulation* 1990, 81:18–27.

59. Jang IK, Gold HK, Leinbach RC, *et al.*: Persistent inhibition of arterial thrombosis by a 1-hour intravenous infusion of argatroban, a selective thrombin inhibitor. *Coron Artery Dis* 1992, 3:407–414.

60. Gold HK, Torres FW, Garabedian HD, *et al.*: Evidence for a rebound coagulation phenomenon after cessation of a 4-hour infusion of a specific thrombin inhibitor in patients with unstable angina pectoris. *J Am Coll Cardiol* 1993, 21:1039–1047.

61. Bock LC, Griffin LC, Latham JA, *et al.*: Selection of single-stranded DNA molecules that bind and inhibit human thrombin. *Nature* 1992, 355:564–566.

62. Tapparelli C, Metternich R, Ehrhardt C, *et al.*: Synthetic low molecular weight thrombin inhibitors: molecular design and pharmacologic profile. *Trends Pharmacol Sci* 1993, 14:366–376.

63. Schror K: Antiplatelet drugs: a comparative review. *Drugs* 1995, 50:7–28.

64. Zoldhelyi P, Fuster V, Chesebro JH: Antithrombins as conjugative therapy in arterial thrombolysis. *Coron Artery Dis* 1992, 3:1003–1009.

65. Kettner C, Mersinger L, Knabb R: The selective inhibition of thrombin by peptides of boroarginine. *J Biol Chem* 1990, 265:18289–18297.

66. Hung DT, Vu TK, Wheaton VI, *et al.*: 'Mirror image' antagonism of thrombin induced platelet activation based on thrombin receptor structure. *J Clin Invest* 1992, 89:444–450.

67. Knapp A, Degenhardt T, Dodt J: Hirudisins: hirudin-derived thrombin inhibitors with desintegrin activity. *J Biol Chem* 1992, 267:24230–24234.

68. Bode C, Hudelmayer M, Mehwald P, *et al.*: Fibrin targeted recombinant hirudin inhibits fibrin deposition on experimental clots more efficiently than recombinant hirudin. *Circulation* 1994, 90:1956–1963.

69. Preisack MB, Karsch KR: The paradigm of restenosis following percutaneous transluminal coronary angioplasty. *Eur Heart J* 1993, 14(suppl I):187–192.

70. Wolinsky H, Thung SN: Use of a perforated balloon catheter to deliver concentrated heparin into the wall of the normal canine artery. *J Am Coll Cardiol* 1990, 15:475–481.

71. Moura A, Lam JYT, Hébert D, *et al.*: Local heparin delivery decreases the thrombogenicity of the balloon injured artery [abstract]. *Circulation* 1994, 90:I-449.

72. Leung WH, Kaplan AV, Grant GW, *et al.*: Local delivery of antithrombin agent by an infusion balloon catheter reduces platelet deposition at the site of balloon angioplasty. *Coron Artery Dis* 1991, 2:699–706.

73. Nunes GL, Hanson SR, King SB, *et al.*: Local delivery of a synthetic antithrombin with a hydrogel-coated angioplasty balloon catheter inhibits platelet-dependent thrombosis. *J Am Coll Cardiol* 1994, 23:1578–1583.

74. Meyer, BJ, Fernández-Oritz A, Mailhac A, *et al.*: Local delivery of r-hirudin by a double-balloon perfusion catheter prevents mural thrombosis and minimizes platelet deposition after angioplasty. *Circulation* 1994, 90:2474–2480.

75. Gimple LW, Gertz SD, Haber HL, *et al.*: Effect of chronic subcutaneous or intramural administration of heparin on femoral artery restenosis after balloon angioplasty in hypercholesterolemic rabbits: a quantitative angiographic and histopathological study. *Circulation* 1992, 86:1536–1546.

76. Oberhoff M, Herdeg C, Shamet K, *et al.*: Delivery of low molecular weight heparin via porous balloon catheter for the prevention of smooth muscle cell proliferation [abstract]. *Circulation* 1993, 88:I-661.

77. Hong MK, Wong C, Haudenschild CC, *et al.*: Efficacy of locally delivered low molecular weight heparin (Enoxaprin) on smooth muscle cell proliferation [abstract]. *J Am Coll Cardiol* 1995, 25:376A.

78. Kaplan AV, Vandormael M, Bartorelli A, *et al.*: Heparin delivery at the site of angioplasty with a novel drug delivery sleeve: initial clinical series [abstract]. *J Am Coll Cardiol* 1995, 25:286A.

79. Camenzind E, Kint PP, Dimario C, *et al*: Intracoronary heparin delivery in humans: acute feasibility and long-term results. *Circulation* 1995, 92:2463–2472.

80. Camenzind E, Reys A, Ligthart J, *et al.*: Local intracoronary delivery of heparin and of a somatostatin analogue (Octreotide) following angioplasty in man: evaluation of efficacy of delivery by radio-isotopic technique [abstract]. *J Am Coll Cardiol* 1995, 25:285A.

81. Camenzind E, van der Giesen W, Ligthart J, *et al.*: Local, low pressure heparin delivery following angioplasty in man: the solution to restenosis? [abstract]. *J Am Coll Cardiol* 1995, 25:376A.

82. Camenzind E, Vrolix M, Hanet C, *et al.*: Local heparin delivery following balloon angioplasty to prevent restenosis: Preliminary results of an open multicenter registry [abstract]. *Circulation* 1995, 92:I-346.

83. Camenzind E, Legrand V, Vrolix M, *et al.* on behalf of the Dispatch investigators: An open multicenter registry to evaluate local heparin delivery following balloon angioplasty for the prevention of restenosis: Preliminary results. *J Am Coll Cardiol* 1996, 27(2 suppl A):321A.

84. Oberhoff M, Hermann T, Maier R, *et al.*: Local drug delivery of low molecular weight heparin after PTCA: first clinical experience using the porous balloon (PILOT-study) [abstact]. *J Am Coll Cardiol* 1996, 27(supp A):14.

85. Sheth S, Park KD, Dev V, *et al.*: Prevention of stent subacute thrombosis by segmented polyurethane urea-polyethylene oxide-heparin coating in the rabbit carotid [abstract]. *J Am Coll Cardiol* 1994, 23:187A.

86. van der Giessen W, Hårdhammer PA, van Beusekom HMM, *et al.*: Reduction of thrombotic events using heparin-coated Palmaz-Schatz stents [abstract]. *Circulation* 1993, 88:I-661.

87. Serruys PW, Emanuelsson H, van der Giessen W, *et al.* on behalf of the Benestent-II Study Group: Heparin-coated palmaz-Schatz stents in human coronary arteries: early outcome of the Benestent-II pilot study. *Circulation* 1996, 93:412–422.

88.•• Serruys PW on behalf of the Benestent-II Study Group: BENESTENT-II pilot study: 6 months follow-up of phase 1, 2 and 3 [abstract]. *Circulation* 1995, 92:I-542.

Description of the landmark trial's long-term results following heparin-coated Palaz-Schatz stent implant.

89. Serruys PW, de Jaegere P, Kiemeneij F, *et al.* for the Benestent Study Group: A comparison of balloon-expandable-stent implantation with balloon angioplasty in patients with coronary artery disease. *N Engl J Med* 1994, 331:489–495.

90. van Beusekom HMM, Serruys PW, van der Giessen WJ: Coronary stent coatings. *Coron Artery Dis* 1994, 5:590–596.

91. Faxon DP, Spiro TE, Minor S, *et al.* and the ERA investigators: Low molecular weight heparin in prevention of restenosis after angioplasty: results of Enoxaparin Restenosis (ERA) Trial. *Circulation* 1994, 90:908–914.

92. Karsch K, Preisack MB, Bonan R, on behalf of the REDUCE study group: Low molecular weight heparin, reviparin, in prevention of restenosis after PTCA: results of the REDUCE trial. *J Am Coll Cardiol* 1996, 27(2 suppl A):113A.

93. Geary RL, Koyama N, Wang TW, *et al.*: Failure of heparin to inhibit hyperplasia in injured baboon arteries. The role of heparin-sensitive and -insensitive pathways in the stimulation of smooth muscle cell migration and proliferation. *Circulation* 1995, 91:2972–2981.

94. Leimgruber PP, Roubin GS, Hollman J, *et al.*: Restenosis after successful coronary angioplasty in patients with single-vessel disease. *Circulation* 1986, 73:710–717.

95. Rupprecht HJ, Brenneke R, Bernhard G, *et al.*: Analysis of risk factors for restenosis after PTCA. *Cathet Cardiovasc Diagn* 1990, 19:151–159.

96. Bourassa MG, Lespérance J, Eastwood C, *et al.*: Clinical, physiologic, anatomic and procedural factors predictive of restenosis after percutaneous transluminal coronary angioplasty. *J Am Coll Cardiol* 1991, 18:368–376.

97. Zoldhelyi P, Bichler J, Owen GO, *et al.*: Persistent thrombin generation in humans during specific thrombin inhibition with hirudin. *Circulation* 1994, 90:2671–2678.

98.• Topol EJ, Califf RM, Weisman HF, *et al.* on behalf of the EPIC investigators: Randomised trial of coronary intervention with antibody against platelet IIb/IIIa integrin for reduction of clinical restenosis: results at six months. *Lancet* 1994, 343:881–886.

Landmark trial indicating the role of c7E3 in restenosis prevention.

99. The EPIC investigators: Use of a monoclonal antibody directed against the platelet glycoprotein IIb/IIIa receptor in high-risk coronary angioplasty. *N Engl J Med* 1994, 330:956–961.

100. Narins CR, Hillegass WB, Nelson CL, *et al.*: Relation between activated clotting time during angioplasty and abrupt closure. *Circulation* 1996, 93:667–671.

101. Schwartz L, Bourassa MG, Lesperance J, *et al.*: Aspirin and dipyridamole in the prevention of restenosis after percutaneous transluminal coronary angioplasty. *N Engl J Med* 1988, 318:1714–1719.

102. Chesebro JH, Webster MWI, Reeder GS, *et al.*: Coronary angioplasty: antiplatelet therapy reduces acute complications but not restenosis [abstract]. *Circulation* 1989, 80(suppl II):64.

103. Bertrand ME, Allain H, LaBlanche JM, on behalf of the TACT study: Results of a randomized trial of ticlopidine versus placebo for prevention of acute closure and restenosis after coronary angioplasty (PTCA): The TACT study [abstract]. *Circulation* 1990, 82:III-190.

104. Ferguson JJ: EPILOG and CAPTURE trials halted because of positive interim results. *Circulation* 1996, 93:637.

Chapter 19

Recent Studies of Hirudin and Its Analogues, Bivalirudin and Hirugen

John A. Bittl

Hirudin and its analogues, bivalirudin and hirugen, are direct thrombin inhibitors that have been extensively investigated as substitutes for heparin during coronary angioplasty. These investigations constitute a direct test of the so-called "thrombin hypothesis," which is based on the recognition that thrombin is the strongest agonist of platelet activation, platelets play a central role in arterial thrombus formation, and heparin has several theoretical limitations as an antithrombotic agent.

In this chapter, we review the evidence for thrombin generation and arterial thrombus formation relevant to the discussion of coronary angioplasty. This serves as a background for interpreting the results of several studies of direct thrombin inhibitors in coronary angioplasty. The results of these studies are summarized to provide new insights into the thrombin hypothesis and new perspectives on the pathogenesis of ischemic complications following angioplasty.

Evidence for Thrombin Activation During Coronary Angioplasty

The development of direct thrombin inhibitors for coronary angioplasty is based on the observation that thrombin-mediated platelet activation plays a central role in arterial thrombus formation [1,2]. Although the lipid-laden atheroma is the most thrombogenic type of plaque studied [3], the lipid composition *per se* does not determine the extent of thrombus formation. Instead, tissue factor protein, which is present in high concentrations associated with monocytes and lipid in atherosclerotic plaque [4], combines with factors VIIa and Xa to form the prothrombinase complex [5] and catalyzes the generation of thrombin from prothrombin (Fig. 19-1). Thrombin not only mediates the conversion of fibrinogen to fibrin but is one of the most potent agonists of platelet activation.

The extent of platelet deposition and thrombus formation during spontaneous plaque rupture or balloon angioplasty is not only related to the thrombogenicity of the underlying substrate but also to rheologic factors producing increased shear stress [6,7]. It has been observed that balloon injury of canine carotid artery increases platelet deposition significantly, but the presence of a constriction induced by a vascular ring increases it further. As compared with spontaneous platelet–thrombus formation within a normal arterial segment, a balloon-injured and dilated segment has a twofold increase in platelet deposition. The superimposition of a stenosis on a segment of arterial injury is associated with an additional threefold increase in platelet deposition. Critical shear rate thresholds, above which thrombus accretion superimposed on a firmly anchored mural platelet thrombus would likely cause vessel occlusion, appear at vessel diameters of 1.5 to 1.6 mm and are associated with shear rates of 5000 s^{-1} [7].

In contrast to the extensive experimental literature on thrombin generation during balloon injury of arterial segments, clinical evidence for thrombin generation during coronary angioplasty remains sparse. In an important study, Marmur and colleagues [8•] measured intracoronary markers of thrombin generation (prothrombin fragment F_{1+2}) and thrombin activity (fibrinopeptide A) in samples of intracoronary blood aspirated from the central lumen of angioplasty balloons. They observed that the intracoronary generation of thrombin, as measured by concentrations of prothrombin fragment F_{1+2}, rose from 0.47 nM (95% CI, 0.40–0.50) before balloon dilatation to 0.55 nM (0.46–0.72) after balloon dilatation (P = 0.001). In the presence of heparin anticoagulation, evidence for thrombin-mediated conversion of fibrinogen to fibrin as determined by the appearance of fibrinopeptide A did not increase in response to balloon dilatation for the entire study group of 26 patients: 2.0 ng/mL (1.3–2.2) before dilatation versus 1.8 ng/mL (1.3–3.0) after dilatation (P value not significant). Increases in fibrinopeptide A, however, were seen in five of seven high-risk patients and were more likely to occur in the setting of ulcerated or thrombus-containing lesions [8•].

Information from several sources leads to a comprehensive view of arterial thrombotic occlusion relevant

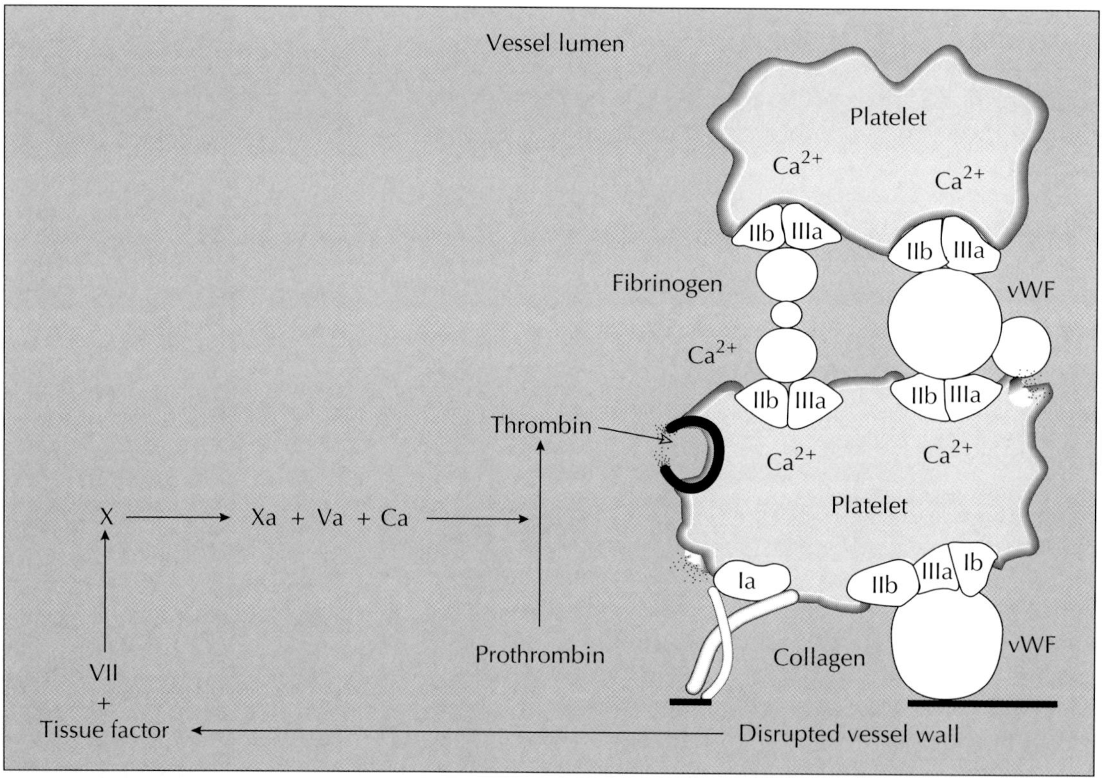

Figure 19-1. Arterial thrombus formation. Balloon dilatation exposes subintimal collagen and tissue factor. Tissue factor, factor Xa, and factor VIIa comprise the prothrombinase complex, which catalyzes the formation of thrombin. In addition to converting fibrinogen to fibrin (not shown), thrombin activates platelets. Activated platelets externalize glycoprotein IIb/IIIa receptors, which bind to adhesive macromolecules such as fibrinogen or von Willebrand Factor (vWF) and thus mediate the process of platelet aggregation. (*From* Stein and colleagues [73]; with permission.)

to coronary angioplasty (*see* Fig. 19-1). This involves platelet-dependent processes occurring in several stages [6]: 1) plaque rupture leads to exposure of tissue factor protein and thrombin-mediated platelet activation; 2) as thrombus grows in the presence of normal flow, shear rates rise and platelet receptor IIb/IIIa-mediated mechanisms predominate; 3) during the final occlusion phase, flow and shear rates fall, resulting in a total occlusion that is dependent on the presence of von Willebrand factor.

Thrombin Inhibitors

Heparin has several theoretical limitations as an anticoagulant for coronary angioplasty. First, heparin binds extensively to endothelial cells and plasma proteins [9], reducing its bioavailability and producing a nonlinear dose-response curve [10]. Although the unpredictability of the anticoagulation response during angioplasty can be reduced by monitoring activated clotting times (ACT), there continues to be wide variability between the incidence of ischemic complications and the level of anticoagulation achieved during angioplasty [11,12•]. The second limitation of heparin involves its neutralization by high local concentrations of platelet factor 4. For example, one milliliter of platelet thrombus extract from a clotted stent removed from a porcine coronary artery contains enough antiheparin activity to neutralize the anticoagulant activity in 140 mL of heparinized blood [13]. A third limitation of heparin involves a conformational change in clot-bound thrombin that renders it inaccessible to inhibition by the heparin–antithrombin III complex yet allows the sequestered thrombin to activate platelets and convert fibrinogen to fibrin [14,15]. Because of localized resistance to heparin during angioplasty, high systemic doses of heparin are commonly administered, which reduce the risk of ischemic complications but increase the risk of bleeding [12•].

The development of direct thrombin inhibitors was based on the observations of the action of native hirudin, a 65-amino-acid polypeptide isolated from the salivary gland of the medicinal leech, that is a potent irreversible inhibitor of thrombin (*see* Chapter 20). Bivalirudin is a 20-amino-acid peptide modeled after native hirudin that also irreversibly inhibits the activity of thrombin [16], and hirugen is a 12-amino-acid peptide that competitively inhibits the fibrinogenolytic and platelet-activating effects of thrombin (*see* Chapter 20).

The direct thrombin inhibitors have several theoretical advantages over heparin. Several investigators have observed that the direct thrombin inhibitors are more potent than heparin in inhibiting clot-bound thrombin [15,17]. Gast and colleagues [17] have reported the effects of hirudin and heparin and observed that hirudin is the more potent inhibitor of both fluid-phase and clot-bound thrombin. Measuring the anticoagulant content at which 50% of thrombin is inhibited (IC_{50}), these investigators observed that hirudin was two times (IC_{50} 8 vs 3 ng/mL) and heparin six times (IC_{50} 1205 vs 200 ng/mL) less active against clot-bound thrombin compared with fluid-phase thrombin [17]. In addition, the direct thrombin inhibitors do not require a cofactor such as antithrombin III and have no known natural inhibitors such as platelet factor 4 [13].

The direct thrombin inhibitors are superior to low molecular weight heparin in their ability to lower D dimer levels in an experimental model of venous thrombosis, suggesting that direct thrombin inhibitors may inhibit thrombin-induced thrombus growth [18]. Thus, by combining antithrombotic activity with specific thrombus-binding properties within a single hybrid molecule, direct thrombin inhibitors may reversibly interrupt the recruitment of platelets and decrease the formation of fibrin. These agents may also lead to a lower risk of bleeding than that observed with heparin. In experimental models, such as the rat carotid endarterectomy model, the use of bivalirudin is associated with significant reductions in ^{111}In-labeled platelet deposition without a significant hemostatic defect [19].

Dose of Direct Thrombin Inhibitors and Measurements of Systemic Anticoagulation

Are the measurements of activated partial thromboplastin times (aPTT) or ACT appropriate tests to compare the direct thrombin inhibitors with heparin? As compared with heparin, the direct thrombin inhibitors produce more predictable levels of systemic anticoagulation with less variable aPTT [20]. Carteaux and colleagues [21] measured the ACT, aPTT, and thrombin-generation tests in a guinea pig carotid thrombosis model treated with hirudin or heparin. In the model, thrombosis was induced by subendothelial damage with subsequent cyclic flow variations. Heparin in a dose of 1 IU/kg/min or hirudin in a dose of 30 μg/kg/min both doubled the aPTT, but heparin was ineffective in reducing the incidence of cyclic flow reductions, whereas hirudin reduced them by 80%. Heparin in a dose of 10 IU/kg/min achieved the same antithrombotic effect as the hirudin dose, but the aPTT was indefinitely prolonged. For a similar prolongation of the ACT, however, heparin and hirudin had identical antithrombotic effects.

Thrombin generation was predictive of the antithrombotic effect of the thrombin inhibitors but not of heparin [21].

High-Risk Coronary Angioplasty

The development of new antithrombotic regimens to improve the results of high-risk angioplasty is based on three assertions: 1) thrombin is generated during high-risk coronary angioplasty; 2) most of the complications of high-risk coronary angioplasty are related to thrombus formation; and 3) direct thrombin inhibitors are superior to heparin in preventing thrombin-mediated ischemic complications of angioplasty. Preliminary studies using direct thrombin inhibitors such as hirudin or bivalirudin as a substitute for heparin have provided new insights into these assertions.

It is an accepted fact from several clinical studies that the outcome of angioplasty performed for unstable angina is related to the severity and acuity of the clinical presentation [22]. Pooled analyses reveal that rates of acute myocardial infarction (AMI) after angioplasty are approximately 6.3% for patients with postinfarction angina [23–30], 6.3% for patients with refractory unstable angina [31–38], 5.1% for patients with unstable angina stabilized on medical therapy [23,36,39–41], 1.6% for patients with stable angina [42–48], and 1% for patients undergoing angioplasty for symptomatic restenosis [49–52].

The relation between clinical presentation and ischemic complications of percutaneous transluminal coronary angioplasty (PTCA) also has important implications for understanding the pathogenesis and optimal treatment of unstable ischemic syndromes. Although unstable angina and myocardial infarction (MI) are commonly linked together as syndromes with a similar pathogenesis involving plaque rupture and arterial thrombus formation, each syndrome is associated with different degrees of thrombus burden accounting for the range of angioplasty-related complications that spans almost an order of magnitude. Several studies have tested the hypothesis that the complications of high-risk angioplasty may be reduced when a direct thrombin inhibitor is used in place of heparin.

Studies of Hirudin in Percutaneous Transluminal Coronary Angioplasty

In an angiographic study evaluating hirudin for unstable angina, 166 patients with ischemic chest pain, abnormal electrocardiograms, and abnormal coronary arteriograms with 60% or greater stenosis with a visual appearance consistent with thrombus were treated with heparin or various doses of hirudin. Overall, the 116 patients treated with hirudin tended to show greater improvement in cross-sectional area of the culprit lesion than the 50 patients treated with heparin, suggesting that the direct thrombin inhibitor was more effective than heparin in reducing the extent of coronary thrombus burden associated with the syndrome of unstable angina [53].

Several experimental studies suggested that hirudin would also be superior to heparin for long-term outcomes. Sarembock and colleagues [54] evaluated the effects of hirudin on neointimal proliferation in a rabbit iliac model of balloon injury. They observed a significant reduction in the amount of neointimal formation and lumen narrowing after treatment with the direct thrombin inhibitor.

Consequently, hirudin was evaluated as a means of reducing restenosis after coronary angioplasty in a randomized, double-blind study known as HELVETICA (Hirudin in a European Trial Versus Heparin in the Prevention of Restenosis after PTCA) [55••], in which 1141 patients were randomly assigned to treatment with aspirin plus heparin (10,000 IU intravenous bolus plus 15 IU/kg intravenously per hour for 24 hours), hirudin infusion (40 mg intravenous bolus plus 0.2 mg/kg intravenously per hour for 24 hours), or hirudin infusion plus prolonged subcutaneous therapy (40 mg intravenous bolus plus 0.2 mg/kg intravenously per hour for 24 hours plus 40 mg subcutaneously twice daily for 72 hours) in an effort to reduce clinical and angiographic restenosis at 7 months. Although the use of hirudin was associated with a significant reduction in the secondary endpoint, which consisted of a composite of death, MI, or need for repeat revascularization at 96 hours (11.0% vs 5.6% in the group of patients treated with prolonged hirudin therapy), hirudin did not improve the primary endpoint of restenosis (Fig. 19-2) [55••].

Studies of Bivalirudin in Percutaneous Transluminal Coronary Angioplasty

In an open-label, dose escalation study involving 258 patients undergoing elective angioplasty [56•], bivalirudin was used as a substitute for heparin. Five groups of approximately 50 patients each were treated with five successive bolus doses (0.15, 0.25, 0.35, 0.45, and 0.55 mg/kg body weight) matched with five successive infusion doses (0.6, 1.0, 1.4, 1.8, and 2.2 mg/kg per hour). Bivalirudin resulted in a dose-dependent anticoagulant effect and no increase in bleeding complications. The incidence of major and minor angioplasty complications, including abrupt vessel closure,

MI, or the need for emergency bypass surgery, was reduced in patients treated with the highest two doses compared with the lower doses (Fig. 19-3). This study [56•] established a dose-response curve for bivalirudin at the lower end of the dosing range, demonstrated for the first time that coronary angioplasty could be performed with a direct thrombin inhibitor in place of heparin, and provided the basis for a controlled comparison of bivalirudin with heparin in patients undergoing coronary angioplasty.

In the Hirulog Angioplasty Study [57••], 4098 patients with postinfarction or unstable angina were randomly assigned to treatment with either bivalirudin or heparin during angioplasty. Aspirin was given to all patients in an oral dose of 300 to 325 mg. In this double-blind study, patients assigned to heparin therapy were given a bolus of 175 U/kg, followed by an 18- to 24-hour infusion of 15 U/kg. The dosing of heparin was based on several factors. First, consensus was reached among investigators in 1992 that the minimum ACT should be 350 seconds during angioplasty and that heparin should be given overnight after angioplasty for high-risk patients with unstable or postinfarction angina. Second, it was also concluded that dosing of heparin should be adjusted by weight in parallel with the weight-adjusted dosing of bivalirudin. Third, observations made in the heparin registry in patients with unstable angina suggested that the standard practice was to achieve a median ACT of 375 seconds with a median 24-hour dose of 41,100 units of heparin, which was equivalent to 178 U/kg bolus plus 15 U/kg/h for 24 hours [58,59]. Fourth, additional observations were made in 90 consecutive unstable patients undergoing angioplasty at three participating institutions that a heparin bolus of 150 to 175 U/kg was required to achieve a minimum ACT of 350 to 400 seconds during the procedure, heparin could be administered at a rate of 1000 U/h overnight, and no bleeding complications were observed. In a subset of 30 patients in whom serial ACT monitoring was obtained, the peak ACT was recorded in the laboratory with a steady decline to approximately 200 seconds 18 to 24 hours after angioplasty.

Patients randomly assigned to bivalirudin therapy were given a bolus of 1.0 mg per kilogram of body weight, followed by a 4-hour infusion of 2.5 mg/kg/h, and a 14- to 20-hour infusion of 0.2 mg/kg/h. The dosing of bivalirudin was based on observations in the phase II study [56•] that a bolus of 0.55 mg/kg followed by 2.2 mg/kg/h resulted in a median ACT of 352 seconds. The bivalirudin concentrations associated with the highest doses in this study resulted in systemic concentrations of drug (10 μM) [56•] that exceeded the expected concentrations of thrombin measured in coronary arterial blood during coronary angioplasty (0.5 nM) [8•] as well as the inhibition con-

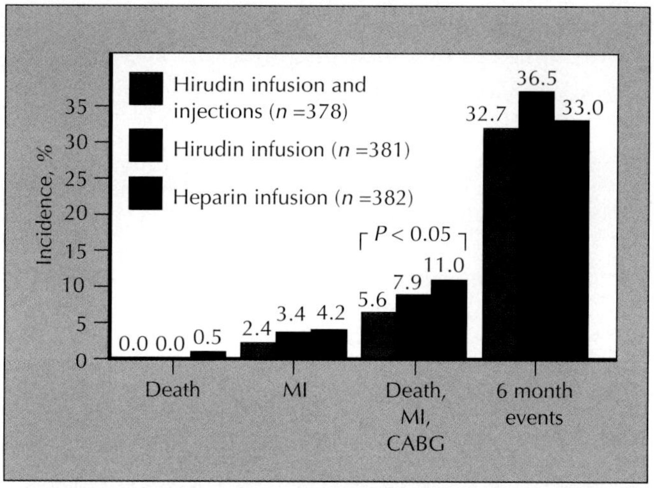

Figure 19-2. Major and minor ischemic complications in patients receiving hirudin or heparin during angioplasty. The incidence of death, myocardial infarction (MI), or the composite at 96 hours is shown. The cumulative incidence of any major complication or need for revascularization at 7 months is presented. The dosing of anticoagulants involved either a hirudin infusion alone (40 mg intravenous bolus plus 0.2 mg/kg intravenously per hour for 24 hours), hirudin infusion plus prolonged subcutaneous therapy (40 mg intravenous bolus plus 0.2 mg/kg intravenously per hour for 24 hours plus 40 mg subcutaneously twice daily for 72 hours), or heparin infusion (10,000 IU intravenous bolus plus 15 IU/kg intravenously per hour for 24 hours). CABG—emergency coronary artery bypass surgery. (*From* Serruys and colleagues [55••]; with permission.)

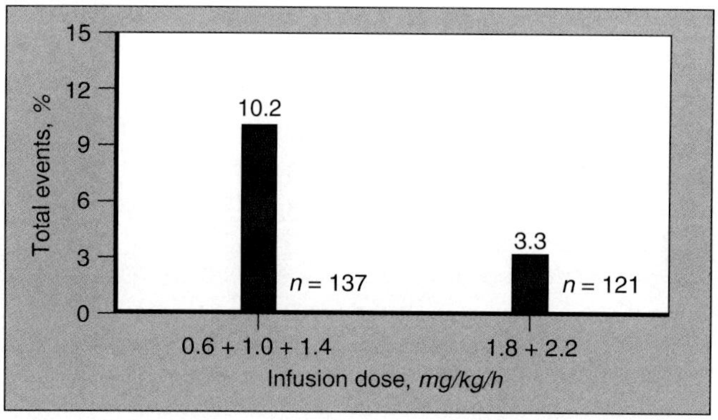

Figure 19-3. Major and minor ischemic complications in patients receiving bivalirudin or heparin during angioplasty. The total incidence of death, myocardial infarction, emergency bypass surgery, or abrupt vessel closure is shown for patients receiving five different infusion doses of bivalirudin during and after angioplasty. The incidence of complications was reduced in patients receiving the highest two doses of the direct thrombin inhibitor. (*Adapted from* Topol and colleagues [56•])

stant of bivalirudin (2 nM) [16] by more than three orders of magnitude. In order to verify that the level of anticoagulation achieved with bivalirudin given overnight matched that achieved with heparin, 12 consecutive patients were treated at one participating institution with the dosing regimen used in the protocol. This produced a median peak ACT of 360 seconds during the procedure, and a median nadir ACT of 190 seconds 24 hours later.

During the study, blinding of personnel was achieved by having the research pharmacist prepare three syringes for bolus administration and two infusion bags for the 4-hour and 14- to 20-hour infusions of study drug. No labeling information revealed whether the syringes or bags contained heparin or bivalirudin. Patients randomly assigned to heparin or to bivalirudin had an infusion bag change at 4 hours, even though no change in dose was made for the heparin-treated patients. ACTs (Hemochron; International Technidyne, Edison, NJ) were measured at 5 minutes and 45 minutes after the first bolus of study drug. If the value was less than 350 seconds, a saline bolus was given to bivalirudin-assigned patients, and a heparin bolus of 60 units per kilogram was given to heparin-assigned patients.

As compared with heparin therapy in the entire cohort of patients, bivalirudin did not reduce the likelihood of in-hospital death (odds ratio [OR] 2.2 [95% CI, 0.7–2.2]; $P = 0.27$), Q-wave or non–Q-wave MI (OR 0.8 [0.6–1.1]; $P = 0.20$), or emergency bypass surgery (OR 1.0 [0.6–1.6]; $P = 1.00$) [57••]. The use of bivalirudin was not associated with a significant reduction in the incidence of abrupt vessel closure, which was defined nonrestrictively as either 1) established closure in the presence of total or subtotal occlusion with TIMI (Thrombolysis In Myocardial Infarction) grade 0 to 1 flow [60,61] or 2) threatened closure in the presence of greater than 50% diameter stenosis and reduced TIMI flow, requiring additional therapy with intracoronary stenting, thrombolytic therapy, or return to the cardiac catheterization laboratory [59,62]. No differences in the cumulative incidence of death, MI, or need for revascularization were seen at 6-month follow-up (Fig. 19-4).

For patients with postinfarction angina, however, bivalirudin produced a significant reduction in the incidence of MI (OR 0.4 [0.2–0.9]; $P = 0.04$) or any complication of death, MI, or emergency bypass surgery (OR 0.4 [0.2–0.9]; $P = 0.03$). This difference, however, had disappeared at the 6-month follow-up evaluation (Fig. 19-5).

In the Hirulog Angioplasty Study, the overall rates of ischemic complications were lower than anticipated from the pilot study using heparin anticoagulation [59]. Of the 2039 heparin-treated patients in the Hirulog Angioplasty Study, 0.2% of the patients died, 1.7% required bypass surgery, and 3.9% experienced Q-wave or non–Q-wave MI. The overall rate of major

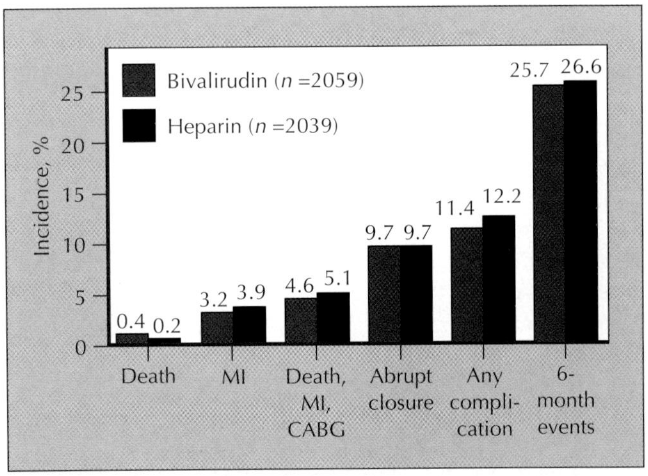

Figure 19-4. Major and minor ischemic complications in patients receiving bivalirudin or heparin during angioplasty performed for unstable angina. The incidence of death, Q-wave or non–Q-wave myocardial infarction (MI), emergency coronary artery bypass surgery (CABG), abrupt vessel closure, or the composite during hospitalization is shown. The cumulative incidence of any major complication or need for revascularization at 6 months is presented. (*Adapted from* Bittl and colleagues [57••]; with permission.)

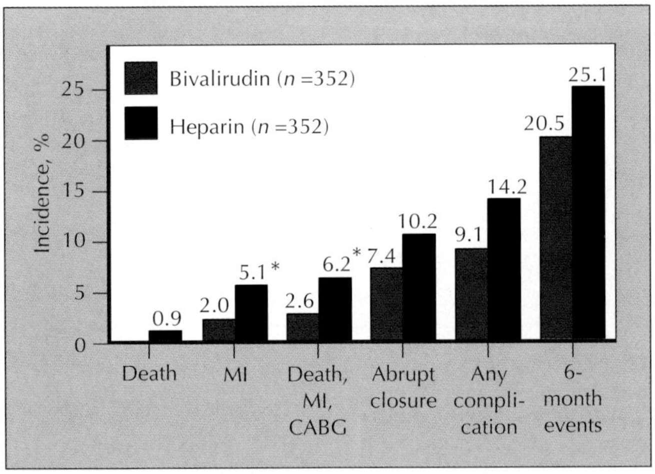

Figure 19-5. Major and minor ischemic complications in patients receiving bivalirudin or heparin during angioplasty performed for postinfarction angina. The incidence of death, Q-wave or non–Q-wave myocardial infarction (MI), emergency coronary artery bypass surgery (CABG), abrupt vessel closure, or the composite during hospitalization is shown. The cumulative incidence of any major complication or need for revascularization at 6 months is presented. *Asterisks* indicate $P < 0.05$. (*Adapted from* Bittl and colleagues [57••]; with permission.)

complications (4.8%) seen in the Hirulog Angioplasty Study was lower than the 7.6% rate seen in the heparin registry using identical definitions and methods for data quality assurance [59] and lower than the rates reported in several other studies of patients with unstable angina [22]. Because the heparin dosing used in the Hirulog Angioplasty Study was associated with a low incidence of MI, the comparison treatment involving new antithrombotic therapy would have to result in a MI rate of less than 2% for statistical significance. It is unlikely that any new antithrombotic therapy could achieve this goal.

Bivalirudin and heparin treatment resulted in identical rates of abrupt vessel closure, an ischemic complication predominantly ascribed to thrombus formation currently attributed to intimal dissection or extrusion of atheromatous plaque in about 80% of cases [59,63,64••,65]. Such mechanical disruption is unlikely to respond to improved anticoagulation regimens but may improve with coronary stenting.

Hemorrhagic Complications With Direct Thrombin Inhibitors During Angioplasty

The large studies comparing the direct thrombin inhibitors with heparin indicate that these new agents can be used safely and reduce the risk of bleeding. In the HELVETICA study, the incidence of hemorrhagic complications was equivalent among the three treatment groups. The rate of overt bleeding with a decrease in hemoglobin of 2 g/dL or greater, transfusion, intracranial hemorrhage or retroperitoneal bleeding was 6.2% in patients treated with heparin, 5.5% in patients treated with intravenous hirudin, and 7.7% in patients treated with intravenous and subcutaneous hirudin [55••].

The large randomized double-blind studies of bivalirudin versus high-dose heparin showed substantial reductions in bleeding rates for patients treated with bivalirudin. As compared with heparin (Fig. 19-6), the use of bivalirudin was associated with lower odds of major bleeding complications such as intracranial hemorrhage (OR 0.5; 95% CI, 0.0–5.5; P = 0.62), retroperitoneal bleeding (OR 0.3 [0.1–0.9]; P = 0.02), or erythrocyte transfusion (OR 0.4 [0.3–0.6]; P < 0.001) [57••]. Bivalirudin therapy was associated with no increase in complications involving pulmonary, neurologic, or other organ systems in the 4098-patient study (Fig. 19-7). This finding was explained in part by the observation that patients treated with bivalirudin had lower levels of systemic anticoagulation than those treated with heparin (median ACT, 346 seconds [interquartile range, 305–405] for bivalirudin-treated patients vs 383 seconds [332–450] for heparin-treated patients; P < 0.001). In addition, the doses of heparin used were the highest reported in any study.

Thrombin "Escape" with Direct Thrombin Inhibitors

Unlike the direct thrombin inhibitors, heparin has a multiplicity of actions against clotting factors. Heparin is active against factor IIa, IXa, Xa, XIa, and XIIa. Although the direct thrombin inhibitors potently block the action of activated thrombin, they do not inhibit the generation of thrombin. Thus, several experts have raised the possibility that discontinuation of direct thrombin inhibitors could be associated with the sudden onset of acute ischemic syndromes precipitated by elevated local concentrations of uninhibited thrombin associated with the persistence of the underlying thrombogenic substrate, dissociation of thrombin-antithrombin complexes, or a reduced clearance of thrombin.

Zoldhelyi and colleagues [66] predicted a higher incidence of ischemic events after stopping a direct thrombin inhibitor than after stopping heparin. Because hirudin does not inhibit the activation of thrombin, evidence of persistent thrombin generation is often seen during treatment with direct thrombin inhibitors [66]. This concern was also raised in a study of the inhibition and generation of thrombin in the presence of thrombin inhibitors carried out in plasma.

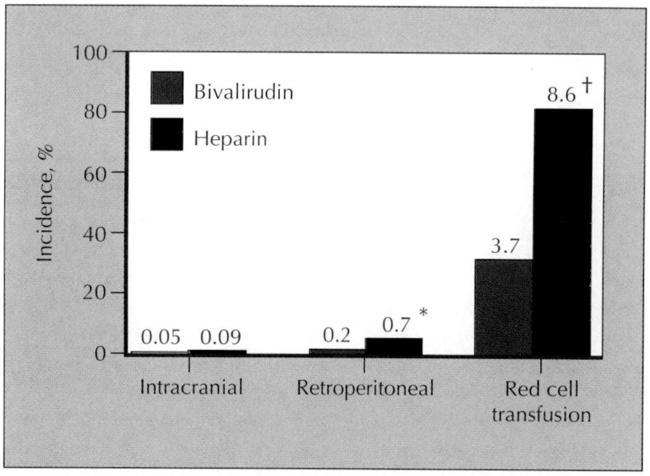

Figure 19-6. Bleeding complications in patients receiving bivalirudin or heparin during angioplasty performed for unstable or postinfarction angina. The incidence of intracranial hemorrhage, retroperitoneal hemorrhage, or red cell transfusion is shown. *Asterisk* indicates P = 0.02; *dagger* indicates P < 0.001. (*Adapted from* Bittl and colleagues [57••]; with permission.)

Activation of citrated plasma was accompanied by the sudden onset of thrombin generation after a delay of about 2 minutes. Addition of 50 ng hirudin/mL or 0.1 U heparin/mL prolonged the clotting time to 3 minutes. Thrombin generation and F_{1+2} was significantly lower in heparinized plasma than in hirudinized plasma, suggesting that heparin was more effective than hirudin in inhibiting the action of factor Xa [67].

Analogous clinical results observed in the biochemical substudy in HELVETICA [55••] provided interesting insights into the comparison of the actions of heparin and hirudin. Heparin therapy was associated with a reduction in the generation of thrombin, as determined by the levels of prothrombin fragment F_{1+2} (1.0 nM before balloon dilatation vs 0.9 nM after dilatation), whereas hirudin administered intravenously and subcutaneously was associated with a slight increase in levels of F_{1+2} (1.0 nM vs 1.3 nM). Although hirudin was at least as effective as heparin in inhibiting activated thrombin, increased thrombin generation at the time of discontinuation of anticoagulant therapy theoretically increased the risk of

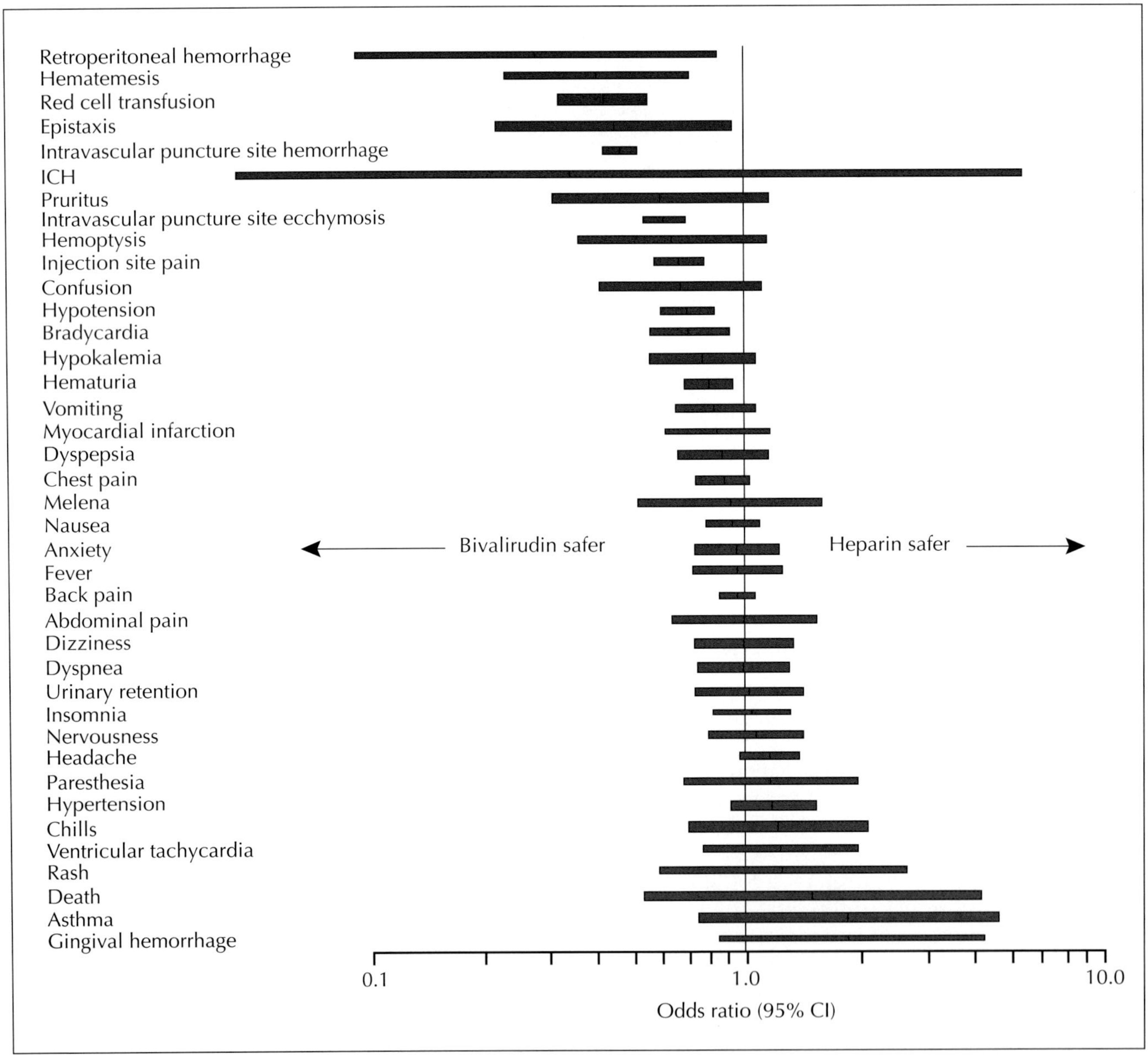

Figure 19-7. Adverse events. The odds of adverse events is given for patients treated with bivalirudin or heparin. The statistical reliability of the odds ratio is given by the 95% CIs. ICH—intracranial hemorrhage. (*From* Bittl and colleagues [74]; with permission.)

"thrombin rebound," but this was not observed in the study [55••].

The possibility of ischemic rebound was directly evaluated in the Hirulog Angioplasty Study [57••]. In the Hirulog Angioplasty Study, the timing of major complications such as death, MI, or emergency bypass was carefully reported by blinded study personnel. After discontinuation of either heparin or bivalirudin at 18 to 24 hours, 25 of 2039 patients (1.2%) who had received heparin therapy experienced a major complication, whereas only seven of 2059 patients treated with bivalirudin (0.3%) experienced a complication [68]. These clinical results are consistent with the absence of ischemic rebound reported after discontinuation of hirudin in TIMI 5 [20].

Heparin-Induced Thrombocytopenia and Thrombosis

Mediated by the action of heparin, platelet factor 4, and IgG, the syndrome of heparin-induced thrombocytopenia is a complex illness that frequently leads to arterial thrombosis, venous thrombosis, or both. The syndrome can be prevented by the use of low molecular weight heparin [69], but once it appears, low molecular weight heparin is no longer recommended. Several studies have suggested that direct thrombin inhibitors are safe in the treatment of patients with this syndrome. Chamberlin and colleagues [70] successfully treated three patients with bivalirudin without ischemic or bleeding complications. Bivalirudin has also been used for heparin-associated thrombocytopenia and deep venous thrombosis [71].

Direct Thrombin Inhibitors and Platelet Glycoprotein IIb/IIIa Inhibitors

Because of the possibility that multiple redundant pathways may lead to platelet activation during coronary angioplasty, arterial thrombus formation may nonetheless proceed in the presence of complete thrombin inhibition. The final common pathway for platelet aggregation is mediated by the exposure of the platelet glycoprotein IIb/IIIa fibrinogen receptor. It is thus reasonable to evaluate the combination of a thrombin inhibitor and simultaneous inhibition of the more distal steps in platelet aggregation mediated by the IIb/IIIa receptor to provide an optimal approach in preventing arterial thrombus formation. In a canine model of intracoronary thrombosis, the combination of tissue plasminogen activator (1 mg/kg over 20 minutes) together with the platelet glycoprotein IIb/IIIa receptor inhibitor Integrelin (Cor Therapeutics, San Francisco, CA) (2.5 μg/kg per minute for 90 minutes) and the direct thrombin inhibitor hirudin (10 μg/kg per minute for 90 minutes) was associated with more complete restoration of coronary flow and reduced the reocclusion rate more than the use of either Integrelin or hirudin alone [72].

Conclusions

Results from several randomized controlled studies establish the principle that the direct thrombin inhibitors hirudin and bivalirudin are safe substitutes for heparin during coronary angioplasty. Therapy with these agents results in at least equivalent efficacy as heparin but a lower risk of bleeding in patients who undergo angioplasty for unstable angina. Hirudin therapy is associated with a lower risk of in-hospital complications in patients undergoing angioplasty for unstable angina. Bivalirudin therapy is associated with a lower risk of ischemic complications than heparin in patients who undergo angioplasty for postinfarction angina, suggesting that the complications of angioplasty performed in this setting are mediated by thrombin.

The treatment effect of the direct thrombin inhibitors appears to be weaker than that for the platelet glycoprotein IIb/IIIa receptor inhibitors (*see* Chapters 13 to 16). This difference is ascribed to the different sites of action between the two classes of drugs. The thrombin inhibitors block only one of many pathways leading to platelet activation, whereas the IIb/IIIa receptor blockers inhibit the final common pathway of platelet aggregation.

As compared with heparin, the use of direct thrombin inhibitors may theoretically improve the clinical outcome and reduce the risk of PTCA for lesions in degenerated saphenous vein grafts, for lesions causing AMI, and for thrombus-containing lesions requiring coronary stenting. Further areas of investigation involving direct thrombin inhibitors in angioplasty should focus on these settings where the consequences of increased thrombus burden are substantial, or where the risk of heparin is unacceptable, as in the syndrome of heparin-associated thrombocytopenia and thrombosis.

REFERENCES AND RECOMMENDED READING

Recently published papers of particular interest have been highlighted as:
- • Of special interest
- •• Of outstanding interest

1. Fuster V, Badimon JJ, Badimon L: Clinical-pathological correlations of coronary disease progression and regression. *Circulation* 1992, 86 (suppl III):1–11.
2. Fuster V, Badimon L, Badimon JJ, *et al.*: The pathophysiology of coronary artery disease and the acute coronary syndromes. *N Engl J Med* 1992, 326:242–250; 310–318.
3. Fernández-Ortiz A, Badimon JJ, Falk E, *et al.*: Characterization of the relative thrombogenicity of atherosclerotic plaque components: implications for consequences of plaque rupture. *J Am Coll Cardiol* 1994, 23:1562–1569.
4. Annex BH, Denning SM, Channon KM, *et al.*: Differential expression of tissue factor protein in directional atherectomy specimens from patients with stable and unstable coronary syndromes. *Circulation* 1995, 91:619–622.
5. Banner DW, D'Arcy A, Chene C, *et al.*: The crystal structure of the complex of blood coagulation factor VIIa with soluble tissue factor. *Nature* 1996, 380:41–46.
6. Strony J, Beaudoin A, Brands D, *et al.*: Analysis of shear stress and hemodynamic factors in a model of coronary artery stenosis and thrombosis. *Am J Physiol* 1993, 265:H1787–H1796.
7. Merino A, Cohen M, Badimon JJ, *et al.*: Synergistic action of severe wall injury and shear forces on thrombus formation in arterial stenosis: definition of a thrombotic shear rate threshold. *J Am Coll Cardiol* 1994, 24:1091–1094.
8. • Marmur JD, Merlinie PA, Sharma SK, *et al.*: Thrombin generation in human coronary arteries after percutaneous transluminal balloon angioplasty. *J Am Coll Cardiol* 1994, 24:1484–1491.

The only study directly assessing the generation of thrombin in coronary angioplasty.

9. Young E, Prins M, Levine MN, *et al.*: Heparin binding to plasma proteins, an important mechanism for heparin resistance. *Thromb Haemost* 1992, 67:639–643.
10. Hirsh J, van Aken WG, Gallus AS, *et al.*: Heparin kinetics in venous thrombosis and pulmonary embolism. *Circulation* 1976, 53:691–695.
11. Ferguson JJ, Dougherty KG, Gaos CM, *et al.*: Relation between procedural activated coagulation time and outcome after percutaneous transluminal coronary angioplasty. *J Am Coll Cardiol* 1994, 23:1061–1065.
12. • Narins CR, Hillegass WB Jr, Nelson CL, *et al.*: Relation between activated clotting time during angioplasty and abrupt closure. *Circulation* 1996, 93:660–671.

A comprehensive analysis of the relation between ischemic complications of angioplasty activated clotting time achieved with heparin.

13. Eitzmann DT, Chi L, Saggin L, *et al.*: Heparin neutralization by platelet-rich thrombi: role of platelet factor 4. *Circulation* 1994, 89:1523–1529.
14. Hogg PJ, Jackson CM: Fibrin monomer protects thrombin from inactivation by heparin antithrombin III: implications for heparin efficacy. *Proc Natl Acad Sci U S A* 1989, 86:3619–3623.
15. Weitz JI, Hudoba M, Massel D, *et al.*: Clot-bound thrombin is protected from inhibition by heparin-antithrombin III but is susceptible to inactivation by antithrombin III-independent inhibitors. *J Clin Invest* 1990, 86:385–391.
16. Maraganore JM, Bourdon P, Jablonski J, *et al.*: Design and characterization of hirulogs: a novel class of bivalent peptide inhibitors of thrombin. *Biochemistry* 1990, 29:7095–7101.
17. Gast A, Tschipp TB, Schmid G, *et al.*: Inhibition of clot-bound and free (fluid-phase thrombin) by a novel synthetic thrombin inhibitor (R0 46-6240), recombinant hirudin and heparin in human plasma. *Blood Coagul Fibrinolysis* 1994, 5:879–887.
18. Monreal M, Angles AM, Monreal L, *et al.*: Effects of recombinant hirudin on D dimer levels before and after experimental venous thrombosis. *Hemostasis* 1994, 24:338–343.
19. Hamelink JK, Tang DB, Barr CF, *et al.*: Inhibition of platelet deposition by combined hirulog and aspirin in a rat carotid endarterectomy model. *J Vasc Surg* 1995, 21:492–498.
20. Cannon CP, McCabe CH, Henry TD, *et al.*: A pilot trial of recombinant desulfatohirudin compared with heparin in conjunction with tissue-type plasminogen activator and aspirin for acute myocardial infarction: results of the Thrombolysis in Myocardial Infarction (TIMI) 5 Trial. *J Am Coll Cardiol* 1994, 23:993–1003.
21. Carteaux JP, Gast A, Tschopp TB, *et al.*: Activated clotting time as an appropriate test to compare heparin and direct thrombin inhibitors such as hirudin or Ro 46-6240 in experimental arterial thrombosis. *Circulation* 1995, 91:1568–1574.
22. de Feyter PJ, Serruys PW: Percutaneous transluminal coronary angioplasty for unstable angina. In *Textbook of Interventional Cardiology*, edn 2. Edited by Topol EJ. Philadelphia: WB Saunders Co; 1994:274–291.
23. de Feyter PJ, Serruys PW, Soward A, *et al.*: Coronary angioplasty for early postinfarction unstable angina. *Circulation* 1986, 74:1365–1370.
24. Holt GW, Sugrue DD, Bresnahan JF, *et al.*: Results of percutaneous transluminal coronary angioplasty for unstable angina pectoris in patients 70 years of age and older. *Am J Cardiol* 1988, 61:994–997.
25. Gottlieb SO, Walford GD, Ouyang P, *et al.*: Initial and late results of coronary angioplasty for early postinfarction unstable angina. *Cathet Cardiovasc Diagn* 1987, 13:93–99.
26. Safian RD, Snyder LD, Snyder BA, *et al.*: Usefulness of percutaneous transluminal coronary angioplasty for unstable angina pectoris after non–Q-wave acute myocardial infarction. *Am J Cardiol* 1987, 59:263–266.

27. Hopkins J, Savage M, Zalewski A, *et al.*: Recurrent ischemia in the zone of prior myocardial infarction: result of coronary angioplasty of the infarct-related artery. *Am Heart J* 1988, 115:14–19.

28. Suryapranata H, Beatt K, de Feyter PJ, *et al.*: Percutaneous transluminal coronary angioplasty for angina pectoris after a non–Q-wave acute myocardial infarction. *Am J Cardiol* 1988, 61:240–243.

29. Morrison DA: Coronary angioplasty for medically refractory unstable angina in patients with prior coronary bypass surgery. *Cathet Cardiovasc Diagn* 1990, 20:174–181.

30. TIMI Study Group Phase II Trial: Comparison of invasive and conservative strategies after treatment with intravenous tissue plasminogen activator in acute myocardial infarction. *N Engl J Med* 1989, 320:618–627.

31. Timmis AD, Griffin B, Crick JC, *et al.*: Early percutaneous transluminal coronary angioplasty in the management of unstable angina. *Int J Cardiol* 1987, 14:25–31.

32. de Feyter PJ, Suryapranata H, Serruys PW, *et al.*: Coronary angioplasty for unstable angina: immediate and late results in 200 consecutive patients with identification of risk factors for unfavorable early and late outcome. *J Am Coll Cardiol* 1988, 12:324–333.

33. Thijs Plokker HW, Ernst SM, Bal ET, *et al.*: Percutaneous transluminal coronary angioplasty in patients with unstable angina pectoris refractory to medical therapy: long-term clinical and angiographic results. *Cathet Cardiovasc Diagn* 1988, 14:15–18.

34. Sharma B, Wyeth RP, Kilath GS, *et al.*: Percutaneous transluminal coronary angioplasty of one vessel for refractory unstable angina pectoris: efficacy in single and multivessel disease. *Br Heart J* 1988, 59:280–286.

35. Perry RA, Seth A, Hunt A, *et al.*: Coronary angioplasty in unstable angina and stable angina: a comparison of success and complications. *Br Heart J* 1988, 60:367–372.

36. Myler RK, Shaw RE, Stertzer SH, *et al.*: Unstable angina and coronary angioplasty [review]. *Circulation* 1990, 82:II-88–II-95.

37. Morrison DA: Percutaneous transluminal coronary angioplasty for rest angina pectoris requiring intravenous nitroglycerin and intra-aortic balloon counterpulsation. *Am J Cardiol* 1990, 66:168–172.

38. Rupprecht HJ, Brennecke R, Kottmeyer M, *et al.*: Short- and long-term outcome after percutaneous transluminal coronary angioplasty in patients with stable and unstable angina. *Eur Heart J* 1990, 11:964–969.

39. Quigley PJ, Erwin J, Maurer BJ, *et al.*: Percutaneous transluminal coronary angioplasty in unstable angina. *Br Heart J* 1986, 55:227–230.

40. Steffenino G, Meier B, Finci L, *et al.*: Follow up results of treatment of unstable angina by coronary angioplasty. *Br Heart J* 1987, 57:416–419.

41. Stammen F, de Scheerder I, Glazier JJ, *et al.*: Immediate and follow-up results of the conservative coronary angioplasty strategy for unstable angina pectoris. *Am J Cardiol* 1992, 69:1533–1537.

42. Bredlau CE, Roubin G, Leimgruber P, *et al.*: In-hospital morbidity and mortality in patients undergoing elective coronary angioplasty. *Circulation* 1985, 72:1044–1052.

43. Hartzler G: Complex coronary angioplasty: multivessel/multilesion dilatation. In *Practice of Coronary Angioplasty.* Edited by Ischinger T. New York: Springer-Verlag; 1986:250–267.

44. Holmes DR Jr, Holubkov R, Vlietstra RE, *et al.*: Comparison of complications during percutaneous transluminal angioplasty from 1977 to 1981 and from 1985 to 1986: The National Heart, Lung, and Blood Institute Percutaneous Transluminal Coronary Angioplasty Registry. *J Am Coll Cardiol* 1988, 12:1149–1155.

45. Tuzcu EM, Simpfendorfer C, Badhwar K, *et al.*: Determinants of primary success in elective percutaneous transluminal coronary angioplasty for significant narrowing of a single major coronary artery. *Am J Cardiol* 1988, 62:873–875.

46. de Feyter PJ, van den Brand M, Serruys PW: Increase of initial success and safety of single-vessel PTCA in 1371 patients: a seven-years' experience. *J Intervent Cardiol* 1988, 1:1–10.

47. O'Keefe JH Jr, Reeder GS, Miller GA, *et al.*: Safety and efficacy of percutaneous transluminal coronary angioplasty performed at time of diagnostic catheterization compared with that performed at other times. *Am J Cardiol* 1989, 63:27–29.

48. Myler RK, Shaw RE, Stertzer SH, *et al.*: Lesion morphology and coronary angioplasty: current experience and analysis. *J Am Coll Cardiol* 1992, 19:1641–1652.

49. Dimas AP, Grigera F, Arora RR, *et al.*: Repeat coronary angioplasty as treatment for restenosis. *J Am Coll Cardiol* 1992, 19:1310–1314.

50. Weintraub WS, Ghazzal ZMB, Douglas JS, *et al.*: Initial management and long-term clinical outcome of restenosis after initially successful percutaneous transluminal coronary angioplasty. *Am J Cardiol* 1992, 70:47–55.

51. Alfonso R, Macaya C, Iniquez A, *et al.*: Repeat coronary angioplasty during the same angiographic diagnosis of coronary restenosis. *Am Heart J* 1990, 119:237–241.

52. Meier B, King SB III, Gruentzig AR, *et al.*: Repeat coronary angioplasty. *J Am Coll Cardiol* 1984, 4:463–466.

53. Topol EJ, Fuster V, Harrington RA, *et al.*: Recombinant hirudin for unstable angina pectoris: a multicenter, randomized angiographic trial. *Circulation* 1994, 89:1557–1566.

54. Sarembock IJ, Gertz SD, Gimple L, *et al.*: Effectiveness of recombinant desulphatohirudin in reducing restenosis after balloon angioplasty of atherosclerotic femoral arteries in rabbits. *Circulation* 1991, 84:232–243.

55.•• Serruys PW, Herrman J-PR, Simon R, *et al.*: A comparison of hirudin with heparin in the prevention of restenosis after coronary angioplasty. *N Engl J Med* 1995, 333:757–763.

A randomized, controlled, double-blind comparison of heparin with hirudin in patients undergoing angioplasty for unstable angina.

56.• Topol EJ, Bonan R, Jewitt D, *et al.*: Use of a direct antithrombin, hirulog, in place of heparin during coronary angioplasty. *Circulation* 1993, 87:1622–1629.

The first demonstration that a direct thrombin inhibitor could be used safely as as substitute for heparin during angioplasty.

57.•• Bittl JA, Strony J, Brinker JA, *et al.*: Treatment with bivalirudin (Hirulog) as compared with heparin during coronary angioplasty for unstable or postinfarction angina. *N Engl J Med* 1995, 333:764–769.

A large randomized, controlled, double-blind comparison of bivalirudin with hirudin in patients undergoing angioplasty for unstable angina.

58. Grassman ED, Leya F, Johnson SA, *et al.*: Percutaneous transluminal coronary angioplasty for unstable angina: predictors of outcome in a multicenter study. *J Thromb Thrombolys* 1994, 1:73–78.

59. Wolfe MW, Roubin GS, Schweiger M, *et al.*: Length of hospital stay and complications after percutaneous transluminal coronary angioplasty: clinical and procedural predictors. *Circulation* 1995, 92:311–319.

60. The TIMI Research Group: Immediate vs delayed catheterization and angioplasty following thrombolytic therapy for acute myocardial infarction: TIMI II A results. *JAMA* 1988, 260:2849–2858.

61. Detre KM, Holmes DR Jr, Holubkov R, *et al.*: Incidence and consequences of periprocedural occlusion: The 1985-1986 National Heart, Lung, and Blood Institute Percutaneous Transluminal Coronary Angioplasty Registry. *Circulation* 1990, 82:739–750.

62. Roubin GS, Cannon AD, Agrawal SK, *et al.*: Intracoronary stenting for acute and threatened closure complicating percutaneous transluminal coronary angioplasty. *Circulation* 1992, 85:916–927.

63. Lincoff AM, Popma JJ, Ellis SG, *et al.*: Abrupt vessel closure complicating coronary angioplasty: clinical, angiographic and therapeutic profile. *J Am Coll Cardiol* 1992, 19:926–935.

64.•• White CJ, Ramee SR, Collins TJ, *et al.*: Coronary angioscopy of abrupt occlusion after angioplasty. *J Am Coll Cardiol* 1995, 25:1681–1684.

This angioscopic study was the first complete evaluation to provide unexpected insights into the pathogenesis of abrupt vessel closure. Only three of 14 patients (18%) had evidence of intracoronary thrombus formation, whereas the majority had large dissection or extruded plaque as the cause of vessel closure.

65. Sassower MA, Abela GS, Koch JM, *et al.*: Angioscopic evaluation of periprocedural and postprocedural abrupt closure after percutaneous coronary angioplasty. *Am Heart J* 1993, 126:444–450.

66. Zoldhelyi P, Bichler J, Owen WG, *et al.*: Persistent thrombin generation in humans during specific thrombin inhibition with hirudin. *Circulation* 1994, 90:2671–2678.

67. Gallistl S, Muntean W: Thrombin-hirudin complex formation, thrombin-antithrombin III complex formation, and thrombin generation after intrinsic activation of plasma. *Thromb Haemost* 1994, 72:387–392.

68. Strony J, Ahmed WH, Meckel CR, *et al.*: Clinical evidence for thrombin rebound after stopping heparin but not Hirulog [abstract]. *Circulation* 1995, 92:I-609.

69. Warkentin TE, Levine MN, Hirsh J, *et al.*: Heparin-induced thrombocytopenia in patients treated with low-molecular weight heparin or unfractionated heparin. *N Engl J Med* 1995, 332:1330–1335.

70. Chamberlin JR, Lewis B, Leya F, *et al.*: Successful treatment of heparin-associated thrombocytopenia and thrombosis using Hirulog. *Can J Cardiol* 1995, 11:511–514.

71. Reid T III: Hirulog therapy for heparin-associated thrombocytopenia and deep venous thrombosis [letter]. *Am J Hematol* 1994, 45:352–353.

72. Nicolini FA, Lee P, Rios G, *et al.*: Combination of platelet fibrinogen receptor antagonist and direct thrombin inhibitor at low doses markedly improves thrombolysis. *Circulation* 1994, 89:1802–1809.

73. Stein B, Furster V, Halperin JL, Chesebro JH: Antithrombotic therapy in cardiac disease. *Circulation* 1989, 80:1501–1513.

74. Bittl JA, on behalf of the Hirulog Angioplasty Study Investigators: Comparative safety profiles of hirulog and heparin in patients undergoing coronary angioplasty. *Am Heart J* 1995, 130:658–665.

Chapter 20

Clinical and Experimental Studies of Newer Antithrombins

Iftikhar J. Kullo
David R. Holmes, Jr.
Robert S. Schwartz

Clinical antithrombotic therapy has changed little during the past few decades, with heparin and warfarin being the mainstays of anticoagulant therapy during this period. These two agents remain the only widely available choices for antithrombotic treatment of the majority of cardiovascular and cerebrovascular diseases. These agents have several limitations (Table 20-1). Treatment of acute coronary syndromes with anticoagulants, thrombolysis, mechanical interventions, or surgery may be marked by resistant thrombotic complications. Thus, 15% to 20% of patients with unstable angina do not respond to conventional therapy with aspirin and heparin and may go on to develop myocardial infarction (MI) and recurrent ischemic pain.

Therapy for such events in the form of coronary artery bypass grafting (CABG) or percutaneous transluminal coronary angioplasty (PTCA) has a high rate of complications. The operative mortality with coronary artery bypass is 3.7% and the incidence of perioperative MI is 10% [1]. PTCA within 1 week of onset of unstable angina was reported to be associated with Q-wave MI in 6.5%, and emergency surgery in 9.4% [2]. The lack of inactivation of clot-bound thrombin by heparin, platelet activation, and a relative resistance to heparin associated with a thrombogenic state may account for some of the complications. Newer antithrombins that do not have these limitations are being studied for use in acute coronary syndromes and as adjuncts to fibrinolysis and angioplasty. These agents have the potential for more effective, more specific, and safer inhibition of the various steps of the coagulation cascade. In this chapter, we review the details of these newer antithrombins with emphasis on clinical and experimental studies.

Biology of Thrombin

Thrombin is a serine protease that plays a central role in thrombogenesis [3] (Figure 20-1). Thrombin cleaves fibrinogen to fibrin monomers, which polymerize to form the matrix of the clot, and activates factor XIII, which stabilizes the clot by cross-linking the fibrin. Additionally, thrombin-induced platelet aggregation contributes to the evolution of thrombus and provides a surface for assembly of protease-cofactor complexes that are involved in the coagulation cascade. Activation of factors V and VIII by thrombin stimulates thrombin generation in a positive feedback loop. Thrombin also initiates a series of reactions to activate endogenous anticoagulant mechanisms. By complexing with thrombomodulin, thrombin activates protein C, and becomes incapable of cleaving fibrinogen and factor V and activating platelets [4].

Besides coagulation, thrombin has effects on the vascular wall cells. Thrombin inhibits endothelial cell proliferation, induces endothelial expression of leukocyte adhesion molecules [5], stimulates vascular smooth muscle cell proliferation [6], and modulates matrix production by smooth muscle cells [7].

Table 20-1. Limitations of Heparin

Pharmacokinetic
Half-life influenced by dose administered
Heparin binds to plasma proteins and the endothelium, resulting in low bioavailability at low doses, variability in dose response, and heparin resistance in certain patients
Hemostatic
Interferes with platelet function
Increases vessel wall permeability
Functional
Inability to catalyze the inactivation of clot-bound thrombin as well as that bound to fibrin degradation products and extracellular matrix
Actions neutralized by platelet factor 4
Clinical
Requires careful laboratory monitoring when given in therapeutic doses
Incidence of major hemorrhage of 2% to 8% when given in therapeutic doses
Heparin-associated thrombocytopenia syndrome
Prolonged use may cause osteoporosis

Direct Thrombin Inhibitors

X-ray crystallography has enhanced our knowledge about the structure and specificity of thrombin and its interactions with substrates and inhibitors. There are three distinct functional domains of the thrombin molecule (Figure 20-2). The active or catalytic binding site is located in a deep, narrow canyon in the surface of the molecule; the anion binding exosite contains the fibrinogen recognition site; and the apolar binding site, located near the active site, may also be important for fibrin binding [8].

Thrombin inhibitors can be characterized as direct or indirect (Table 20-2). Direct inhibition involves interaction with one or more domains of thrombin (Table 20-3). Indirect inhibitors either interfere with thrombin generation or require a cofactor to inhibit the thrombin molecule. Heparin and warfarin, the two most widely used anticoagulants, are indirect thrombin inhibitors.

Hirudin

Hirudin is a 65-amino-acid protein originally isolated from the medicinal leech [9]. Initially extracted from homogenized leech heads, hirudin is now generated by the use of recombinant DNA technology. Recombinant hirudin is weakly allergenic [10].

Hirudin consists of two domains that interact with thrombin over an extended surface area (Figure 20-3). The N-terminal domain is a compact structure that binds to the active site region, whereas the extended negatively charged carboxy terminal domain binds along a groove leading to the anion-binding exosite. These domains have been identified and sequenced, leading to the synthesis of hirudin-like peptides with similar biologic properties.

Hirudin is absolutely specific for thrombin and does not inhibit other serine proteases. The inhibition is direct, does not require any cofactors, and is not influenced by systemic factors.

Hirudin is administered intravenously and is also well absorbed by the subcutaneous and intramuscular routes. Excretion is mostly renal and follows first-order kinetics, with a plasma half-life of approximately 40 minutes. Dose reduction is recommended in patients with renal insufficiency. Intravenous hirudin causes a rapid, dose related, reproducible prolongation of the activated partial thromboplastin time (APTT), clotting time, and thrombin time. Plasma levels can be assessed by radioimmunobioassay, enzyme-linked immunosorbent assay, and by thrombin inhibition.

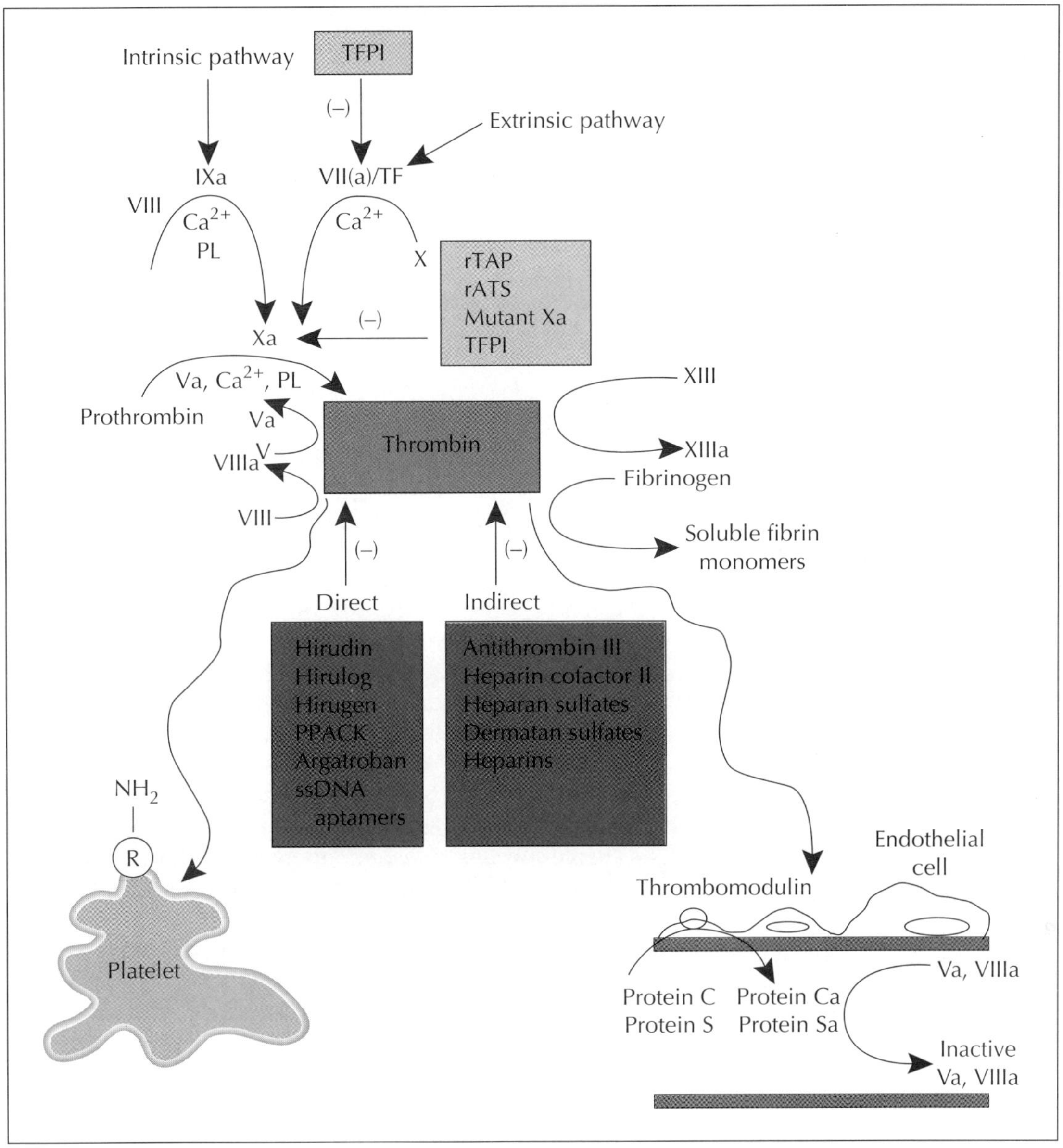

Figure 20-1 The mechanism of thrombin generation and the different drugs that interfere with this process. PPACK—D-Phe-Pro-Arg-chloromethyl ketone; rATS—recombinant peptide antistatin; rTAP—recombinant tick anticoagulant peptide; TFPI—tissue factor pathway inhibitor. (*Adapted from* Scharfstein and colleagues [64]; with permission.)

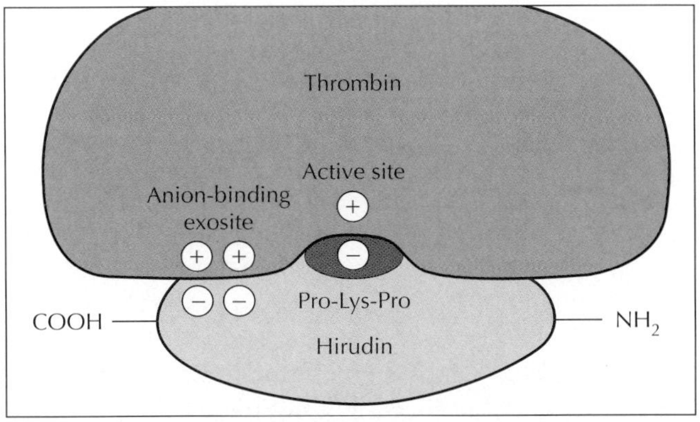

Figure 20-2. The hirudin–thrombin interaction, illustrating the trivalent binding of hirudin to thrombin. The amino terminal region of hirudin binds to the apolar region of thrombin, hirudin's Pro 46-Lys 47-Pro 48 region binds to thrombin's active site, and the highly acidic carboxy terminal region of hirudin binds to thrombin's anion binding exosite. PPACK—D-Phe-Pro-Arg-chloromethyl ketone. (*Adapted from* Scharfstein and Loscalzo [65].)

Hirudin has been used in the management of unstable angina, MI, and as an adjunct to thrombolysis and PTCA. The clinical studies with hirudin are discussed briefly below and summarized in Tables 20-4 through 20-6.

Management of unstable angina and myocardial infarction

Topol and colleagues [11] in a multicenter open-label pilot trial, randomly assigned 166 patients with unstable angina and angiographic thrombus to a 72- to 120-hour infusion of heparin or recombinant hirudin at five escalating doses. All patients received aspirin and anti-ischemic therapy. At similar APTT prolongations,hirudin improved angiographic endpoints compared with high-dose heparin. However, the improvement in TIMI (Thrombosis In Myocardial Infarction) flow grade was not significant and clinical outcomes at 30 days did not differ, although MI developed in 2% of hirudin and 8% of heparin recipients ($P < 0.11$).

In the open-label TIMI-5 pilot study, patients with acute myocardial infarction (AMI) were treated with front-loaded recombinant tissue plasminogen activator (t-PA) plus aspirin and randomly assigned to either heparin or hirudin [12]. A higher rate of reperfusion and a decreased reocclusion rate in the hirudin group resulted in a significantly improved TIMI flow grade at 18 to 26 hours, although there had been no difference at 90 minutes. Incidence of major bleeding was 4.7% in the heparin group and 1.2% in the hirudin group.

In the TIMI-6 pilot trial, patients with MI were treated with streptokinase and aspirin and were randomly assigned to heparin or one of three doses of hirudin. Patients treated with higher dose hirudin (0.1 to 0.2 mg/kg/h) did better than those treated with lower dose hirudin (0.05 mg/kg/h) and heparin [13]. The incidence of major hemorrhage was similar between the heparin group and all hirudin groups. At hospital discharge, the occurrence of death, nonfatal reinfarction, congestive heart failure, or cardiogenic shock was greater in patients receiving the lowest dose of hirudin (21.6%) than in those receiving the higher doses of hirudin (dose 2, 9.7%; dose 3, 11.4%).

In the HIT-III (Hirudin for Improvement of Thrombolysis) trial, patients were randomly assigned to a 48- to 72-hour infusion of either hirudin (0.4 mg/kg bolus, followed by 0.15 mg/kg/h infusion) or heparin after front-loaded t-PA and aspirin [14].

Table 20-2. Thrombin Inhibitors

Direct inhibitors
Hirudin
Hirulog
Hirugen
Argatroban
PPACK
Thrombin aptamers
DUP-714
Hirudisins
Thrombin receptor blockers
Receptor antagonist peptides
Thrombin generation inhibitors
Factor Xa inhibitors
Antistasin
Tick anticoagulant peptide
Inactivated factor X
Tissue factor pathway inhibitor
Antithrombin dependent
Heparin
Low molecular weight heparins
Heparinoids
Recombinant and endogenous anticoagulants
Activated protein C
Antithrombin III
Heparin cofactor I
Tissue factor pathway inhibitor

PPACK—D-Phe-Pro-Arg-chloromethyl ketone.

Table 20-3. Three Sites of Action for Direct Thrombin Inhibitors

Anion binding exosite
Hirudin
Hirulog
Hirugen
Active site
Hirudin
Hirulog
PPACK
Argatroban
Apolar region
Hirudin

PPACK—D-Phe-Pro-Arg-chloromethyl ketone.

This trial was stopped because of an excess of hemorrhagic stroke in the hirudin arm. A trend toward higher APTT was noted in the hirudin group, suggesting that dosage may have been the problem. This trial has been restarted and results will be soon reported.

In the GUSTO (Global Use of Strategies to Open Occluded Coronary Arteries)-IIA, patients with acute coronary syndromes who also received thrombolytics and aspirin were randomly assigned to 3 to 5 days of intravenous fixed-dose hirudin (0.2 mg/kg/h) or weight-adjusted heparin [15]. Although recruitment of 12,000 patients was planned, the trial was stopped early because of excess intracerebral hemorrhagic events after 2564 patients were enrolled. At the dose of hirudin tested, there was a trend toward excess of hemorrhagic stroke compared with heparin. Heparin itself was accompanied by a twofold risk of hemorrhagic stroke in patients receiving thrombolytic therapy. With both thrombin inhibitors, the APTT was a useful index for predicting the risk of hemorrhagic stroke. The trial was restarted as GUSTO-IIB, recruiting 12,142 patients with acute coronary syndromes

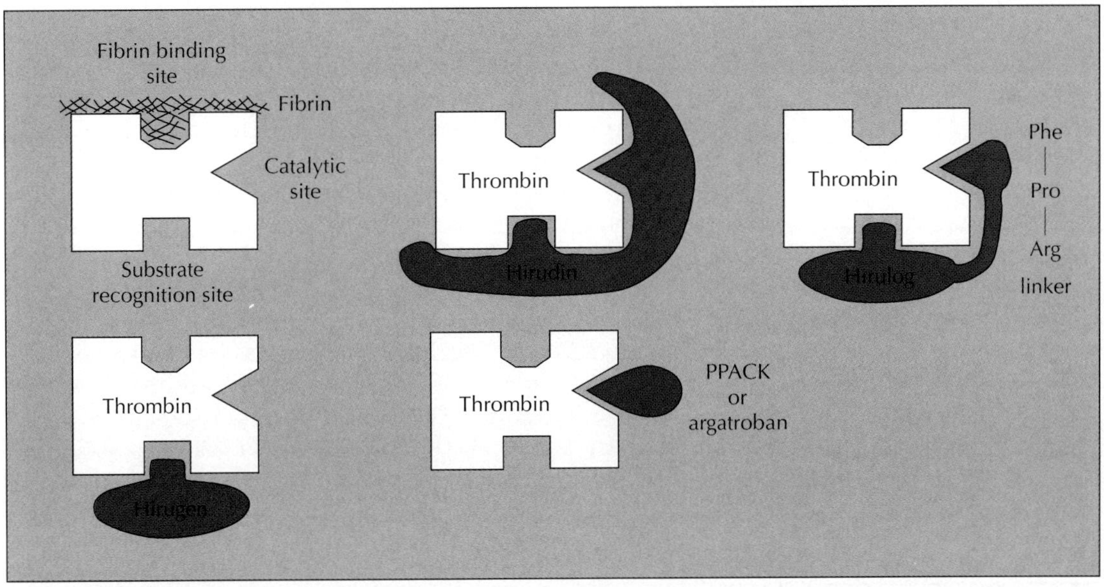

Figure 20-3. The thrombin molecule, with its key binding sites. Thrombin interactions with the direct thrombin inhibitors hirudin, hirulog, hirugen, PPACK (D-Phe-Pro-Arg-chloromethyl ketone), and argatroban are illustrated. (*Adapted from* Lefkovitz and Topol [66••].)

TABLE 20-4. RESULTS OF VARIOUS STUDIES USING DIRECT THROMBIN INHIBITORS IN UNSTABLE ANGINA

Study	Drug	Patients, *n*	Design	Endpoints	Results
Lidon *et al.* [23]	Hirulog	40	Dose ranging	Clinical efficacy	95% success rate with 1 mg/kg/h
Sharma *et al.* [60]	Hirulog	20	Observational	Clinical efficacy Angiographic findings	Intractable angina (5%) Coronary thrombus (5%)
Gold *et al.* [61]	Argatroban	43	Dose ranging	Clinical efficacy Rebound	100% success 21% rebound
Fuchs and Cannon [24]	Hirulog	410	Dose ranging	Clinical efficacy	Decreased death or nonfatal MI at discharge and 6-wk follow-up
Topol *et al.* [62]	Hirudin	140	Dose ranging Randomized with heparin control	Angiographic findings	Improved minimal luminal diameter as compared with heparin

MI—myocardial infarction.

from 13 countries [16]. Patients were randomly assigned to 72 hours of therapy with either heparin (5000 U bolus followed by 1000 U/h) or hirudin (0.1 mg/kg bolus followed by 0.1 mg/kg/h). About one third of the patients had Q-wave MI (ST elevation on the electrocardiogram), and the remainder had either unstable angina or non–Q-wave MI. There was a significant reduction in death and MI at 24 hours in the hirudin-treated group. At 30 days, there was a lower incidence of death and nonfatal myocardial (re)infarction in the hirudin treated group (P = 0.058). There was a slightly more proportionate benefit in the group with ST elevation. There were no significant differences in serious or life-threatening bleeding complications, but hirudin led to an excess of moderate bleeding events (8.8% vs 7.7%; P = 0.03).

The TIMI-9 trial, a randomized, double-blinded study conducted in 150 clinical centers, was designed to compare the efficacy and safety of intravenous heparin versus hirudin in patients with AMI (< 12 hours from onset) treated with a thrombolytic agent (streptokinase or t-PA) [17]. The TIMI-9A study (n = 757) was suspended in April 1994 because of excessive bleeding in both heparin and hirudin groups. TIMI-9B was restarted with lower doses of both heparin and hirudin [18]. The primary endpoint of the study (n = 3002) was the 30-day incidence of death, MI, congestive heart failure, and shock. At 30 days there was no significant difference in the primary endpoint between heparin (11.8%) and hirudin (12.8%) and no difference in the incidence of death and MI (9.3% in the heparin group, 9.6% in the hirudin group). Moreover, there was no difference in major bleeding events, including intracranial hemorrhage, between treatment groups. The investigators concluded that hirudin was as effective but not superior to heparin as an adjunct to thrombolysis in the treatment of MI.

Use of hirudin in percutaneous transluminal coronary angioplasty

In a double-blind pilot trial, 113 low-risk patients with stable angina undergoing PTCA were randomly assigned to a 24-hour infusion of either hirudin or heparin, with doses adjusted to a target APTT of 85 to 120 seconds [19]. Acute closure, leading to MI or coronary bypass surgery, occurred in 10.3% of patients randomly assigned to heparin, but only 1.4% of patients receiving hirudin. None of the differences in this small pilot trial reached statistical significance.

In the HELVETICA (Hirudin in a European Trial vs Heparin in the Prevention of Restenosis after PTCA) trial [20], 1141 patients with unstable angina scheduled for angioplasty were randomly assigned to 1) 10,000 IU of heparin followed by an intravenous infusion for 24 hours and subcutaneous placebo twice daily for 3 days; 2) a bolus dose of 40 mg of hirudin followed by an intravenous infusion of hirudin for 24 hours and subcutaneous placebo twice daily for 3

TABLE 20-5. RESULTS OF VARIOUS STUDIES USING DIRECT THROMBIN INHIBITORS WITH PERCUTANEOUS TRANSLUMINAL CORONARY ANGIOPLASTY

Study	Drug	Patients, *n*	Design	Endpoints	Results
van den Bos *et al.* [19]	Hirudin	113	Randomized Heparin control	MI CABG	1% vs 10% for heparin
Topol *et al.* [11]	Hirulog	291	Dose ranging	Abrupt closure	6.2% (3.9% at high doses vs 11.3% at low doses; P = 0.052)
Serruys *et al.* [20]	Hirudin	1154	Randomized Heparin control	Early complications Restenosis	Significant reduction in early cardiac events; event-free survival at 7 mo not significantly different
Topol *et al.* [11]	Hirulog	291	Dose ranging	Abrupt closure	3.9% to 11.3% incidence

CABG—coronary artery bypass grafting; MI—myocardial infarction.

days; or 3) the same hirudin regimen except that 40 mg of hirudin was given subcutaneously instead of placebo twice daily for 3 days. The primary endpoint was event-free survival at 7 months. Hirudin administration was associated with a significant reduction in early cardiac events occurring in 11%, 7.9%, and 5.6% of patients in the respective groups. At 7 months, however, the event-free survival was not significantly different in the three groups.

Hirulog

Hirulog is a synthetic 20-amino-acid peptide containing the two terminal domains of hirudin joined by a linker domain formed by four glycines [21]. Like hirudin, hirulog blocks the active catalytic site and the anion binding site of the thrombin molecule. Half-life after intravenous administration is 15 to 20 minutes and only 20% is recovered from the urine, suggesting extensive extrarenal metabolism [22].

Management of unstable angina and myocardial infarction

Lidon and colleagues [23] evaluated the efficacy and safety of hirulog in 55 patients with unstable angina in a dose-escalation protocol. With dosages up to 1 mg/kg/h, only one of 20 patients experienced chest pain. In a second dose-finding study [24], hirulog at 0.25 to 1 mg/kg/h given for 72 hours significantly

Table 20-6. Results of Various Studies Using Direct Thrombin Inhibitors in Myocardial Infarction

Study	Drug	Patients, *n*	Design	Endpoints	Results
Tabata *et al.* [63]	Argatroban	22	Heparin control	Angiographic reocclusion	0% vs 15% with heparin
Lidon *et al.* [23]	Hirulog	45	Heparin control	Angiographic patency and reocclusion	80% vs 33% with heparin; no reocclusion
Neuhaus *et al.* [14]	Hirudin	7000 planned	Randomized Heparin control	Mortality and reinfarction	Terminated in July 1994 because of excessive bleeding with hirudin
Cannon *et al.* [12]	Hirudin	260	Randomized Heparin control	Angiographic patency and reocclusion	66% TIMI-3 at 90 min vs 56% with heparin; 2% vs 7% reocclusion; 14% vs 22% bleeding
Lee [13]	Hirudin	193	Randomized Heparin control	Death, MI	Trend toward lower event rates in the hirudin group
Antman [17]	Hirudin	3000 planned	Randomized Heparin control	Mortality	Trial stopped prematurely because of excessive bleeding with heparin and hirudin; restarted with lower doses
GUSTO IIa [15]	Hirudin	12,000 planned	Randomized Heparin control	Mortality	Trial stopped prematurely because of excessive bleeding with heparin and hirudin; restarted with lower doses

MI—myocardial infarction; rHirudin—recombinant hirudin; TIMI—Thrombosis In Myocardial Infarction.

reduced the rate of death or nonfatal reinfarction compared with a dose of 0.02 mg/kg/h. In 45 patients with MI randomly assigned to hirulog (0.5 mg/kg/h) or heparin as an adjunct to streptokinase [23], hirulog had significantly better TIMI-3 patency rates at 90 and 120 minutes. Bleeding complications were similar in the two groups.

Use of hirulog in percutaneous transluminal coronary angioplasty

Topol and colleagues [11] were the first to report use of an anticoagulant other than heparin during coronary angioplasty. Using hirulog, a rapid onset, dose-dependent anticoagulant effect was obtained with minimal bleeding complications. Acute closure at 24 hours was inversely related to the hirulog dosage: 11.3% in patients receiving the three lower doses and 3.9% in those receiving the two higher doses.

Bittl and colleagues [13] randomly assigned 4098 patients with unstable or postinfarction angina to either heparin or hirulog immediately before angioplasty [25]. Hirulog did not significantly reduce the primary endpoint of death, MI, abrupt vessel closure, or rapid clinical deterioration of clinical origin, but did reduce the incidence of bleeding ($P < 0.001$). In a subgroup of postinfarction angina patients, hirulog reduced the risk of immediate ischemic complications, but this difference was no longer apparent after 6 months.

Hirugen

Hirugen, a synthetic hirudin derivative, is a dodecapeptide fragment of the C-terminal region of hirudin. This peptide binds the anion-binding exosite and inhibits thrombin-mediated cleavage of fibrinogen. The catalytic site remains free and hence the antithrombotic activity is weaker than that of hirudin and hirulog [26]. Owing to the weak potency of hirugen, no clinical studies are underway at present.

Argatroban

Argatroban, an arginine derivative and a potent direct thrombin inhibitor, blocks the active site of thrombin. The mode of inhibition is competitive. Argatroban is effective in preventing thrombosis in various animal models and has been licensed in Japan for human use [27]. In a rabbit femoral artery thrombosis model, argatroban (100 µg/kg/min; APTT 2.5 to 3.0 times baseline) accelerated reperfusion compared with heparin (200 IU/kg, APTT > fivefold), although reflow was not increased [28]. In a whole-blood clot thrombus model in stenotic canine coronary arteries, pretreatment with argatroban significantly reduced the time to lysis by t-PA to 23 minutes compared with 40 minutes in the aspirin group. The addition of aspirin to argatroban did not shorten time to lysis, but reduced the incidence of reocclusion by platelet-rich thrombi from 75% to 20%, relative to argatroban alone [29]. In a platelet-rich coronary thrombus model after endothelial injury created by electric current, acceleration of lysis with t-TPA was observed in dogs pretreated with argatroban at a lower dose. Abolition of cyclic flow reduction due to intermittent platelet aggregates required the addition of aspirin [30]. These results suggest that platelet inhibition may help prevent reocclusion when lower affinity antithrombins are used as adjuncts to thrombolysis. Argatroban has been used in the clinical setting in the treatment of thrombotic complications in patients on dialysis and management of heparin-associated thrombocytopenia [27].

PPACK (D-Phe-Pro-Arg-chloromethyl Ketone)

D-Phe-Pro-Arg-chloromethyl ketone (PPACK) specifically inhibits the catalytic site of thrombin by irreversibly alkylating a histidine residue at the active site. Unlike argatroban, PPACK is a noncompetitive thrombin inhibitor. Like other direct thrombin inhibitors, PPACK inhibits both clot-bound and free thrombin with equal potency. The chlormethylketone group is reactive and alkylates cysteine residues in the plasma, hence precluding the use of this agent in clinical studies. PPACK was significantly better than heparin in inhibiting platelet deposition in an ex vivo model of balloon-injured rabbit aortas [31]. A continuous PPACK infusion was significantly better than heparin in abolishing platelet deposition and preventing thrombosis in freshly implanted vascular arterial grafts in primates [32].

In a thrombogenic arteriovenous vascular graft in a porcine model, local delivery of the PPACK effectively inhibited platelet-dependent thrombosis at doses that were several orders of magnitude less than the systemic dose required for an equivalent antithrombotic effect [33]. Similarly, local delivery of PPACK with a hydrogel-coated balloon angioplasty catheter was used to inhibit thrombus formation in a chronic porcine arteriovenous shunt model [34]. In contrast to systemic administration, local delivery of PPACK thus produces maximal inhibition of thrombosis without alterations in hemostasis.

Thrombin Aptamers

Thrombin aptamers are single-stranded DNA oligonucleotides developed after a novel in vitro amplification and selection technique [35]. Aptamers bind the fibrinogen recognition site of the thrombin molecule and have been shown to have potent antithrombotic effects in vitro and in animal models of thrombosis. Thrombin-induced platelet aggregation is specifically inhibited. There is a linear relationship between the infusion rate and the prolongation of the prothrombin time. The aptamers have a rapid onset of action (within 10 minutes) and a short half-life (less than 2 minutes), and may be useful for anticoagulation in extracorporeal circuits and in acute coronary syndromes [36].

DUP-714

DUP-714 is a boroarginine tripeptide that binds thrombin with moderately high affinity and inhibits thrombin-mediated platelet activation and fibrinogen cleavage [37]. Although the compound is an effective anticoagulant in experimental models, it has caused hepatotoxicity in animals, and human studies have not been pursued.

Hirudisins

Hirudisins are hirudin derivatives that combine blockade of platelet IIb/IIIa receptor with thrombin inhibition. Residues 32-35 of hirudin have been replaced by the integrin motif RGDS and KGDS, creating a potent thrombin inhibitor with additional disintegrin activity [38].

Other Thrombin Inhibitors

Low Molecular Weight Heparins

Low molecular weight heparins (LMWH) are fragments of commercial heparin that have been produced by chemical or enzymatic depolymerization of the polysaccharide chains. Mean molecular weights range from 3000 to 6000 D. They possess the pentasaccharide sequence for binding to antithrombin III, but have fewer longer 16-saccharide chains to bind thrombin. Consequently, they selectively catalyze the inhibition of factor Xa by antithrombin III. Advantages over standard heparin include 1) greater bioavailability owing to less binding to plasma proteins and to endothelial cells, 2) longer half-life independent of dose (and hence more predictable results), 3) they are not neutralized by platelet factor 4, and 4) there is less bleeding, at an equivalent antithrombotic effect [39]. Table 20-7 compares LMWH with heparin and hirudin [40].

In the FRISC (Fragmin During Instability in Coronary Artery Disease Study Group) study, 1506 patients with acute coronary syndromes were randomly assigned to subcutaneous dalteparin (Fragmin;

Table 20-7. Comparison of Some Properties of Unfractionated Heparin, Low Molecular Weight Heparin, and Hirudin

Unfractionated heparin	LMWH	Hirudin
Inhibits thrombin and VIIa to the same extent	Inhibits mainly Xa and, to some extent, thrombin	Specific and potent inhibitor of thrombin
Antithrombin III dependent	Antithrombin III dependent	Antithrombin III independent
Neutralized by heparinase, several plasma proteins, platelet activator 4, and endothelium	Neutralized by heparinase; weak endothelial binding	Not neutralized by heparinase, endothelium, macrophages, fibrin monomers, proteins, and platelet activator 4
Does not inactivate clot-bound thrombin and factor VII	Dose not inactivate clot-bound thrombin and factor VII	Inactivates clot-bound thrombin
Inhibits platelet function	Inhibits platelet function	Prevents platelet aggregation induced by thrombin but not other platelet agonists
Induced thrombocytopenia is not rare	Can induce thrombocytopenia	Does not induce thrombocytopenia
Bioavailability after subcutaneous injection is 30%	Bioavailablity after subcutaneous injection is 90%	Good bioavailability (≈ 80%) after subcutaneous injection
Poor dose-effect response	Fair dose-effect response	Fair dose-effect response
Not immunogenic	Not immunogenic	Not or barely immunogenic
Increases vascular permeability	No increases in vascular permeability	No increases in vascular permeability

LMWH—low molecular weight heparin.

Pharmacia, Dublin, OH), 120 IU/kg twice daily for 6 days, and then 7500 IU once daily for the next 35 to 45 days or placebo injections [41••]. The primary endpoints were death and MI in the first 6 days after the event. Secondary events were the rates of death and new MI after 40 and 150 days, the frequency of revascularization procedures, and the need for heparin infusion and a composite endpoint. The primary, secondary, and composite endpoints were favorably affected by dalteparin. Four months after the end of treatment, there were no significant differences in the rate of death, new MI, or revascularization. The authors recommended a combination of dalteparin and aspirin for at least 6 days in patients with unstable coronary artery disease.

Antistasin

Antistasin, a 119-amino-acid polypeptide derived from the salivary gland of the Mexican leech, binds specifically and reversibly to factor Xa. The cDNA for antistasin has been used to generate the recombinant peptide, rATS. A single subcutaneous injection has potent anticoagulant activity for more than 30 hours. Antistatin has been found superior to heparin in preventing platelet-rich thrombi in dacron-grafted arteriovenous femoral grafts in the baboon [42]. Even at fully antithrombotic doses, template bleeding times were not significantly increased. These results demonstrated that selective inhibition of coagulation factor Xa by rATS can completely prevent vascular graft thrombus formation without significantly compromising primary hemostasis as measured by template bleeding time. When used as an adjunct to alteplase in a canine model of femoral artery thrombosis, the time to reperfusion was dramatically reduced with a 2.5 μg/kg/min dose [43]. Clinical studies have been precluded by the high immunogenicity of the compound.

The recombinant peptide rATS reduces neointimal formation after balloon angioplasty in rabbits [44]. Focal femoral atherosclerosis was induced by air dessication and a high-cholesterol diet in 38 New Zealand white rabbits. rATS was administered by intravenous bolus at the time of balloon angioplasty and followed by a 2-hour infusion; control arteries received bolus heparin alone (150 U/kg). Therapeutic prolongation of the APTT occurred in all animals. Restenosis defined as a reduction in angiographic luminal diameter (in mm) from 2 hours after angioplasty to 28 days after angioplasty, was less in the rATS group.

Tick Anticoagulant Peptide

Tick anticoagulant peptide (TAP) is a single polypeptide consisting of 60 amino acids. It was isolated from the soft tick *Ornithodoros moubata* in 1990 and later produced in recombinant form (rTAP). It is a potent and selective inhibitor of factor Xa with the several interesting and potentially clinically useful properties. It has the ability to inhibit factor Xa already assembled in the prothrombinase complex. Also like other factor Xa inhibitors, rTAP blocks an early step in the coagulation cascade and inhibits the generation of thrombin rather than the activity of thrombin already present. Finally, the binding of rTAP to factor Xa is long lasting, suggesting that short-term therapy with rTAP may achieve long-term inhibition at the site of arterial injury [45]. rTAP has shown efficacy in several animal models of thrombosis. In a rabbit model of venous thrombosis, in which internal jugular vein thrombosis is induced with rabbit brain thromboplastin, rTAP caused a dose-dependent decrease in clot weight and was superior to heparin in this respect [46]. In a canine coronary artery model of platelet-rich thrombosis and stenosis, the time to reperfusion by alteplase was shortened from 40 minutes in animals receiving heparin 200 IU/kg compared with 23 minutes with TAP 6 mg/kg/h. The incidence of reocclusion in this model was lower in the TAP group than in the hirudin group (three of eight vs six of eight animals). Thus, TAP and hirudin both significantly increased the incidence of reperfusion and accelerated its rate compared with a saline control and rTAP also showed a trend toward reducing the incidence of reocclusion compared with control, hirudin, and heparin [47].

In a porcine coronary artery injury model, rTAP, when given in fully anticoagulant doses for 60 hours after the injury, resulted in a long-term decrease in neointimal thickness at 28 days [48••]. Like the previous studies mentioned with Xa inhibitors, this study implicates thrombin generation in neointimal formation. Short-term administration of a potent antithrombotic agent may therefore influence the long-term outcome of the coronary arterial injury by a decreasing neointima formation.

TAP may be useful in the management of heparin-resistant thrombosis and as an adjunct to thrombolysis. The therapeutic window is broader than with direct thrombin inhibitors and immunogenicity is low. However, high cost is a limitation.

Mutant Factor Xa

Mutant Factor Xa (Asn_{322}-Ala_{419}) competes with native factor Xa for assembly in the prothrombinase complex, forming an inactive product and inhibiting thrombin generation. To date there are no published clinical investigations involving this agent.

Tissue Factor Pathway Inhibitor

Tissue factor pathway inhibitor (TFPI) is a serum protein with protease activity that has an inhibitory effect on tissue factor [49•]. It inhibits the extrinsic pathway of coagulation by forming a quarternary complex with tissue factor, factor VIIa, and calcium. It also has a direct inhibitory action on factor Xa. TFPI has an affinity for heparin and potentiates its anticoagulant effects [50]. Recombinant TFPI (rTFPI) is an effective antithrombotic drug in an ex vivo model of thrombogenesis [51]. In a canine model of femoral artery thrombosis produced by transluminal electric injury, rTFPI significantly decreased the incidence of reocclusion after rt-PA–induced thrombolysis. However, if the injury was caused by implantation of copper wires—which causes minimal damage to the vessel wall—and produced fibrin-rich rather than platelet-rich thrombi, rTFPI had no significant effect on the incidence of reocclusion [52]. rTFPI has dose-related antithrombotic activity in experimental venous thrombosis induced in rabbits by a combination of endothelial damage and restricted blood flow [53]. In a rabbit model of vascular trauma, topical application of TFPI prevented thrombosis [54]. These studies underline the importance of tissue factor in triggering thrombosis and the potential of rTFPI as an antithrombotic agent. Treatment with TFPI for 3 days in a rabbit atherosclerotic femoral artery injury model reduced angiographic restenosis and decreased neointimal hyperplasia compared with controls, highlighting the importance of early initiators of the extrinsic coagulation pathway, especially factor VII and tissue factor, in the response to arterial injury [55].

Protein C

The protein C–thrombomodulin-protein S system provides a negative feedback regulation of coagulation. Recombinant activated protein C (rAPC) infusions in experimental animals have had antithrombotic effects in the absence of APTT prolongation. In a primate model of arterial thrombosis, rAPC significantly reduced the incidence of graft occlusion and platelet deposition compared with controls [56].

Antithrombin III

Antithrombin III serves as a cofactor for the endogenous glycosaminoglycan, heparan sulfate, as well as for heparin. The resulting complex inhibits thrombin and thrombin-mediated activation of factors V and VIII as well as factors IXa, Xa, and XIIa. Although primarily given as replacement for states of congenital antithrombin III deficiency, recombinant antithrombin III has potential for use as an antithrombotic agent.

Adverse Effects of Direct Thrombin Inhibitors

Risk of Bleeding

Bleeding is the major adverse effect of direct thrombin inhibitors, although theoretically the incidence of bleeding should be low because of their specificity, lack of direct platelet effects, and short half-life. Early experience suggests acceptable bleeding rate profiles both in the normal population as well as in patients with coronary artery disease. In large-scale trials like GUSTO-II and TIMI-9, however, an excess of hemorrhagic stroke was seen in patients simultaneously receiving thrombolytic therapy. High bolus doses have been incriminated in a higher incidence of bleeding. Lack of an effective antidote to rapidly terminate the effects of thrombin inhibitors is a disadvantage.

Problems with laboratory monitoring may contribute to the risk of bleeding. There are several problems with the use of the APTT as a marker for antithrombotic effect after the use of antithrombins. The recent interruption of clinical trials because of excessive bleeding in patients with acute coronary syndromes suggests that patients treated with hirudin were over-anticoagulated despite APTT in the 85- to 100-second range [14,15]. The APTT, unlike prothrombin time (PT), shows considerable interassay variations. Various pharmocokinetic studies suggest that the dose response of hirudin to the APTT is flat and might make it a relatively inaccurate monitoring test [57]. In the GUSTO-IIB trial [16], however, hirudin achieved a consistent anticoagulation as monitored by the APTT. The value of the activated clotting time (ACT) to predict the antithrombotic effect of direct thrombin inhibitors has been demonstrated in an arterial thrombosis model in the guinea pig [58]. The appropriate laboratory ranges of APTT and other in vitro anticoagulant tests need to be established in large scale trials evaluating these agents over wide dosage ranges and in varied clinical settings.

Rebound

No rebound phenomena have been noted thus far with the use of hirudin or hirulog. This may be due to concomitant aspirin ingestion, which has been shown to protect against heparin-associated rebound. Rebound occurred in 23% of patients in a study of argratroban for unstable angina. This suggests the possibility of renewed thrombin activity and thrombus generation with diminishing plasma levels of direct antithrombins. In several recent trials of newer antithrombins, including GUSTO-IIB and the FRISC study [16,20,43], the benefits are seen early on and diminish with time. This phenomenon may be due to continued thrombin generation and possibly platelet activation.

Cost

A major disadvantage of the direct thrombin inhibitors is the cost. A 3-day course of hirudin costs more than $1000. Because heparin performs quite well as an anticoagulant in most trials, it is still the standard therapy, and the routine use of newer antithrombins at present is not justified. The convenience in monitoring therapy, the small clinical benefit seen in several trials, and the somewhat increased bleeding risk need to be thought of when considering the newer antithrombins in select patients. Further studies, including cost-benefit analyses, need to be done to determine indications for the use of these agents in acute coronary syndromes and as adjuncts during coronary interventions.

Future Directions

The newer antithrombins allow a strong and specific inhibition of thrombin with acceptable safety profiles. Efforts to increase selectivity and activity of thrombin inhibitors continue. Lack of effect on thrombin generation with the direct inhibitors remains a problem. Continuing platelet activation may also occur in the face of thrombin inhibition, owing to the multiple pathways of platelet activation other than thrombin. A combination of direct thrombin inhibition and platelet IIb/IIa blockade may circumvent this. Such an approach is efficacious in experimental models [59] and has potential as a therapy in the future. Developing specific inhibitors of thrombin receptors may allow inhibition of platelet and vascular smooth muscle cell activation without affecting the coagulatory function of thrombin. Such substances may have potential use in limiting restenosis.

References and Recommended Reading

Recently published papers of particular interest have been highlighted as:
- • Of special interest
- •• Of outstanding interest

1. Kaiser B, Fareed J, Hoppensteadt D, *et al.*: Influence of recombinant hirudin and unfractionated heparin on thrombin and factor Xa generation in extrinsic and intrinsic activated systems. *Thromb Res* 1992, 65:157–164.
2. Myler R, Shaw R, Sterzer SH: Unstable angina and coronary angioplasty. *Circulation* 1990, 82(suppl II):88–95.
3. Maraganore J: Thrombin, thrombin inhibitors, and the arterial thrombotic process. *Thromb Haemost* 1993, 70:208–211.
4. Esmon CT: The protein C anticoagulant pathway. *Arterioscler Thromb* 1992, 12:135–145.
5. Libby P, Warner S, Friedman G: Interleukin 1: a mitogen for human vascular smooth muscle cells that induces the release of growth-inhibitory prostanoids. *J Clin Invest* 1988, 81:487–498.
6. McNamara C, Sarembock I, Gimple L, *et al.*: Thrombin stimulates proliferation of cultured rat aortic smooth muscle cells by a proteolytically activated receptor. *J Clin Invest* 1993, 91:94–98.
7. Graham D, Alexander J, Miguel R: Aortic endothelial and smooth muscle cell co-culture: an in vitro model of the arterial wall. *J Clin Invest* 1992, 90: 190–194.
8. Stubbs M, Oschkinat H, Mayr I, *et al.*: The interaction of thrombin with fibrinogen: a structural basis for its specificity. *Eur J Biochem* 1992, 206:187–195.
9. Markwardt F: The development of hirudin as an antithrombotic drug. *Thromb Res* 1994, 74:1–23.
10. Close P, Bichler J, Kerry R, *et al.*: Weak allergenicity of recombinant hirudin CGP 39393 (REV ASC) in immunocompetent volunteers: The European Hirudin in Thrombosis Group (HIT Group). *Coronary Artery Disease* 1994, 5:943–949.
11. Topol E, Bonan R, Jewitt D, *et al.*: Use of a direct antithrombin, hirulog, in place of heparin during coronary angioplasty. *Circulation* 1993, 87:1622–1629.
12. Cannon C, McCabe C, Henry T, *et al.*: A pilot trial of recombinant desulfatohirudin compared with heparin in conjunction with tissue-type plasminogen activator and aspirin for acute myocardial infarction: results of the Thrombolysis in Myocardial Infarction (TIMI) 5 trial. *J Am Coll Cardiol* 1994, 23:993–1003.
13. Lee L: Initial experience with hirudin and streptokinase in acute myocardial infarction: results of the Thrombolysis in Myocardial Infarction (TIMI) 6 trial. *Am J Cardiol* 1995, 75:7–13.
14. Neuhaus K, von Essen R, Tebbe U, *et al.*: Safety observations from the pilot phase of the randomized r-Hirudin for Improvement of Thrombolysis (HIT-III) study: a study of the Arbeitsgemeinschaft Leitender Kardiologischer Krankenhausarzte (ALKK). *Circulation* 1994, 90:1638–1642.
15. GUSTO IIa Investigators: Randomized trial of intravenous heparin versus recombinant hirudin for acute coronary syndromes: the Global Use of Strategies to Open Occluded Coronary Arteries (GUSTO) IIa Investigators. *Circulation* 1994, 90:1631–1637.
16. Gusto IIB Investigators: A comparision of recombitant hirudin with heparin for the treatment of acute coronary syndromes. *N Eng J Med* 1996, 335:775–782.

17. Antman EM for the TIMI 9B Investigators: Hirudin in acute myocardial infarction: Thrombolysis and Thrombin Inhibition in Myocardial Infarction (TIMI) 9B Trial. *Circulation* 1996, 94:911–921.

18. Ferguson JJ: Meeting highlights. American Heart Association 68th Scientific Sessions, Anaheim, CA, November 13 to 15, 1995. *Circulation* 1996, 93:843–846.

19. van den Bos, Deckers JW, Heyndrickx GR, *et al.*: Safety and efficacy of recombinant hirudin (CGP 39 393) versus heparin in patients with stable angina undergoing coronary angioplasty. *Circulation* 1993, 88:2058–2066.

20. Serruys PW, Herrman JP, Simon R, *et al.*: A comparison of hirudin with heparin in the prevention of restenosis after coronary angioplasty: Helvetica Investigators. *N Engl J Med* 1995, 333:757–763.

21. Maraganore J, Chao B, Joseph M, *et al.*: Anticoagulant activity of synthetic hirudin peptides. *J Biol Chem* 1989, 264:8692–8698.

22. Maraganore J: Pre-clinical and clinical studies on hirulog: a potent and specific direct thrombin inhibitor. *Adv Exp Med Biol* 1993, 340:227–236.

23. Lidon R, Theroux P, Juneau M, *et al.*: Initial experience with a direct antithrombin, hirulog, in unstable angina: anticoagulant, antithrombotic, and clinical effects. *Circulation* 1993, 88(4 pt 1):1495–1501.

24. Fuchs J, Cannon C: Hirulog in the treatment of unstable angina: results of the Thrombin Inhibition in Myocardial Ischemia (TIMI) 7 trial. *Circulation* 1995, 92:727–733.

25. Bittl J, Strony J, Brinker J, *et al.*: Treatment with bivalirudin (hirulog) as compared with heparin during coronary angioplasty for unstable or postinfarction angina: Hirulog Angioplasty Study Investigators. *N Engl J Med* 1995, 333:764–769.

26. Skrzypczak J, Carperos V, Ravichandran K, *et al.*: Structure of the hirugen and hirulog 1 complexes of α-thrombin. *J Mol Biol* 1991, 221:1379–1393.

27. Matsuo T, Kario K, Kodama K, Okamoto S: Clinical application of the synthetic thrombin inhibitor, argatroban (MD-805). *Semin Thromb Hemost* 1992, 18:155–160.

28. Jang I, Gold HK, Zikind AA, *et al.*: Prevention of platelet rich thrombosis by selective thrombin inhibition. *Circulation* 1990, 81:219–225.

29. Yasuda T, Gold H, Yaoita H, *et al.*: Comparative effects of aspirin, a synthetic thrombin inhibitor, and a monoclonal antibody on coronary artery reperfusion, reocclusion, and bleeding with recombinant tissue type plasminogen activator in a canine preparation. *J Am Coll Cardiol* 1990, 16:714–722.

30. Gold H, Yasuda T, Jang K, *et al.*: Animal models for arterial thrombolysis and prevention of reocclusion: erythrocyte-rich versus platelet-rich thrombus. *Circulation* 1991, 83 (suppl 6):26–40.

31. Kaplan A, Leung L, Leung W, *et al.*: Roles of thrombin and platelet membrane glycoprotein IIb/IIIa in platelet-subendothelial deposition after angioplasty in an ex vivo whole artery model. *Circulation* 1991, 84:1279–1288.

32. Hansen SR, Harker L: Interruption of acute platelet-dependent thrombosis by the synthetic antithrombin D-phenylalanine-L-prolyl-L-arginyl chloromethyl ketone. *Proc Natl Acad Sci U S A* 1988, 85:3188–3194.

33. Scott N, Nunes G, King S, *et al.*: Local delivery of an antithrombin inhibits platelet-dependent thrombosis. *Circulation* 1994, 90:1951–1955.

34. Nunes G, Hanson S, King S, *et al.*: Local delivery of a synthetic antithrombin with a hydrogel-coated angioplasty balloon catheter inhibits platelet-dependent thrombosis. *J Am Coll Cardiol* 1994, 23:1578–1583.

35. Bock L, Griffin L, Latham J, *et al.*: Selection of single-stranded DNA molecules that bind and inhibit human thrombin. *Nature* 1992, 355:564–566.

36. Griffin L, Tidmarsh G, Bock L, *et al.*: In vivo anticoagulant properties of a novel nucleotide-based thrombin inhibitor and demonstration of regional anticoagulation in extracorporeal circuits. *Blood* 1993, 81:3271–3276.

37. Kettner C, Mersinger L, Knabb R: The selective inhibition of thrombin by peptides of boroarginine. *J Biol Chem* 1990, 265:18289–18297.

38. Knapp A, Degenhardt T, Dodt J: Hirudisins: hirudin-derived thrombin inhibitors with disintegrin activity. *J Biol Chem* 1992, 267:24230–24234.

39. Cosmi B, Hirsh J: Low molecular weight heparins. *Curr Opin Cardiol* 1994, 9:612–618.

40. Zoldhelyi P, Verstraete M: Novel antithrombotic drugs in development. *Drugs* 1995, 49:860–884.

41.•• FRISC Study: Fragmin in unstable coronary artery disease. *Lancet* 1996, 390:452–452.

This randomized, placebo-controlled trial is the first study evaluating a LMWH in the management of acute coronary syndromes. The study demonstrates a substantial early benefit of dalteparin with a 63% reduction in death and MI at 6 days. The authors propose the routine use of dalteparin with aspirin in the early management of acute coronary syndromes to reduce the risk of new cardiac events while allowing risk stratification and selection of a long-term treatment strategy.

42. Schaffer LW, Davidson JT, Vlasuk GP, *et al.*: Selective factor Xa inhibition by recombinant antistasin prevents vascular graft thrombosis in baboons. *Arterioscler Thromb* 1992, 12:879–885.

43. Mellott M, Holahan M, Lynch J, *et al.*: Acceleration of recombinant tissue-type plasminogen activator-induced reperfusion and prevention of reocclusion by recombinant antistasin, a selective factor Xa inhibitor, in a canine model of femoral arterial thrombosis. *Circ Res* 1992, 70:1152–1160.

44. Ragosta M, Gimple L, Gertz S, *et al.*: Specific factor Xa inhibition reduces restenosis after balloon angioplasty of atherosclerotic femoral arteries in rabbits. *Circulation* 1994, 89:1262–1271.

45. Waxman L, Smith D, Arcuri K, Vlasuk G: Tick anticoagulant peptide is a novel inhibitor of blood coagulation factor Xa. *Science* 1990, 248:593–596.

46. Vlasuk GP, Ramjit D, Fujita T, *et al.*: Comparison of the in vivo anticoagulant properties of standard heparin and the highly selective factor Xa inhibitors antistasin and tick anticoagulant peptide (TAP) in a rabbit model of venous thrombosis. *Thromb Haemost* 1991, 65:257–265.

47. Sitko G, Ramjit D, Stabilito I, *et al.*: Conjunctive enhancement of enzymatic thrombolysis and prevention of thrombotic reocclusion with the selective factor Xa inhibitor, tick anticoagulant peptide: comparison to hirudin and heparin in a canine model of acute coronary artery thrombosis. *Circulation* 1992, 85:805–815.

48.•• Schwartz R, Holder D, Holmes DJ, *et al.*: Neointimal thickening after severe coronary artery injury is limited by short term administration of a factor Xa inhibitor. *Circulation* 1996, 93:1542–1548.

This study demonstrates the efficacy of thrombin inhibition in reducing neointima in a porcine coronary artery injury model. The importance of thrombin in the pathogenesis of neointima formation in an animal model, which is relevant to human coronary restenosis, is thereby highlighted.

49.• Broze GJ Jr: Tissue factor pathway inhibitor and the revised theory of coagulation. *Thromb Haemost* 1995, 74:90–93.

This article reviews the role of tissue factor pathway inhibitor in a revised theory of coagulation. The role of tissue factor in the pathogenesis of several vascular disease states including plaque thrombosis and atherogenesis is becoming apparent.

50. Lindahl A, Abildgaard U, Staalesen R: The anticoagulant effect in heparinized blood and plasma resulting from interactions with extrinsic pathway inhibitor. *Thromb Res* 1991, 64:155–168.

51. Lindahl AK, Sandset PM, Thune WM, *et al.*: Tissue factor pathway inhibitor prevents thrombus formation on procoagulant subendothelial matrix. *Blood Coagul Fibrinolysis* 1994, 5:755–760.

52. Haskel E, Torr S, Day K, *et al.*: Prevention of arterial reocclusion after thrombolysis with recombinant lipoprotein-associated coagulation inhibitor. *Circulation* 1991, 84:821–827.

53. Holst J, Lindblad B, Bergqvist D, *et al.*: Antithrombotic effect of recombinant truncated tissue factor pathway inhibitor (TFPI1-161) in experimental venous thrombosis: a comparison with low molecular weight heparin. *Thromb Haemost* 1994, 71:214–219.

54. Khouri R, Koudsi B, Kaiding F, *et al.*: Prevention of thrombosis by topical application of tissue factor pathway inhibitor in a rabbit model of vascular trauma. *Ann Plast Surg* 1993, 30:398–402.

55. Jang Y, Guzman L, Lincoff A, *et al.*: Influence of blockade at specific levels of the coagulation cascade on restenosis in a rabbit atherosclerotic femoral artery injury model. *Circulation* 1995, 92:3041–3050.

56. Gruber A, Harker A, Hanson S, *et al.*: Antithrombotic effects of combining activated protein C and urokinase in nonhuman primates. *Circulation* 1991, 84:2454–2462.

57. Tripodi A, Chantarangkul V, Arbini A, *et al.*: Effects of hirudin on activated partial thromboplastin time determined with different reagents. *Thromb Haemost* 1993, 70:286–288.

58. Carteaux J, Gast A, Tschopp T, Roux S: The activated clotting time (ACT) as an appropriate test to compare heparin and direct thrombin inhibitors such as hirudin or Ro-46-6240 in experimental arterial thrombosis. *Circulation* 1995, 91:1568–1574.

59. Nicolini FA, Lee P, Rios G, Kottke-Marchant K, Topol EJ: Combination of platelet fibrinogen receptor antagonist and direct antithrombin inhibitor at low doses markedly improves thrombolysis. *Circulation* 1994, 89:1802–1809.

60. Sharma G, Lapsley D, Vita J, *et al.*: Usefulness and tolerability of hirulog, a direct thrombin-inhibitor, in unstable angina pectoris. *Am J Cardiol* 1993, 72:1357–1360.

61. Gold HK, Torres FW, Garabedian HD, *et al.*: Evidence for a rebound coagulation phenomenon after cessation of a 4-hour infusion of a specific thrombin inhibitor in patients with unstable angina pectoris. *J Am Coll Cardiol* 1993, 21:1039–1047.

62. Topol E, Fuster V, Harrington R, *et al.*: Recombinant hirudin for unstable angina pectoris. A multicenter, randomized angiographic trial. *Circulation* 1994, 89:1557–1566.

63. Tabata H, Mizuno K, Miyamoto A, *et al.*: The effect of a new thrombin inhibitor (Argatroban) in the prevention of reocclusion after reperfusion therapy in patients with acute myocardial infarction. *Circulation* 1993, 86 (suppl I):260.

64. Scharfstein JS, Gold HK, Loscalzo J: New antithrombotic strategies in thrombosis and hemorrhage. Edited by Loscalzo J, Schafer AI. Cambridge, MA: Blackwell Scientific Publications; 1994:1207–1223.

65. Scharfstein J, Loscalzo J: Molecular approaches to antithrombotic therapy. *Hosp Pract (Off Ed)* 1992, 27:77–86.

66.•• Lefkovits J, Topol E: Direct thrombin inhibitors in cardiovascular medicine. *Circulation* 1994, 90:1522–1536.

Excellent review on the clinical use of the newer antithrombins.

INDEX

Page numbers followed by a t *or* f *indicate tables or figures, respectively.*

A

B

C

F

G

H

I

K

L

M

N

O

P

R

S

T

U

V

W

X